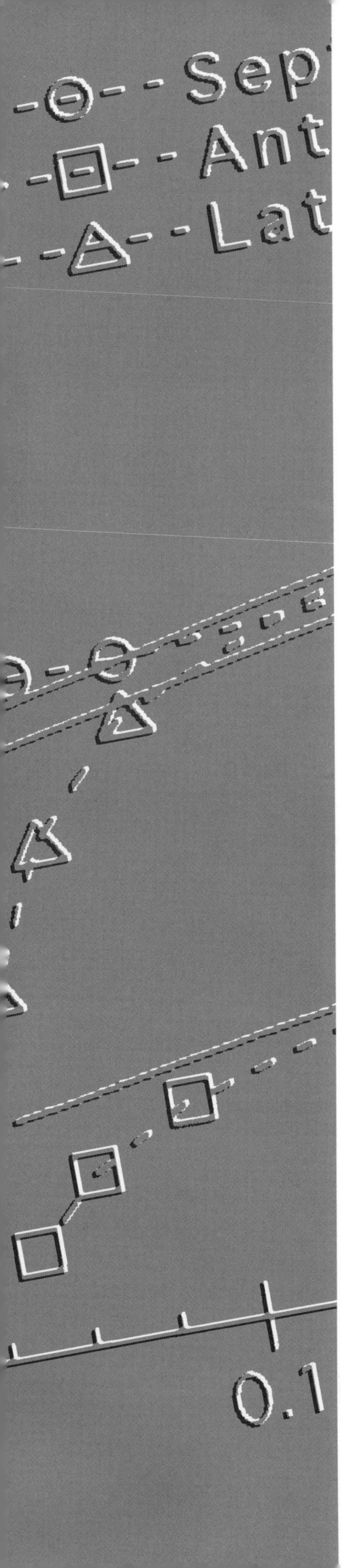

REVIEW OF NUCLEAR MEDICINE TECHNOLOGY

SECOND EDITION

Ann M. Steves, MS, CNMT
Associate Professor and Director
Nuclear Medicine Technology Program
University of Alabama at Birmingham
School of Health Related Professions
Birmingham, Alabama

Published by
SOCIETY OF NUCLEAR MEDICINE
1850 Samuel Morse Drive, Reston, VA 22090-5316

Society of Nuclear Medicine, Inc.
1850 Samuel Morse Drive, Reston, VA 22090-5316

Made in the United States of America

Library of Congress Cataloging-in-Publicaton Data

Steves, Ann M., 1947-
Review of nuclear medicine technology/Ann M. Steves, 2nd ed.
p. cm.
Includes bibliographical references and index.
ISBN 0-932004-45-8 (pbk.)
1. Nuclear medicine—Examinations—Study guides. I. Title.
[DNLM: 1. Nuclear Medicine—examination questions. 2. Technology, Radiologic—examination questions. WN 18.2 S848r 1996]
R896.S74 1996
616.07′575—dc20
DNLM/DLC
for Library of Congress 96-578
CIP

This book is dedicated to Cal Pabst, my husband, who has always supported my professional endeavors with fortitude and patience.

Preface to the First Edition

For some time now, candidates have been seeking a study guide to assist them in preparing for nuclear medicine technology certification examinations. This book was written with that objective in mind. It is intended as a summary of basic nuclear medicine technology practice and it covers the material usually included on national certification examinations. The book is not designed to provide in-depth instructional content but rather to review the familiar concepts and principles and to emphasize their relation to clinical practice.

Certain topics are not included in this text. First, nuclear medicine technology certification examinations do not address all content areas included in an organized curriculum. Second, some subjects are better covered in other texts, for example, basic nursing care and computers.

The movement to replace the centimeter-gram-second (CGS) system with the meter-kilogram-second (MKS) system, also known as the Système International d'Unité (SI) units, in scientific work has not been completed.Therefore, CGS units as well as MKS (or SI) units are used throughout the text wherever possible. Since CGS units are cited in NRC and DOT regulations, only CGS units are quoted when referring to these regulations. Factors to convert from one system of units to another appear in Appendix F.

A publication of this kind is not possible without the hard work and cooperation of many individuals. Most obvious, of course, are the writers. Since "a picture is worth a thousand words," the colleagues who contributed the nuclear medicine images that appear in this book saved the authors much writing by illustrating their points. Certain individuals gave their permission to reprint previously published images; others such as Bob Bowen, Jackie Bridges and the technical staff at Baptist Memorial Hospital East, Brad Pounds and Debora Reimers, scoured their patient files to find suitable images. Other colleagues also unselfishly gave their time to review this work and make helpful suggestions. Thanks to the typists and graphic artists who worked behind the scenes to make the book attractive and appealing. Special recognition goes to Lisa Morgan who accepted the challenge and formatted the entire text using a desktop publishing package.

The confidence and support demonstrated by the Publications Committee and the leadership of the Technologist Section during the time it took to complete this project are sincerely appreciated. I am especially grateful to the directors of the Nuclear Medicine Technology Certification Board for their important contribution to this book. Lastly, to the publications staff of the Society of Nuclear Medicine who offered both technical and moral support, go my appreciation and thanks.

A.M.S.

Preface to the Second Edition

There are numerous changes and additions to this new edition. Many of them resulted from the comments and suggestions of individuals who used the first edition. Others occurred because of the innovations and alterations that have occurred in our profession. First, problem sets have been added to Chapter 1, Radiation Protection, and Chapter 3 Radiopharmacy. Solutions to problems are shown in detail in Appendix A. Second, NRC regulations have been updated throughout the text. Also, additional material has been added concerning pharmacologic stress testing, myocardial imaging protocols and new radiopharmaceuticals such as ^{99m}Tc-sestamibi, ^{99m}Tc-bicisate, ^{89}Sr -chloride, [^{131}I]MIBG, Octreoscan®, and OncoScint®, among other topics.

Book publication is a detailed and laborious process. It is not possible without the hard work and cooperation of many talented and dedicated individuals.

I would like to acknowledge all those who participated in making the first edition a success. To all those who purchased this book and took the time to contact me with their constructive criticism, I extend my thanks. I appreciated the compliments, but particularly valued the recommendations for the second edition.

I also would like to acknowledge all those who worked to make the second edition a reality. I am particularly grateful to the contributors to the first edition who deemed this endeavor important enough to have a second go at it, and to Tim Baker who agreed to write a chapter after being accepted into medical school. Sheila Cooley and Maria Tyson performed most capably and efficiently as typists. There are many other individuals, illustrators, photographers and other production staff, who also deserve my thanks and appreciation for their efforts.

Finally, I thank the Publications Committee of the Technologist Section for their support of this project and the publications staff of the Society of Nuclear Medicine for their sage advice and assistance.

A.M.S.

Contents

Contributors

Timothy D. Baker, CNMT
Formerly, Supervisor
Nuclear Medicine
Walker Baptist Medical Center
Jasper, Alabama
Formerly, Research Technologist
Division of Cardiology
The University of Alabama at Birmingham
Birmingham, Alabama

Helen H. Drew, CNMT
Chief Technologist, In-Patient Services
Nuclear Medicine and Nonimaging
Division of Nuclear Medicine
Johns Hopkins Hospital
Baltimore, Maryland

Robert L. Gladding, CNMT
Staff Technologist
Department of Nuclear Medicine
Hospital of the University of Pennsylvania
Philadelphia, Pennsylvania

John D. Praither, MS, MT
Technical Director
Radioimmunoassay Department
American Medical Laboratories
Fairfax, Virginia

Charles G. Stephenson, CNMT
Formerly, Staff Technologist
Department of Nuclear Medicine
Mariner's Hospital
Islamorada, Florida

Ann M. Steves, MS, CNMT
Associate Professor and Director
Nuclear Medicine Technology Program
School of Health Related Professions
The University of Alabama at Birmingham
Birmingham, Alabama

1 Radiation Protection

Ann M. Steves

There are few activities a nuclear medicine technologist engages in that do not include elements of radiation protection. Prevention of unnecessary radiation exposure to oneself, co-workers, patients and the general public is a routine part of competent clinical practice. This chapter reviews the principles of radiation protection and the implementation of these principles in the nuclear medicine department.

PRACTICAL METHODS FOR REDUCING EXPOSURE

There are three factors involved in reducing external radiation exposure: time, distance and shielding.

Time

Minimizing the amount of time spent in a radiation field will limit the total radiation received. Practical applications of the time factor include working efficiently when handling radioactive materials and practicing new procedures with nonradioactive materials until the desired speed and accuracy are attained.

Distance

Increasing the distance from a radiation source will decrease the amount of radiation received. The radiation dose rate (the dose per unit time) from a small volume radiation source varies inversely with the square of the distance from the source. This relationship is called the inverse square law.

By doubling the distance, the radiation dose rate is reduced to one-fourth of the original. If the distance is halved, the dose rate is increased to four times the original. Table 1-1 outlines the steps taken to ascertain the new radiation dose resulting from a given change in distance.

The formula for the inverse square law is expressed as:

*

$$\frac{I_1}{I_2} = \frac{(d_2)^2}{(d_1)^2},$$

where I_1 = dose rate (intensity) at distance d_1 from the source and I_2 = dose rate (intensity) at distance d_2 from the source.

Example 1. If 10 milliroentgen/hour (mR/hr) is measured at 3 meters (m), what is the dose rate at 0.5 m?

$$\frac{10\ \text{mR/hr}}{I_2} = \frac{(0.5\ \text{m})^2}{(3.0\ \text{m})^2}$$

$$I_2 \times 0.25\ \text{m}^2 = 10\ \text{mR/hr} \times 9\ \text{m}^2$$

$$I_2 = \frac{10\ \text{mR/hr} \times 9\ \text{m}^2}{0.25\ \text{m}^2} = 360\ \text{mR/hr}$$

Example 2. If 150 mR/hr is measured at 20 cm, at what distance will 95 mR/hr be measured?

$$\frac{150\ \text{mR/hr}}{95\ \text{mR/hr}} = \frac{(d_2)^2}{(20\ \text{cm})^2}$$

$$(d_2)^2 = \frac{150\ \text{mR/hr} \times 400\ \text{cm}^2}{95\ \text{mR/hr}}.$$

$$d^2 = \sqrt{632\ \text{cm}^2} = 25\ \text{cm}$$

Practical applications of the distance factor include using tongs to handle large quantities of radioactivity, storing radioactive materials away from high occupancy areas and using restraint devices to hold patients in position.

Shielding

Shielding involves the use of a material, usually lead, to absorb the radiation transmitted from a source. The type of radiation determines the type of shielding to be used. Alpha particles, which are not used clinically, can be completely stopped by a sheet of paper. Complete absorption of beta particles can be achieved with only a few millimeters of plastic. Therefore, a syringe provides adequate shielding of beta emissions.

Lead vial and syringe shields should not be used to shield a pure beta emitter such as phosphorous-32 (^{32}P) because bremsstrahlung will be produced. Bremsstrahlung is radiation that results from the deceleration of the beta particles

Table 1.1
Application of Inverse Square Law

Distance factor	Distance factor squared	Inverse of square
2	$(2)^2 = 4$	$\frac{1}{4}$
$\frac{1}{2}$	$\left(\frac{1}{2}\right)^2 = \frac{1}{4}$	4

as they approach the nuclei of the lead atoms in the shield. As the beta particles slow down, they lose energy that is released in the form of x-rays. The amount of bremsstrahlung increases with the density of the material through which the beta particles pass. Consequently, a low density material, such as plastic or lucite, is recommended to absorb beta particles and to reduce the amount of bremsstrahlung produced in the shielding material.

For gamma and x-rays, lead shielding is used to reduce, rather than completely absorb, the radiation emitted from a source. The ability of a material to absorb or attenuate x- and gamma rays is expressed as the half-value layer (HVL). The HVL is defined as the thickness of a material required to reduce the radiation intensity to half its original value. Thus, one HVL reduces the radiation intensity to 50%, two HVLs reduce the intensity to 25% and so on (Fig. 1-1). A specific HVL is related to the photon energies of the x- or gamma radiation as well as the type of shielding material (Table 1-2). Vial and syringe shields, lead bricks and leaded-glass L-blocks are shielding devices that effectively reduce personnel radiation exposure.

Table 1.2
Half-Value Layer (HVL) of Lead for Selected Radionuclides

Radionuclide	Primary photon energy (keV)	HVL of lead (mm)
^{125}I	27.5	0.04
^{99m}Tc	140	0.27
^{51}Cr	320	2.0
^{131}I	364	3.0
^{18}F	511	4.1
^{137}Cs	662	6.5

Internal Exposure

Internal radiation exposure can result when radionuclides are inhaled, ingested or absorbed through the skin. The following steps are recommended practices to minimize the possibility of internal contamination while working in the nuclear medicine department.

1. Refrain from eating, drinking or smoking in areas where radionuclides are used.
2. Use automatic pipettes to measure or transfer radioactive solutions.
3. Wear protective clothing such as lab coats and gloves when handling radionuclides or objects that may be radioactive.
4. Monitor hands, clothing and shoes after working with radionuclides.
5. Clean up radioactive spills promptly.
6. When working with iodine-131 (^{131}I) solutions, keep vials tightly capped and open them only in a fume hood.
7. When performing lung ventilation studies with radioactive gases, ensure that the gas trapping and room ventilation systems are working efficiently.

PERSONNEL MONITORING

External radiation exposure levels received by nuclear medicine personnel can be documented with various dosimeter devices. The following types of dosimeters are most commonly used to measure personnel exposure.

Film Badges

The film badge consists of a plastic holder in which a strip of photographic film is held between a set of filters. Following development, the amount of darkening (density) on the film is proportional to the amount of radiation absorbed. The three or four filters are each made of a different material (lead, copper, aluminum, plastic) so that the energy range and penetration of the radiation striking the badge can be assessed. The film badge holder also has an opening where the film can be exposed to beta particles and low-energy photons. Film badges are effective in measuring radiation exposures of 10 mrem to several hundred rems.

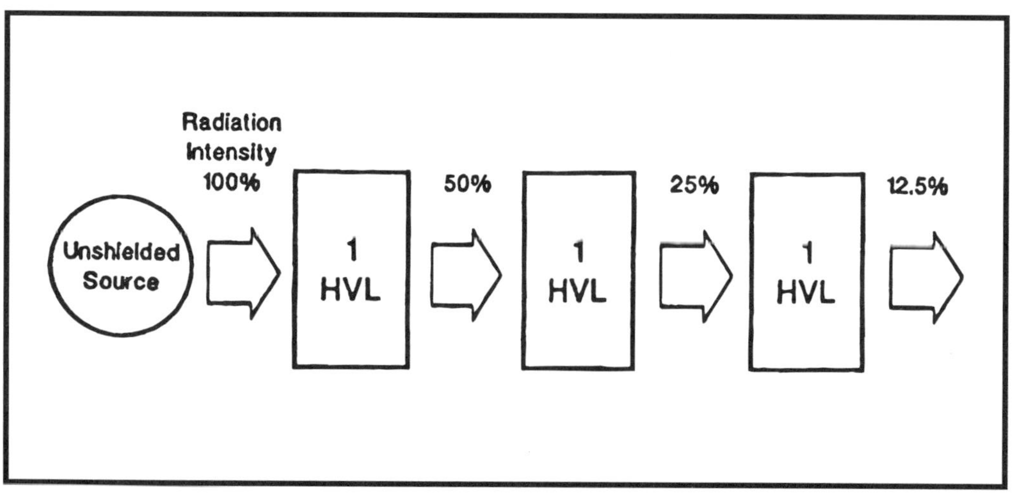

Figure 1.1 One HVL of shielding material reduces radiation intensity to one-half of the original intensity. An additional HVL will halve radiation intensity again and so on.

Film badges should be worn between the waist and the shoulder at the site of the highest exposure rate to the body. Because the latent image on the film tends to fade over time, it is recommended that film badges be processed monthly.

Thermoluminescent Dosimeters

A thermoluminescent dosimeter (TLD) uses special material, typically lithium fluoride crystals, that emit a quantity of light proportional to the amount of radiation absorbed by the crystals. The light is released and measured when the crystals are heated to an extremely high temperature. Filters may also be used in TLDs to distinguish nonpenetrating from penetrating radiation.

Although this type of dosimeter is more expensive than a film dosimeter, it is less affected by environmental conditions such as humidity and temperature. Due to the small size of the crystals, it is possible to use TLDs in the form of rings to monitor hand exposure. Ring badges should be worn on the forefinger of the dominant hand with the crystal facing the palm of the hand.

Pocket Ionization Chambers

Pocket ionization chambers are useful supplementary monitoring devices. Immediate radiation exposure measurements are provided through a scale in the dosimeter itself or through a separate reading device. The amount of ionization is directly related to the amount of radiation exposure. Pocket dosimeters are expensive compared to film badges and TLDs and require careful handling to prevent inaccurate readings.

NRC REGULATIONS

Occupational Dose Limits

The Nuclear Regulatory Commission (NRC) has established the maximum upper limits of radiation exposure that radiation workers may receive. These occupational dose limits are based on the concept of "acceptable risk." That is, the dose levels cited in the regulations are levels below which the likelihood of an individual developing radiation-induced diseases such as cancer or genetic changes is negligible.

Occupational dose limits, formerly called maximum permissible doses, are now called total effective dose equivalent (TEDE) limits. TEDE is defined as the sum of the deep dose equivalent (DDE) and the committed effective dose equivalent (CEDE). The DDE refers to external exposure, whereas the CEDE refers to internal exposure. Since instances of internal exposure are rare in nuclear medicine technologists, the TEDE is essentially equivalent to the DDE. Table 1-3 lists the TEDE limits for occupationally workers, the general public and the embryo/fetus.

ALARA

To increase awareness of radiation protection techniques and to reduce occupational radiation exposure, the NRC subscribes to a philosophy called ALARA (as low as reasonably achievable). Individuals who practice the ALARA concept attempt to keep their radiation exposure as low as possible using reasonable cost and effort.

Table 1.3
Annual Radiation Exposure Limits
Set by the NRC

	TEDE rem (mSv)
Occupational exposures	
Whole body	5 (50)
Lens of eye	15 (150)
Gonads	50 (500)
Hands/Forearms	50 (500)
Skin	50 (500)
Red marrow	50 (500)
Public exposure	0.1 (1)
Embryo/Fetus exposure	0.5 (5)

Radiation Areas

For purposes of radiation control, the NRC defines restricted and unrestricted areas. An unrestricted area is one in which access is not limited by or under the control of the radioactive materials licensee. Radiation levels in an unrestricted area must be such that anyone who is in the area will receive less than 2 mrem (0.02 mSv) in any 1 hr. If this radiation limit is exceeded, then the area is considered restricted and access to that area must be controlled. For example, in a nuclear medicine department, reception and waiting areas are unrestricted, whereas imaging rooms are restricted.

The NRC requires that restricted areas be posted with specific signs depending on the radiation level present. Such signs display the conventional magenta radiation symbol on a yellow background with one of the following phrases.

Caution: Radioactive Materials. These words are used to indicate any area in which certain quantities of radioactive materials are used or stored. Table 1-4 lists some radionuclides commonly used in the nuclear medicine department with the amounts that require posting.

Caution: Radiation Area. These words are used to denote areas in which an individual could receive more than 5 mrem (0.05 mSv) in 1 hr.

Caution: High Radiation Area. These words are used to designate areas in which an individual could receive more than 100 mrem (1 mSv) in 1 hr.

Grave Danger: Very High Radiation Area. These words are used to post an area in which an individual could receive an absorbed dose of more than 500 rads (5 grays) in 1 hr.

Table 1.4
Quantities of Selected Radionuclides Requiring Posting with Caution: Radioactive Materials Sign (NRC)

Radionuclide	Quantities exceeding (mCi)
^{57}Co	1
^{67}Ga	10
^{89}St	0.1
^{99}Mo	1
^{99m}Tc	10
^{123}I	1
^{133}Xe	10
^{137}Cs	0.1

The NRC also requires that surveys be performed to monitor for external radiation exposure and surface contamination in locations where radioactivity is routinely stored or used. Daily surveys must be conducted in radiopharmaceutical preparation and administration areas; storage sites must be monitored weekly. Either an ionization chamber or a Geiger-Mueller counter may be used for surveying and the instrument should be sensitive enough to detect 0.1 mrem/hr. Sites that show a higher than normal level of background radiation should be considered contaminated. Wipe tests should be performed at these locations to determine if contamination is removable.

A piece of filter paper or a cotton swab is used to wipe a 10-cm^2 (4 square inch) area. The wipe is then counted in a scintillation counter. If radioactivity is detected on the wipe, decontamination of the area should be undertaken until background levels are achieved, or until no more contamination can be removed. If the contamination cannot be completely removed, taping a piece of paper over the site will serve as a reminder to personnel and deter them from walking or working in that area.

NRC regulations state that the area survey and wipe records must be retained for three years. The record must include the following:

1. Date survey was performed.
2. Initials of individual performing survey.
3. Instruments used to make survey.
4. Diagram of area surveyed.
5. Measured dose rates (mrem/hr) and/or removable contamination (dpm/cm^2) keyed to locations on the diagram of the area surveyed.

RECEIPT AND STORAGE OF RADIOACTIVE MATERIALS

Receipt

The NRC requires that all shipments of radioactive materials displaying a radioactive label (White I, Yellow II or Yellow III) be wipe tested. The procedure for monitoring and opening radioactive shipments includes the following steps:

1. Visually inspect the package for signs of damage or moisture.
2. Measure exposure rates at the package surface and at a distance of 1 m from the surface. If the exposure rates exceed 200 mrem/hr at the surface or 10 mrem/hr at 1 m from the surface, notify the NRC and the carrier delivering the shipment. Notification may best be accomplished through the institution's radiation safety officer (RSO).
3. After opening the package, verify that the contents match the packing slip and check the integrity of the radionuclide container.
4. Wipe the external surface of the container, assay the wipe and decontaminate the container's exterior surface as required. If removable contamination exceeds 22 dpm/cm^2 $\times$ 300 cm^2 (6600 dpm or 0.003 μCi) of container surface, notify the NRC and the carrier through the RSO.
5. Monitor the packaging material for contamination and remove the radiation labels before discarding the packaging material. If the materials are contaminated, dispose of them as radioactive waste.

Storage

Radioactive materials that are being stored for later use should be shielded to minimize radiation levels in the work area. Vial shields and lead bricks usually provide sufficient protection. Containers should be clearly and completely labeled so that a technologist can locate the desired material quickly, thereby minimizing radiation exposure. Storage areas should be posted with the appropriate radiation signs. If access to these areas cannot be limited, then these areas should be locked.

Certain radioactive materials may have additional storage requirements. Volatility of liquid radioactive sodium iodide can be minimized if the solution is kept refrigerated. Radioactive gases, such as ^{133}Xe, are best stored in a fume hood. If leaks should occur, the radioactivity will be vented through the hood rather than spreading throughout the work area.

RADIOACTIVE WASTE DISPOSAL

Decay in Storage. License requirements for radioactive waste disposal have become more stringent and burial of waste has become the most costly disposal method. For these reasons, decay in storage is an easier, inexpensive method for the low-level radioactive waste generated in nuclear medicine. In this method, radioactive waste is separated according to half-life; technetium-99m (^{99m}Tc) waste typically is segregated from other longer lived waste such as thallium-201 (^{201}Tl) ($T_{1/2}$ = 3.0 days), gallium-67 (^{67}Ga) ($T_{1/2}$ = 3.3 days), etc. After the waste has been allowed to decay to background radiation levels, the radiation symbols are defaced and the waste is disposed of along with other nonradioactive trash. If the waste contains potentially biohazardous materials (used needles, syringes, etc.), then it should be incinerated after the radioactivity has decayed to background levels.

According to the NRC, only radionuclides with a half-life of less than 65 days may be decayed in storage. Materials must be held for a minimum of 10 half-lives and be monitored to ascertain that there is no measurable radiation emitted from the waste before final disposal.

Sewage Disposal. The amount of soluble waste that may be discharged into the sewer system is based on the rate of waste-water discharge from a facility. NRC regulations specify the maximum concentrations and total annual amounts that may be disposed of by this method. It is important to note that radioactive urine or feces are exempt from any limitations and may be discarded through the sewer system.

Incineration. Special permission is required to dispose of radioactive materials by incineration.

Transfer to Authorized Recipient. Long-lived radioactive waste can be disposed of by transferring the material to an authorized commercial waster handler. Such companies either bury the material at an approved site or incinerate the waste. Any radioactive materials transferred for disposal must be packaged and labeled according to the U.S. Department of Transportation (DOT) requirements.

Release to Atmosphere. Radioactive gases may be discharged directly into the atmosphere in limited quantities. Maximum airborne concentrations are specified in the NRC regulations.

Whatever method of waste disposal, records of the disposal must be maintained to document compliance with regulations.

Decontamination

Minor radioactive spills involving a small area or relatively low radiation dose rate occasionally occur. The procedure for handling minor contamination is as follows:

1. Clear the area where the spill has occurred and notify other personnel in the immediate vicinity.
2. Don disposable, protective clothing such as shoe covers, gloves and lab coats.
3. Contain the spill in a limited area. Place absorbent material over liquids as soon as possible.
4. Place all materials used to mop up the spill into plastic bags.
5. Monitor the area and initiate decontamination as necessary.
6. Remove any contaminated clothing or protective gear and discard with other contaminated materials.
7. Label all radioactive materials and dispose of them properly with other contaminated materials.
8. Report the spill to the RSO.

Contaminated personnel should be decontaminated as quickly as possible to prevent internal absorption or inhalation of the radioactivity. Contaminated clothing should be removed immediately, before leaving the area of the spill. Mild soap and warm water should be used to remove contamination on the skin. The use of abrasive cleansers and brushes to clean the skin should be avoided. The treatment of serious injuries always takes precedence over decontamination.

Major spills involving widespread areas of contamination or a high radiation dose rate are managed differently. Precautions for dealing with major contamination include:

1. To prevent the spread of airborne contamination, shut off fume hoods, ventilation, heating and air conditioning equipment.
2. Remove contaminated articles before leaving the area.
3. Evacuate and close all doors to the area.
4. Lock the doors and post warning signs.
5. Begin decontamination of personnel involved.
6. Notify the RSO immediately. Cleanup and decontamination of major spills should be conducted under the supervision of the RSO.

EXERCISES

Solutions to exercises may be found in Appendix A.

1. What is the radiation intensity of a source at 1.5 m that measures 6 mR/hr at 4.5 m?
2. If the radiation intensity of a source at 0.4 m measures 2.6 mR/hr, at what distance will the intensity be halved?
3. The exposure rate measured at 0.5 inches from the surface of a radiopharmaceutical vial is 175 mR/hr. If the technologist uses 12-inch tongs to move the source into the dose calibrator, what is the exposure rate to the technologist's hands?
4. If the radiation intensity measured at 1 m from an ^{131}I therapy patient is 96 mR/hr, at approximately what distance should a visitor stand to receive an exposure rate of no more than 2 mR/hr?
5. If the exposure rate from a point source is 200 mR/hr at 3 m from the source, at what distance will the exposure rated be reduced by 75%?
6. The HVL for ^{99m}Tc (140 keV) in lead is 2.6 mm. (a) What percentage of photons is transmitted by 5.2 mm thickness of lead? (b) What thickness of lead is required to reduce the exposure rate of a ^{99m}Tc source from 30 mR/hr to no more than 2 mR/hr?
7. The HVL for ^{60}Co in lead is 1.25 cm. (a) If the intensity of a ^{60}Co source is decreased to 5 mR/hr from 40 mR/hr, how many HVLs of lead were used to shield the source? (b) What percentage of ^{60}Co photons is absorbed by 3.75 cm thickness of lead?

REFERENCES

1. Early PJ, Sodee DB. *Principles and practice of nuclear medicine,* 2nd ed. St. Louis: Mosby-Year Book; 1995:65–80, 323–326.

2. Eichling JO, Izzo LM, Moore MM. Radiation safety in nuclear medicine. In: Bernier DR, Christian PE, Langan JK, eds. *Nuclear medicine technology and techniques*, 3rd ed. St. Louis: Mosby-Year Book; 1994:162–187.

3. Steves AM. Radiation protection in nuclear medicine. In: Dowd SB. *Practical radiation protection and applied radiobiology*. Philadelphia: WB Saunders; 1994:204–226.

4. Thompson MA, Hattaway MP, Hall JD, et al. *Principles of imaging science and protection*. Philadelphia: WB Saunders; 1994:453–474.

5. U.S. Nuclear Regulatory Commission. Federal Regulations, Title 10, Chapter 1, Energy, Parts 20 and 35. Washington, DC: U.S. Government Printing Office; January 1, 1995.

2 Federal Regulatory Agencies

Ann M. Steves

Various federal, state and local government agencies have authority to regulate the use of radioactive materials. Jurisdiction over certain aspects of regulation is shared by more than one agency. Technologists need to be familiar with regulations at all levels that affect the practice of nuclear medicine technology. Since, however, the national certification examinations test knowledge only of federal regulations, this chapter will discuss the three major federal agencies that control the use of radioactive materials in nuclear medicine practice.

NUCLEAR REGULATORY COMMISSION

In 1974, the NRC was created to assume responsibility from the Atomic Energy Commission for regulation of the purchase, receipt, use and disposal of radioactive materials. Radioactive materials produced by a nuclear reactor (by-product material) and certain special radionuclides such as uranium, thorium and plutonium come under the jurisdiction of the NRC.

By agreement with the NRC, some states, known as agreement states (Table 2-1), accept responsibility for the regulation of radioactive materials. The regulations established by agreement states must be consistent with those of the NRC. Federal facilities within the agreement states are regulated by the NRC. Such facilities include Veterans Administration hospitals and military installations.

Authorization to use reactor by-product material is granted by the NRC or agreement state in the form of a license. There are several categories of licenses; each specifies what radioactive material is authorized for what purposes and who the authorized users are.

Table 2.1
Agreement States

Alabama	Nevada
Arizona	New Hampshire
Arkansas	New Mexico
California	New York
Colorado	North Carolina
Florida	North Dakota
Georgia	Oregon
Idaho	Rhode Island
Kansas	South Carolina
Kentucky	Tennessee
Louisiana	Texas
Maryland	Utah
Mississippi	Washington
Nebraska	

NRC authority extends to the remaining 23 states, the District of Columbia and several U.S. territories.

DEPARTMENT OF TRANSPORTATION

The DOT controls the packaging and interstate movement of hazardous materials including radioactivity. Transportation of radioactive materials is permitted if there are adequate safeguards to contain the radiation emitted by the material as well as the material itself. The type of packaging used to ship radioactive materials is classified as Type A or Type B. Type A is adequate for normal transport. Type B packaging is more accident-resistant and is used for very large quantities of radioactive material. Most radiopharmaceuticals used in routine nuclear medicine practice are transported in Type A packaging.

Type A packages are labeled according to one of three categories based on the measured dose rate, in millirem per hour, at the package surface and at 1 m from the surface (Fig. 2-1). The dose rate measured at 1 m from the surface is called the transport index (TI) and it must appear on the label. The label must also specify the radionuclide and the amount of radioactivity contained in the package.

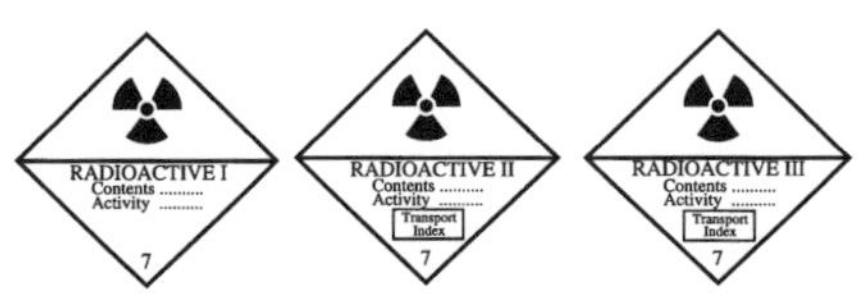

DOT Class	I (white)	II (yellow)	III (yellow)
Exposure rate at package surface cannot exceed (mR/hr)	0.5	50	200
Exposure rate at 1 meter from package surface cannot exceed (mR/hr)	No detectable radiation	1	10

Figure 2.1 The label types and exposure limits for packages containing radioactive materials. Category I labels have a white background. Categories II and III labels have a yellow background on the upper half and a white background on the lower half.

FOOD AND DRUG ADMINISTRATION

Since 1975, the manufacture, distribution, safety and effectiveness of radiopharmaceuticals have been regulated and monitored by the Food and Drug Administra-tion (FDA). Only approved radiopharmaceuticals, those that have a new drug authorization (NDA), can be distributed for sale in the United States. All radiopharmaceuticals must be submitted for review by the FDA before an NDA is issued. A drug that is under investigation by the FDA for future approval is called an investigational new drug (IND) and may only be used in patients under very controlled conditions, which are specified by the FDA. Before an investigational drug is used, the patient must give informed, written consent.

FEDERAL REGULATIONS

Selected federal regulations of the NRC, DOT and FDA pertinent to nuclear medicine technologist (NMT) certification appear in Appendix B.

REFERENCES

1. Early PJ, Sodee DB. *Principles and practice of nuclear medicine,* 2nd ed. St. Louis: Mosby-Year Book; 1995:94–95, 323–336.
2. Eichling JO, Izzo LM, Moore MM. Radiation safety in nuclear medicine. In: Bernier DR, Christian PE, Langan JK. *Nuclear medicine technology and techniques,* 3rd ed. St. Louis: Mosby-Year Book; 1994:162–187.
3. Phan T, Ling M, Wasnich R. *Practical nuclear pharmacy,* 3rd ed. Honolulu: Banyan Press; 1987:1–2, 6–11.
4. Saha GB. *Fundamentals of nuclear pharmacy,* 3rd ed. New York: Springer-Verlag; 1992:202–218.
5. U.S. Regulatory Commission. *Federal Regulations,* Title 10, Chapter 1, Energy, Parts 20 and 35. Washington, DC: U.S. Government Printing Office; January 1, 1995.

(2) NDA -
New DRUG Application

(1) IND
INVESTIGATIONAL NEW DRUG

3 Radiopharmacy

Ann M. Steves

Most, if not all, of the radiopharmaceuticals compounded on site by the nuclear medicine technologist are labeled with ^{99m}Tc. Therefore, most of the concepts presented in this chapter will be applied to the ^{99}Mo/^{99m}Tc generator and ^{99m}Tc radiolabeling. The principles of unit dose preparation discussed at the end of the chapter pertain to any radiopharmaceutical administered to a patient.

RADIONUCLIDE GENERATORS

Radionuclide generators provide a convenient source of short-lived radionuclides. In a radionuclide generator, a longer-lived radionuclide called the parent decays to a shorter-lived radionuclide called the daughter. The daughter can be removed periodically as it is replenished by decay of the parent. Examples of parent-daughter systems used in radionuclide generators include germanium-68/gallium-68 (^{68}Ge/^{68}Ga), rubidium-81/krypton-81m (^{81}Rb/^{81m}Kr) and ^{99}Mo/^{99m}Tc. Some of these systems have been developed commercially and are supplied as sterile, shielded, automatically operated devices.

Molybdenum-99/Technetium-99m Generator

A ^{99}Mo/^{99m}Tc generator consists of a column containing aluminum trioxide (alumina) onto which the parent radionuclide, ^{99}Mo, is absorbed (Fig. 3-1). A porous glass disk holds the alumina in place but allows saline to pass through it. The daughter radionuclide, ^{99m}Tc, is removed or eluted from the column when a sterile, evacuated vial is placed at the opposite end of the saline eluant. The vacuum in the collection vial causes the saline to be pulled through the alumina column, which removes the loosely bound ^{99m}Tc. Due to the different chemical properties of the parent and the daughter, ^{99}Mo remains on the column while ^{99m}Tc is collected as the generator eluate in the form of [^{99m}Tc]sodium pertechnetate.

A ^{99}Mo/^{99m}Tc generator is designated as either a "wet" column or "dry" column type. A wet column generator contains a supply of sterile saline within the generator itself. To elute this type of generator, the technologist chooses the appropriate size collection vial (such as 5, 10, 20 or 30 ml) to obtain the volume and activity concentration desired. Because no air follows the saline as it flows over the column, the column remains wet. A dry column generator requires that saline be added to the column for each elution. A vial of sterile saline, provided by the generator manufacturer, is placed on the charging port, a needle connected to tubing that carries the saline to the alumina column. An evacuated vial is then placed onto the needle on the collection port. The vacuum pulls the saline over the column, removing the ^{99m}Tc activity. Using an evacuated vial with a volume larger than the saline volume causes air to be pulled over the column, completely removing any saline. Hence, the name dry column generator. With this type of generator, the activity concentration of the eluate depends on the volume of saline used to elute the generator. After eluting a wet or dry column generator, the eluate activity and volume should be recorded.

All commercially available ^{99}Mo/^{99m}Tc generators contain ^{99}Mo produced from the fission of uranium-235 (^{235}U). The advantage of using ^{99}Mo fission molybdenum (FM) is its high specific activity. Specific activity refers to the amount of radioactivity per unit mass of a radionuclide or radiopharmaceutical and is expressed in such units as millicuries per milligram (mCi/mg), megabecquerels per milligram (MBq/mg), curies per mole (Ci/mole) or gigabecquerels per mole (GBq/mole). Due to the high specific activity, large amounts of ^{99}Mo (FM) can be bound onto a small ion-exchange column, which leads to higher activity concentration in the eluate.

It is extremely important to maintain the sterility of a generator. Manufacturers may place millipore filters between the column and the collection vial to ensure sterility, but aseptic technique must be observed during the elution process. The septa of eluate and saline vials should be swabbed with alcohol. Needles used to deliver saline or to collect the eluate should be replaced with new, sterile needles following each elution.

The shielding surrounding commercially manufactured generators is designed to meet DOT requirements. This means that generators are adequately shielded for transport purposes. Additional shielding may be necessary to reduce radiation exposure to personnel responsible for eluting the generator. In addition, the eluate collection vial should also be shielded. Standing at a distance from the generator after elution has been initiated will further reduce radiation exposure.

Generator Yields

The amount of ^{99m}Tc activity eluted from a generator is proportional to the amount of ^{99}Mo activity present on the column and to the time elapsed since the last elution. Following an elution, the amount of ^{99m}Tc activity on the column increases due to ^{99}Mo decay. When the ^{99m}Tc in a generator is eluted once a day, the maximum ^{99m}Tc activity and yield is obtained approximately every 24 hr as shown in Table 3-1. A second or third elution may be performed with-

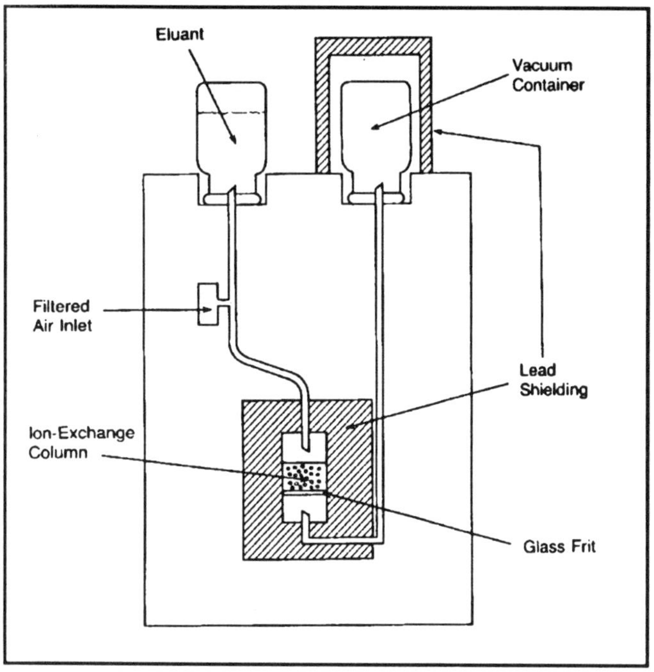

Figure 3.1 Cross-section of a typical commercial radionuclide generator. Reprinted with permission from: Chilton HM, Witcofski RL. *Nuclear pharmacy.* Philadelphia: Lea and Febiger; 1986:27.

out severely decreasing the yield of the next morning's elution, depending on the length of time since the last elution.

In determining ^{99m}Tc yields, the elution efficiency of the generator also needs to be considered. The entire ^{99m}Tc activity present on the column will not be eluted. A typical elution efficiency is 70%–90%. There is a sophisticated method of calculating expected generator yields. A simplified, useful rule of thumb when elution is performed only once every 24 hr is that the eluate yield will be 80% of the previous yield. For example, if the ^{99m}Tc yield on Day 1 is 800 mCi (29.6 GBq), the yield on Day 2 will be approximately 640 mCi (23.7 GBq).

The amount of ^{99m}Tc eluted from a generator may vary for several reasons. A mechanical problem such as an air leak in the tubing may prevent the saline from being drawn out of the column into the collection vial. In addition, "channeling" of the alumina column causes only a portion of the column to be exposed to saline, leaving ^{99m}Tc on that part of the column not washed with eluant. Finally, chemical reduction of ^{99m}Tc from the +7 valence state to other reduced states occurs when reducing agents are formed by the radiolysis of water. The reduced ^{99m}Tc remains bound onto the column and is not eluted.

Eluate Assay and Quality Control

Concentration. Immediately following elution, the eluate is assayed in a dose calibrator to determine the total ^{99m}Tc activity in the collection vial. The eluate concentration ([^{99m}Tc]pertechnetate) is calculated using the formula:

$$\text{Concentration} = \frac{\text{Total } ^{99m}\text{Tc activity (mCi)}}{\text{Elution volume (ml)}}.$$

Table 3.1
Percent of Technetium-99m Activity Present on Generator Column at Selected Times Following Elution

Time since elution (hr)	^{99m}Tc activity (% ^{99}Mo activity)
1	9.4
2	18
3	26
4	32
5	39
6	44
7	49
8	54
9	58
10	61
11	65
12	68
18	80
24	87

The total eluate activity, time of assay and elution volume should be recorded in the appropriate logbook.

Molybdenum-99 Content. Although ^{99}Mo is tightly bound to the alumina column, a tiny quantity of ^{99}Mo will be present in the generator eluate. The appearance of ^{99}Mo in generator eluate is called "molybdenum (or moly) breakthrough." Because ^{99}Mo is a radionuclide other than the one desired (^{99m}Tc), the ^{99}Mo in the eluate is considered a radionclidic impurity. When administered to patients, ^{99}Mo is taken up by the parenchymal cells of the liver and delivers an unnecessary radiation dose to that organ. For this reason, limits have been established for allowable quantities of ^{99}Mo in generator eluate.

Each generator eluate must be assayed for ^{99}Mo content to ensure that maximum allowable limits are not exceeded. The NRC states that the amount of ^{99}Mo in ^{99m}Tc generator eluate may not exceed 0.15 μCi (5.55 kBq) per 1 mCi (37 MBq) ^{99m}Tc at the time of administration to the patient. One of two assaying methods may be used. With either method, the total ^{99m}Tc activity in the eluate should first be measured using a dose calibrator.

Lead Shield (or Moly Shield) Method. A lead container is used, which is designed to absorb ^{99m}Tc photons (140 keV) as well as permit the passage of higher energy (740, 780 keV) ^{99}Mo photons. The generator eluate is placed in the moly shield and assayed in a dose calibrator to determine the ^{99}Mo content. Sometimes it is necessary to apply a correction factor to the ^{99}Mo assay. Instructions supplied with the moly shield should be consulted. To determine the amount of ^{99}Mo contamination in the eluate, divide the

^{99}Mo assay results by the total number of millicuries of ^{99m}Tc in the eluate measured with the dose calibrator.

$$^{99}\text{Mo breakthrough} = \frac{\mu\text{Ci } ^{99}\text{Mo}}{\text{mCi } ^{99m}\text{Tc}}.$$

Mock Moly Method. This method compares the unknown ^{99}Mo activity to that of a cesium-137 (^{137}Cs) reference standard of known activity. A well-type scintillation counter is used. The pulse-height analyzer window is set to accept counts within a range of 600–1000 keV, which will include the principle photons of ^{99}Mo (740, 780 keV) and ^{137}Cs (662 keV). A shielded eluate sample (for absorbing ^{99m}Tc photons) and an identically shielded ^{137}Cs standard are counted using the same geometry. The amount of ^{99}Mo contamination is determined using the formula:

$$\mu\text{Ci } ^{99}\text{Mo} = \frac{\text{net counts } ^{99m}\text{Tc eluate}}{\text{net counts } ^{137}\text{Cs standard}} \times \mu\text{Ci } ^{137}\text{Cs standard.}$$

Then the ^{99}Mo breakthrough equation displayed above is used.

Radionuclidic purity changes with time. Because ^{99}Mo ($T_{1/2} = 66$ hr) decays more slowly than ^{99m}Tc ($T_{1/2} = 6$ hr), the ^{99}Mo/^{99m}Tc ratio increases with time. The time at which ^{99}Mo contamination in ^{99m}Tc eluate will exceed acceptable limits can be calculated using the following equation. This time may be shorter than the generator manufacturer's stated expiration time of the ^{99m}Tc eluate:

$$t = \frac{-\ln \text{Mo}_0 / \text{Tc}_0}{0.1052} - 18.03,$$

where t equals the time in hours after the initial ^{99}Mo assay and Mo_0/Tc_0 equals the initial number of microcuries of ^{99}Mo divided by the initial number of millicuries of ^{99m}Tc.

Example. The initial ^{99}Mo contamination in an eluate of ^{99m}Tc was determined to be 32.5 μCi (1.2 MBq) ^{99}Mo in 500 mCi (18.5 GBq) ^{99m}Tc immediately following elution at 0700. At what time will the eluate contain a ^{99}Mo level exceeding the established limits?

$$\text{Mo/Tc} = \frac{32.5\ \mu\text{Ci } ^{99}\text{Mo}}{500\ \text{mCi } ^{99m}\text{Tc}} = 0.065$$

$$t = \frac{-\ln(\text{Mo/Tc})}{0.1052} - 18.03$$

$$t = \frac{-\ln(0.065)}{0.1052} - 18.03$$

$$t = \frac{(2.73337)}{0.1052} - 18.03$$

$$t = 8 \text{ hr.}$$

The eluate will contain ^{99}Mo levels exceeding the limit of 0.15 μCi ^{99}Mo/mCi ^{99m}Tc (5.55 kBq ^{99}Mo/37 MBq ^{99m}Tc) at 1500, eight hours following elution.

Aluminum Ion Content. Aluminum ions from the generator column appearing in the ^{99m}Tc eluate are a chemical impurity. Such impurities can affect the biodistribution of radiopharmaceuticals. Although alumina (Al^{+3}) breakthrough rarely occurs, it is important to ascertain that the established United States Pharmacopeia (USP) Al^{+3} concentration limit of 10 μg Al^{+3}/ml eluate is not exceeded.

Commercially available test kits for determining Al^{+3} concentration contain specially treated indicator paper and a standard Al^{+3} (10 μg/ml). Similar size drops of ^{99m}Tc eluate and the standard Al^{+3} solution are placed adjacent to one another on the indicator paper. The color intensities of both spots are compared. As long as the intensity of the eluate sample is less than that of the standard, the eluate contains less than 10 μg Al^{+3}/ml of eluate.

PREPARATION OF TECHNETIUM-99m RADIOPHARMACEUTICALS

Commercially prepared kits are available for compounding a wide variety of ^{99m}Tc-labeled radiopharmaceuticals. Such kits have a long shelf-life and can be kept in the nuclear medicine department until a specific ^{99m}Tc-labeled agent is required. Technetium-99m-sodium pertechnetate eluted from a ^{99}Mo/^{99m}Tc generator is combined with the appropriate kit reagents to form a tissue-specific compound after only a brief incubation period.

Kit instructions include specific information about the amount of activity and volume of generator eluate to be added. Depending on the day's schedule, a range of activities and volumes may be prepared to meet specific scheduling needs. It is, however, important to add only those activities and volumes within the ranges stated in the directions. Failure to do so may change the formulation of the compound and alter its distribution in the body. Information about incubation periods and special procedures (such as heating) necessary to ensure complete radiolabeling are also included in the package insert.

Example. What activity and what volume should be added to the following gluceptate kit at 0800 if four patients will receive 15 mCi (555 MBq) each, sometime between 0800 and 1200?

Gluceptate Kit:
Maximum ^{99m}Tc activity to be added: 300 mCi (11.1 GBq)
Reconstituting volume: 2–10 ml
[^{99m}Tc]pertechnetate:
Concentration: 25 mCi/ml (925 MBq/ml)
Total volume: 20 ml
Calibration time: 0800.

Solution: Technetium-99m-gluceptate is prepared by adding the appropriate volume and activity of ^{99m}Tc to the lyophilized ("freeze-dried") gluceptate reagent supplied in the sterile reaction vial. To ensure that there will be sufficient activity, assume that all four injections will be given at noon. How much activity will be needed at the time of preparation (0800) if 60 mCi (2.22 GBq) will be needed at 1200?

$$\frac{\text{activity at noon}}{\text{4 hr decay factor}} = \text{activity at 0800}$$

$$\frac{\text{60 mCi}}{0.63} = \text{95 mCi (or 3.51 GBq)}.$$

Calculate the volume of [^{99m}Tc]pertechnetate to be added to the kit at 0800:

$$\frac{\text{95 mCi}}{\text{25 mCi/ml}} = \text{3.8 ml}.$$

Therefore, 95 mCi (3.51 GBq) in 3.8 ml should be added to the gluceptate kit.

Most ^{99m}Tc-labeled compounds, with the exception of ^{99m}Tc-sulfur colloid, are prepared with chemically reduced ^{99m}Tc, a more chemically a ctive form of technetium. For this reason, ^{99m}Tc labeling is accomplished in the presence of stannous chloride, a reducing agent. The stannous ion (Sn^{+2}) reduces the valence state of the technetium in the pertechnetate ion from +7 to +4, or another reduced valence state. The reduced ^{99m}Tc (IV) is a more reactive species, capable of combining with a variety of compounds such as macroaggregated albumin (MAA), methylene diphosphonate (MDP), diethylenetriamine penta-acetic acid (DTPA), 2, 3-dimercaptosuccinic acid (DMSA), gluceptate and disofenin. To prepare kits such as this, the technologist injects the appropriate activity and volume of [^{99m}Tc]pertechnetate into the reaction vial and agitates the vial to dissolve the lyophilized reagent. Some kits may require a brief incubation period or heating for complete labeling to occur.

Technetium-99m-MAA is prepared with reduced ^{99m}Tc. There is, however, one additional consideration in preparing ^{99m}Tc-MAA related to the number of MAA particles that will be administered to the patient. The recommended number of MAA particles to be administered is 200,000–700,000 particles. It is extremely important to observe the volume requirements stated in the kit package insert. The volume added to the kit governs the number of particles in each milliliter of radiopharmaceutical and therefore the number of particles a patient will receive. If too few particles are administered, the perfusion lung image may be technically unsatisfactory and may have the appearance of decreased uptake. Administering more than the recommended number of particles may pose a danger to the patient if too many small arterioles are blocked with MAA particles. Likewise, it is important to observe the expiration time of the MAA preparation if the recommended number of particles is not to be exceeded. As ^{99m}Tc decays, the number of radioactive particles decreases, while the total number of particles in a milliliter remains constant. Therefore, as time passes, more particles must be administered to obtain the same amount of activity.

Technetium-99m-sulfur colloid incorporates ^{99m}Tc in the unreduced, +7 valence state. Therefore, a reducing agent such as stannous chloride is not required. Instead, sulfur colloid kits contain an acid, sodium thiosulfate, a buffer and gelatin. The labeled compound is prepared in two steps. First, the [^{99m}Tc]pertechnetate, acid and sodium thiosulfate are heated in a sterile reaction vial in a shielded, boiling water bath for several minutes. During the heating, elemental sulfur precipitates out of the solution, condensing to form colloidal size particles. The ^{99m}Tc is contained within the colloidal particles. After the vial is vented, buffer is added to neutralize the pH. Gelatin is used to maintain particle size at 0.01–1 micron. Larger particles may become trapped in the lung capillaries before reaching the liver. Undesirably large particles can be caused by excessive heating during preparation or high levels of aluminum in the [^{99m}Tc]pertechnetate used to prepare the labeled colloid.

Radiopharmaceutical Quality Control

In reduced ^{99m}Tc agents, ^{99m}Tc is present in three different chemical forms: (a) bound ^{99m}Tc agent, (b) unbound (free) [^{99m}Tc]pertechnetate and (c) hydrolyzed, reduced ^{99m}Tc (HR-Tc). The proportions of these three chemical forms may vary from one preparation to the next. Because the bound ^{99m}Tc agent is the desired form, the others should be present in only very small quantities.

Technetium-99m-pertechnetate and HR-Tc are radiochemical impurities. Radiochemical purity is defined as the fraction of total radioactivity present in its desired chemical form. If radiochemical impurities exceed certain limits in a given preparation, the distribution of radiopharmaceutical in the patient will be altered. Free pertechnetate can be visualized on images as increased tracer concentration in the stomach, thyroid and salivary glands. Unexpected uptake in the reticuloendothelial system, especially the liver, indicates significant amounts of HR-Tc.

Following radiolabeling, the radiochemical purity of a preparation can be determined using radiochromatography. In this method, a drop of the radiopharmaceutical to be tested is placed at a point called the origin, near one end of the paper strip (Fig. 3-2). The strip is then immersed into a solvent. By capillary action, the solvent travels up the strip carrying with it the soluble components in the sample.

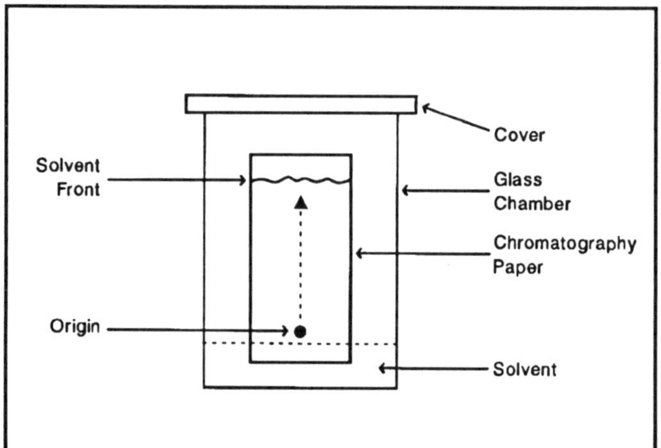

Figure 3.2 Radiochromatography apparatus for determining radiochemical purity.

Insoluble components remain at the origin. As the solvent nears the top of the strip, the strip is removed, dried and cut in half. Each half is counted in a well counter or dose calibrator and the labeling or tagging efficiency, the fraction of radioactivity incorporated into the desired radiolabeled agent, is calculated (Fig. 3-3).

For reduced ^{99m}Tc agents, the labeling efficiency is determined as follows:

$$\text{labeling efficiency} = 100\% - (\%\ \text{free}\ ^{99m}\text{Tc})\ \text{pertechnetate} + \text{HR} - {}^{99m}\text{Tc}.$$

As shown in Figure 3-3, each half of the strip contains either the labeled compound and/or one of the radiochemical impurities. The solvent and support media required (paper or fiberglass/silica gel strip) depend on the radiopharmaceutical to be tested. Table 3-2 shows examples of solvent/support media systems for certain radiopharmaceuticals. The R_f value refers to the distance the component travels from the origin compared to the distance traveled by the solvent (Fig. 3-4).

$$R_f \text{ value} = \frac{\text{distance component travels from origin}}{\text{distance of solvent front from origin}}.$$

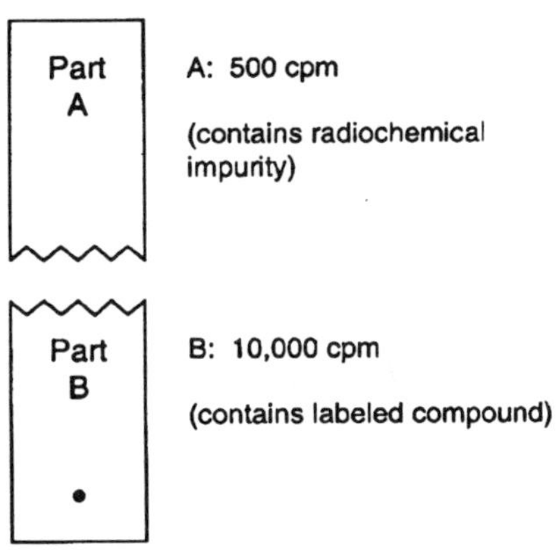

$$\%\ \text{Radiochemical Impurity} = \frac{\text{cpm in Part A}}{\text{cpm in Part A} + \text{cpm in Part B}} \times 100\ \%$$

$$= \frac{500\ \text{cpm}}{500\ \text{cpm} + 10{,}000\ \text{cpm}} \times 100\ \%$$

$$= 4.8\ \%$$

$$\%\ \text{Labeling efficiency} = 100\ \% - \%\ \text{radiochemical impurity}$$

$$= 100\ \% - 4.8\ \% = 95.2\ \%$$

Figure 3.3 Calculation of labeling efficiency or radiochemical purity.

Therefore, R_f values of zero indicate that the component remains at the origin; R_f values of 1 indicate that the component is at the solvent front. These values are characteristic for a given radiochemical component in a given solvent/support media system (Table 3-2).

Minimum radiochemical purity values for selected radiopharmaceuticals are shown in Table 3-3.

UNIT DOSE PREPARATION

When liquid radiopharmaceuticals are received in multidose vials, the technologist must determine the volume containing the desired amount of radioactivity to be administered. The first step in preparing a unit dose is to carefully examine the label on the radiopharmaceutical vial and note the following information.

1. Radionuclide and chemical form of radiopharmaceutical. A radionuclide such as ^{99m}Tc may be tagged to a variety of chemical compounds (MDP, DTPA, MAA), so care should be taken to choose the correct radiopharmaceutical for a given nuclear medicine procedure.
2. Expiration time/date. The time at which the radiopharmaceutical should no longer be administered to patients.
3. Volume (in milliliters). The total amount of liquid in the vial.
4. Total activity (in mCi, MBq, μCi or kBq). The total amount of radioactivity present in the vial at the time of assay or calibration.
5. Concentration (in mCi/ml, MBq/ml, μCi/ml or kBq/ml). The amount of activity per unit volume at the time of assay or calibration. Concentration is obtained by dividing the total activity in the vial by the total volume:

$$\text{Concentration} = \frac{\text{total activity}}{\text{total volume}}.$$

6. Assay or calibration time/date. The time and/or date when the total activity and concentration were determined.
7. Specific activity (in mCi/mg, MBq/mg, μCi/mg or kBq/mg). The amount of activity per unit mass of a radionuclide or radiopharmaceutical. Do not confuse specific activity with concentration. A specific activity may not appear on all radiopharmaceutical labels.
8. Lot number. A number assigned by the manufacturer to each batch of radiopharmaceutical. The number can be used to trace problems associated with the radiopharmaceutical.

After the technologist secures the correct radiopharmaceutical and ascertains that the expiration time has not passed, the amount of radioactivity to be administered to the patient is determined. For adults, a standard dose range has usually been established by the nuclear medicine physician. Occasionally an adult dose may be based on the patient's body weight. There are several methods that can be used to calculate pediatric doses (Table 3-4). To achieve images of similar quality and counting statistics as those of adults, the method based upon body surface area is recommended. For example, based on this method, a child weigh-

Table 3.2
Radiochromatography Techniques for Selected Technetium-99m Radiopharmaceuticals

Radiopharmaceutical	Support media	Solvent	Rf value*: Radiopharmaceutical	Rf value*: Free $^{99m}TcO_4$	Rf value*: HR ^{99m}Tc†
^{99m}Tc-sulfur colloid	Gelman ITLC-SG	0.9% NaCl	0.0	0.9	N.A.
^{99m}Tc-macroaggregated albumin	Gelman ITLC-SG	0.9% NaCl	0.0	0.9	N.A.
^{99m}Tc-sodium pertechnetate	Whatman 31 ET	Acetone	0.0‡	0.9	0.0
^{99m}Tc-pentetate (DTPA)	Whatman 31 ET	Methyl ethyl ketone	0.0	0.9	0.0
	Gelman ITLC-SG	0.9% NaCl	1.0	1.0	0.0
^{99m}Tc-pyrophosphate	Whatman 31 ET	Methyl ethyl ketone	0.0	1.0	0.0
	Gelman ITLC-SG	0.9% NaCl	1.0	1.0	0.0
^{99m}Tc-medronate (MDP)	Whatman 31 ET	Methyl ethyl ketone	0.0	0.9	0.0
	Gelman ITLC-SG	0.9% NaCl	1.0	1.0	0.0
^{99m}Tc-oxidronate (HMDP)	Whatman 31 ET	Acetone	0.0	0.9	0.0
	Gelman ITLC-SG	0.9% NaCl	1.0	1.0	0.0
^{99m}Tc-gluceptate	Whatman 31 ET	Acetone	0.0	0.9	0.0
	Gelman ITLC-SG	0.9% NaCl	1.0	1.0	0.0
^{99m}Tc-succimer (DMSA)	Gelman ITLC-SA	Acetone	0.0	1.0	0.0
^{99m}Tc-2,6-diisopropyl IDA (disofenin)	Gelman ITLC-SA	Saturated NaCl	0.0	1.0	0.0
	Gelman ITLC-SG	Distilled H_2O	1.0	1.0	0.0

$$^*Rf\text{ value} = \frac{\text{distance component travels from origin}}{\text{distance of solvent front from origin}}.$$

†HR ^{99m}Tc = hydrolyzed, reduced ^{99m}Tc and includes all colloidal species of reduced ^{99m}Tc.

‡Methyl ethyl ketone (MEK) may be used in place of acetone and vice versa.

Reprinted with permission from: Chilton HM, Witcofski RL. *Nuclear pharmacy.* Philadelphia: Lea & Febiger; 1986:79.

ing 30 kg should receive 62% of the recommended adult dose. Therefore, if the adult dose is 20 mCi (740 MBq), a child weighing 30 kg should receive 0.62 × 20 mCi (740 MBq) or 12.4 mCi (459 MBq).

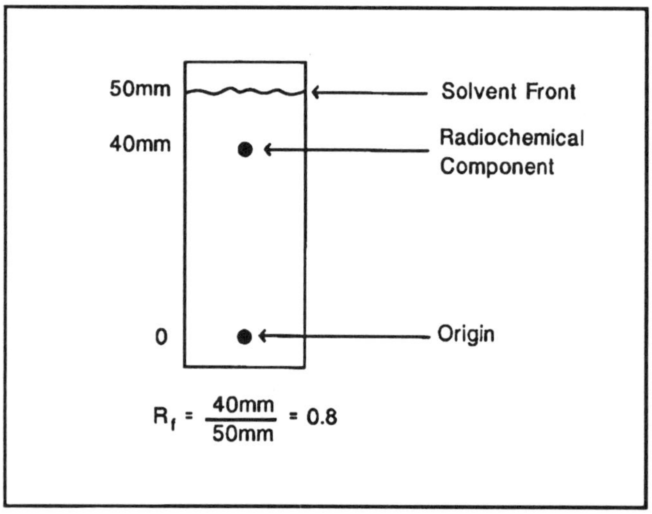

Figure 3.4 Calculation of R_f value.

Next, the initial radiopharmaceutical concentration is decay-corrected for the time of administration and the volume to be administered is determined as follows:

$$C_0 \times DF = C_t,$$

where C_0 equals the initial concentration, DF equals the decay factor and C_t equals the concentration at time t:

$$\frac{\text{patient dose}}{C_t} = \text{volume to be administered.}$$

Example. A technologist needs to administer 3 mCi (111 MBq) ^{99m}Tc-MAA to a patient at 1000. If the concentration of the radiopharmaceutical is 15 mCi/ml (555 MBq/ml) at 0600, what volume should be administered to the patient?

Solution: Decay correct the initial concentration for 1000. From a table of decay factors for ^{99m}Tc, the decay factor for 4 hr (0600–1000) is 0.631.

$$C_0 \times DF = C_t$$

$$15\text{ mCi/ml} \times 0.631 = 9.5\text{ mCi/ml (or 351 MBq/ml)}.$$

Table 3.3
Minimum Radiochemical Purity Values for Selected Radiopharmaceuticals (from USP XXII)*

Minimum purity	Radiopharmaceutical
85%	^{99m}Tc-succimer (DMSA)
90%	^{99m}Tc-pentetate (DTPA)
	^{99m}Tc-sodium pertechnetate
	^{99m}Tc-py rophosphate
	^{99m}Tc-macroaggregated albumin
92%	^{99m}Tc-sulfur colloid
97%	[^{131}I]orthoiodohippuric acid (OIH)

*Values shown are minimum percentages of radioactivity present in desired radiochemical form.

Reprinted with permission from: Chilton HM, Witcofski RL. *Nuclear pharmacy.* Philadelphia: Lea & Febiger; 1986:80.

Determine the volume to be administered:

$$\frac{\text{patient dose}}{C_t} = \text{volume to be administered}$$

$$\frac{3\ \text{mCi}}{9.5\ \text{mCi/ml}} = 0.32\ \text{ml.}$$

Example. A technologist needs 3.5 mCi (129 MBq) of [^{201}Tl]thallous chloride to perform myocardial imaging on September 6. If the concentration of the radiopharmaceutical is 2 mCi/ml (74 MBq/ml) on September 8, what volume should be administered to the patient?

Solution. Decay-correct the September 8 concentration for September 6. From a table of decay factors for ^{201}Tl, the decay factor for 2 days (September 6–8) is 0.634. In this instance, the radiopharmaceutical is being administered before the calibration time. Therefore, the initial concentration is the unknown.

$$C_0 \times DF = C_t$$

$$C_0 = C_t/DF$$

$$C_0 = \frac{2.0\ \text{mCi/ml}}{0.634}$$

$$= 3.2\ \text{mCi/ml (or 118 MBq/ml) on September 6.}$$

Determine the volume to be administered:

$$\frac{\text{patient dose}}{C_0} = \text{volume to be administered}$$

$$\frac{3.5\ \text{mCi}}{3.2\ \text{mCi/ml}} = 1.1\ \text{ml.}$$

Pertinent information such as the name of the radiopharmaceutical, lot number, activity and volume administered, time and date and patient's name should be entered into the appropriate records.

With the appropriate size syringe and a 20–22-gauge needle, the technologist withdraws the calculated volume into the syringe in accordance with aseptic and radiation protection techniques. Aseptic technique includes maintaining the sterility of the needle hub as it is attached to the syringe and the needle itself and cleansing the top of the radiopharmaceutical vial with alcohol. Radiation protection includes wearing disposable gloves, using syringe and vial shields, working behind a lead shield and using tongs as appropriate. Working quickly and efficiently minimizes radiation exposure as well. The stability of the radiopharmaceutical can be prolonged if the technologist refrains from injecting air into the radiopharmaceutical vial.

The syringe containing the radiopharmaceutical should then be assayed in a dose calibrator to ascertain that the activity is within the prescribed dose range. To prevent misadministration, the technologist should label the syringe with the patient's name or ID number, radiopharmaceutical name, activity and time and date of assay.

Table 3.4
Methods for Calculating Pediatric Radiopharmaceutical Dosages

1. Clark's Rule (weight)	2. Webster's Rule (age)	3. Young's Rule (age)
$\frac{\text{weight in lb} \times \text{adult dose}}{150 \text{ lb}}$	$\frac{\text{age (yr)} + 1}{\text{age} + 7} \times \text{adult dose}$	$\frac{\text{age (yr)}}{\text{age} + 12} \times \text{adult dose}$

4. Body Surface Area*

Weight		Surface area	Fraction of
kg	lb	(m^2)	adult dose†
2	4.4	0.15	0.09
4	8.8	0.25	0.14
6	13.2	0.33	0.19
8	17.6	0.40	0.23
10	22.0	0.46	0.27
15	33.0	0.63	0.36
20	44.0	0.83	0.48
25	55.0	0.95	0.55
30	66.0	1.08	0.62
35	77.0	1.20	0.69
40	88.0	1.30	0.75
45	99.0	1.40	0.81
50	110.0	1.51	0.87
55	121.0	1.58	0.91

*Based on average adult surface area of 1.73 m^2.

†Reprinted with permission from Modell W, ed. *Drugs of choice 1958–1959.* St. Louis: C V Mosby; 1958:42.

Reprinted with permission from: Chilton HM, Witcofski RL. *Nuclear pharmacy.* Philadelphia: Lea and Febiger; 1986:47.

EXERCISES

Solutions to exercises may be found in Appendix A.

1. If 378 mCi [^{99m}Tc]pertechnetate are eluted from a ^{99}Mo/^{99m}Tc generator and contained in 20 ml, what is the concentration of the eluate?
2. If 15 ml ^{99m}Tc eluate are assayed to contain 10.6 μCi ^{99}Mo and 598 mCi ^{99m}Tc, what is the ^{99}Mo concentration in the eluate?
3. The ^{99}Mo assay results shown below were obtained at 0600, immediately following generator elution. Can this eluate be used in patients at 1600?

^{99}Mo	6.1 μCi
^{99m}Tc	279 mCi

4. If the following reagents are available, what is the maximum amount of ^{99m}Tc-oxidronate, in gigabecquerels, that can be prepared from one kit?

Oxidronate Kit

Maximum ^{99m}Tc activity to be added:	5.55 GBq
Reconstituting volume:	0.5–5.0 ml

[^{99m}Tc]pertechnetate

Concentration:	925 MBq/ml
Total volume:	10 ml

5. What is the final concentration of ^{99m}Tc-sulfur colloid if the maximum activity is prepared with the following reagents?

Sulfur Colloid Kit

Reaction vial:	3 ml sodium thiosulfate mixture
Syringe A:	2 ml hydrochloric acid
Syringe B:	2 ml buffer solution
Maximum ^{99m}Tc activity to be added:	250 mCi
^{99m}Tc volume to be added:	1–3 ml

[^{99m}Tc]Pertechnetate

Concentration:	38.5 mCi/ml
Total volume:	10 ml

6. At 0900, Patient A receives 1 ml ^{99m}Tc-MAA containing 3 mCi and 300,000 particles. If Patient B receives 3 mCi from the same preparation at 1500, how many particles does Patient B receive?

7. Based on the R_f values and chromatography results shown below, what is the radiochemical purity of this preparation?

	R_f values cpm	Chromatography Results	
Free $^{99m}TcO_4^-$	0.9	Top half of strip	1563 cpm
^{99m}Tc-pentetate	0.0	Bottom half of strip	27,695 cpm

8. Based on the chromatography results shown below, determine the tagging efficiency of the preparation.

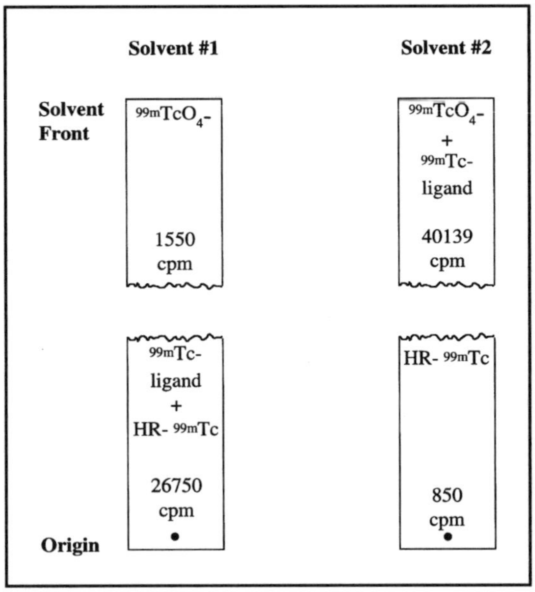

9. A technologist needs to obtain 29.6 MBq ^{111}In-oxine at 1200 on July 15. The label on the radiopharmaceutical vial contains the following information:

Total activity:	74 MBq
Volume:	1.0 ml
Assay time/date:	1200, July 12

What volume is required to obtain the necessary activity on July 15?

10. A technologist must administer 1.0 mCi [^{201}Tl]thallous chloride at 1400 on September 7. If the concentration of the radiopharmaceutical is 3.0 mCi/ml at 1200 on September 10, what volume should be administered to the patient on September 7?

REFERENCES

1. Chilton HM, Witcofski RL. *Nuclear pharmacy: an introduction to the clinical application of radiopharmaceuticals.* Philadelphia: Lea & Febiger; 1986:26–28, 54–66,71–82.

2. Early PJ, Sodee DE. *Principles and practice of nuclear medicine,* 2nd ed. Mosby Year-Book, Inc.; 1995:56–59, 96, 104–117, 747–749.

3. Eliot AT. Radionuclide generators. In: Sampson CB, ed. *Textbook of radiopharmacy: theory and practice.* New York: Gordon and Breach Science Publishers; 1990:33–51.

4. Kowalsky RJ, Perry JR. *Radiopharmaceuticals in nuclear medicine practice.* Norwalk, CT: Appleton & Lange; 1987:59–74.

5. Marchant T, ed. *A guide to radiopharmaceutical quality control.* North Billerica, MA: Du Pont Company, 1985.

6. Phan T, Ling M, Wasnich R. *Practical nuclear pharmacy,* 3rd ed. Honolulu, HI: Banyan Press; 1987.

7. Ponto JA. Expiration times for ^{99m}Tc. *J Nucl Med Technol* 1981; 9:40–41.

8. Ponto JA, Swanson DP, Freitas JE. Clinical manifestations of radiopharmaceutical formulation problems. In: Hladik WB III, Saha GP, Study KT, eds. *Essentials of nuclear medicine science.* Baltimore: Williams & Wilkins; 1987:268–289.

9. Robbins PJ. *Chromatography of technetium-99m radiopharmaceuticals— a practical guide.* Reston, VA: Society of Nuclear Medicine; 1984.

10. Saha GB. *Fundamentals of nuclear pharmacy,* 3rd ed. New York: Springer-Verlag; 1992.

11. Schwarz SW, Anderson CJ, Welch MJ. Radiochemistry and radiopharmacology. In: Bernier DR, Christian PE, Langan JK, eds. *Nuclear medicine technology and techniques,* 3rd ed. St. Louis: Mosby Year-Book, Inc.; 1994:145–152.

12. Steves AM. *Nuclear medicine—radiopharmacy series* (six computer-assisted instruction programs). Edwardsvillle, KS: Educational Software Concepts, Inc.; 1995.

13. *The United States Pharmacopoeia XXII.* Rockville, MD: United States Pharmacopoeial Convention, Inc.; 1990.

4 Instrumentation Quality Assurance

Ann M. Steves

Regulatory agencies require that quality control testing be performed on instrumentation to ensure patient safety and diagnostic accuracy. The term quality control refers to the testing designed to identify equipment problems. Quality assurance refers to a system designed to identify problems, propose solutions and monitor results to achieve the desired level of performance.

SCINTILLATION CAMERA

Table 4-1 lists the quality control tests to be performed on scintillation cameras and the optimum testing frequency.

Field Uniformity

Field uniformity is the ability of a scintillation camera to produce a uniform image when the source provides a uniform distribution of photons over the detector (Fig. 4-1). Clinically, it is the ability of the instrument to produce accurate images of a radionuclide distribution in patients.

Field uniformity measurements may be intrinsic or extrinsic. Intrinsic testing monitors the condition of the sodium iodide crystal and electronics associated with the scintillation camera detector and is performed without a collimator attached to the detector. The extrinsic method, performed with a collimator in place, assesses the instrument as it is used clinically. Both methods have advantages and disadvantages. However, once a particular method is adopted, it should be used consistently by everyone performing quality control testing in the nuclear medicine department. Table 4-2 compares the testing procedure for the two methods.

Uniformity images should be inspected carefully for areas of nonuniformity and compared to previous flood images (Fig. 4-2). The possibility of subtle changes requires comparison of current images with those acquired several weeks or months previously. Causes of field nonuniformity are listed in Table 4-3. One of the most common and easily remedied sources of nonuniformity is photopeak misadjustment (i.e., the photopeak is not correctly positioned within the window, or the wrong energy setting is chosen for the radionuclide being imaged). Uniformity that changes noticeably from one day to the next often indicates a photopeaking problem. The size and shape of the flood field image should also be consistent from day to day.

Spatial Resolution

Spatial resolution is the ability of a scintillation camera to reproduce small differences in radionuclide concentration in closely spaced areas. Clinically, resolution affects the ability to visualize small defects.

As with field uniformity, spatial resolution can be measured intrinsically or extrinsically with an appropriate bar or multihole phantom (Fig. 4-3). The smallest bar and space width or hole size should be matched to the resolution limits of the camera system specified by the camera manufacturer.

Table 4.1
Scintillation Camera Quality Control

Test	Testing frequency
Field uniformity	Daily
Spatial resolution	Weekly
Spatial linearity	Weekly
Sensitivity	Semiannually

These tests should also be performed following repair or adjustment of the instrument.

Figure 4.1 Normal field uniformity image. Courtesy of Department of Veterans Affairs Medical Center, Birmingham, AL.

Table 4.2
Comparison of Intrinsic and Extrinsic Scintillation Camera Quality Control

	Intrinsic	Extrinsic
Collimator	None	Low-energy, parallel-hole
Radiation source	^{99m}Tc point source	^{99m}Tc liquid flood
	^{99m}Tc liquid flood	^{57}Co solid sheet
	^{57}Co solid sheet	
Source distance	Point source placed 4–5 crystal diameters away from detector	Flood source placed directly on face of collimator
	Flood source placed on crystal face	

Table 4.3
Causes of Scintillation Camera Field Nonuniformities

Misadjusted photopeak
Damaged crystal
Collimator defect
"Mistuned" photomultiplier tube
Photomultiplier tube malfunction
Radioactive contamination on crystal or collimator
Scratched, dirty CRT screen or multiformatter lenses
Film processing artifacts

Hine-Duley Phantom. The Hine-Duley phantom consists of lead bars and spaces of three different widths; the bars are embedded in plastic (Fig. 4-3A). Since resolution is not measured equally over all areas with this phantom, multiple images must be acquired to assess resolution for the entire detector area.

Figure 4.2 Nonuniform field source image collected following a power failure. Note photomultiplier tubes. Courtesy of Department of Veterans Affairs Medical Center, Birmingham, AL.

Four-Quadrant Bar Phantom. The four-quadrant bar phantom contains spaces and lead bars of four different widths (Fig. 4-3B). The spaces and bars in each quadrant are of equal width. Four images, acquired at 90° to one another, are required to assess resolution over the entire detector.

Parallel-Line Equal-Space (PLES) Phantom. All lead bars and spaces are of equal width in the PLES phantom (Fig. 4-3C). Two images acquired at 90° to one another are necessary to monitor resolution over the entire crystal.

Orthogonal-Hole Phantom. The orthogonal-hole phantom consists of a lead sheet containing holes of equal diameter arranged at right angles to one another (Fig. 4-3D). Only one image is needed to determine resolution over all areas of the detector.

Resolution phantom images should be carefully examined to detect changes in resolution by comparing current images to previous ones. As with uniformity testing, sudden changes from one day to the next usually are caused by improper photopeak adjustment. Subtle changes over time are expected as the crystal ages. Factors that can affect spatial resolution are listed in Table 4-4.

Spatial Linearity

Spatial linearity is the ability of a scintillation camera to produce a uniform image with straight lines corresponding to straight lines in a phantom. Clinically, it is the accurate portrayal of true organ shape. Linearity can be assessed along with resolution by examining the straightness of a set of parallel bars or, in the case of the orthogonal-hole phantom, the straightness of parallel rows of holes. Current images should be compared with those obtained when the scintillation camera was installed.

Sensitivity

Sensitivity is the ability to detect ionizing events in a sodium iodide crystal expressed in counts per second per microcurie (cps/μCi). It can be measured simultaneously when uniformity is performed if the activity of the source and the room background is known. The activity in the source must be carefully measured and corrected for decay, then the count rate obtained per unit activity can be calculated.

$$\text{Sensitivity} = \frac{(\text{counts} - \text{backround})/\text{time}}{\text{activity of source}} = \text{cps}/\mu\text{Ci or cpm}/\mu\text{Ci.}$$

The calculated sensitivity is then compared to previous values. Sensitivity can be affected by incorrect energy settings, incorrect collimation, if extrinsic sensitivity is performed, or improper detector-source distance.

DOSE CALIBRATOR

Table 4-5 lists the dose calibrator quality control tests and the testing frequency required by the NRC.

Constancy

Constancy testing determines the reproducibility of measurements of a source of known activity from day to day. A long-lived standard is measured at each of the commonly used radionuclide settings. Each measurement is compared to the calculated (decay-corrected) value for the standard at that setting on that day. An outline of the constancy testing procedure is as follows:

1. Count a long-lived standard, such as ^{57}Co or ^{137}Cs, of known activity on the appropriate dose calibrator setting.

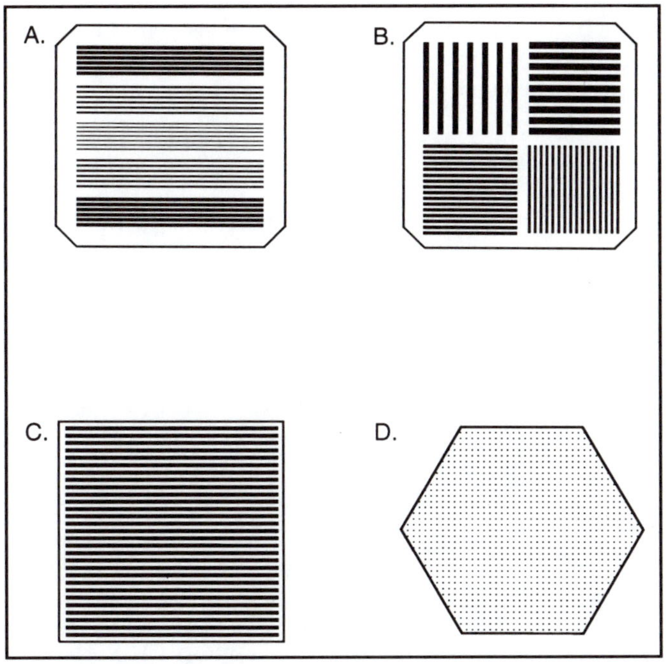

Figure 4.3 Transmission phantoms used to measure the spatial resolution of a scintillation camera. (A) Hine-Duley phantom. (B) Four-quadrant bar phantom. (C) Parallel-line equal-space (PLES) phantom. (D) Orthogonal hole phantom.

Table 4.4
Factors Affecting Scintillation Camera Spatial Resolution

Photopeak adjustment
PHA window width
Source-detector distance
Gamma-ray energy
Collimator type
Crystal degradation

2. Obtain a background at the same setting to determine net activity.
3. Correct the known activity for decay and determine the $\pm 10\%$ range of this value.
4. The measured value should be within 10% of the decay-corrected activity (Fig. 4-4).
5. Using the same reference source, repeat the measurement for all commonly used radionuclide settings.
6. Again correcting for background and decay, determine the $\pm 10\%$ range of each calculated value. Compare each measured value to the range of calculated values for that radionuclide setting.
7. Each measured value should be within $\pm 10\%$ of the decay-corrected value at each setting.

According to the NRC, if the constancy error is greater than 10%, the instrument should be repaired or replaced.

Activity Linearity

A linearity test ascertains how accurately a dose calibrator measures activities over a wide range, from millicurie to microcurie amounts. The test involves assaying a source with a relatively short half-life over a period of several days and comparing the predicted and measured results. Linearity testing is conducted as follows:

1. Assay an aliquot of ^{99m}Tc at 2–3-hr intervals over 3 or more days. According to the NRC, the starting activity should approximate the highest activity that will be administered to a patient. The starting activity must be assayed until it reaches 30 μCi (1.1 MBq).

Table 4.5
Dose Calibrator Quality Control (NRC)

Test	Testing frequency
Constancy	Daily
Activity linearity	At installation and quarterly
Accuracy	At installation and annually
Geometry dependence	At installation

These tests should also be performed after adjustment or repair of the instrument.

2. Correct all measurements for background.
3. Calculate the predicted activity for each time the sample was measured.
4. Plot both the calculated and measured activities on semi-log paper (activity versus time) as shown in Figure 4-5.
5. Measured activities should be within ±10% of calculated activities.

According to the NRC, if linearity errors exceed 10%, mathematically corrected dose calibrator readings should be calculated for activities greater than 10 μCi (0.37 MBq).

An alternate method of performing an activity linearity test is to use the commercially available systems "Calicheck" (Calcorp, Inc., Cleveland, OH) or "Lineator" (Biodex Medical Systems, Shirley, NY). These systems consist of a series of lead tubes that absorb ^{99m}Tc photons by a known amount. After the source is assayed initially, it is measured several more times after each of the lead tubes is placed in sequence around the source. Measurements of the shielded source simulate radioactive decay. This method saves time and decreases personnel exposure. The source used to perform the test may also be used in patients after linearity data collection.

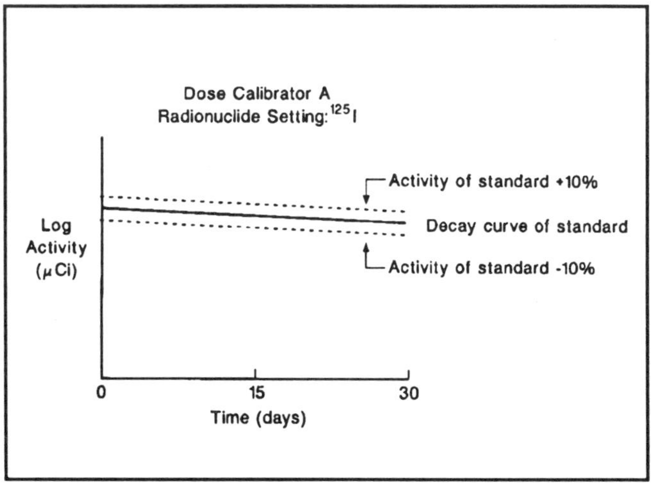

Figure 4.4 Graph of dose calibrator constancy.

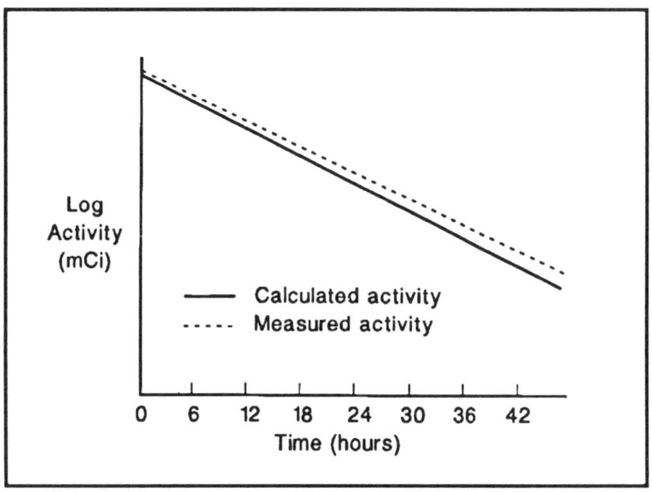

Figure 4.5 Dose calibrator activity linearity graph.

Accuracy

Accuracy testing assesses the ability of a dose calibrator to accurately measure the activity of radionuclides of different gamma energies. According to the NRC, at least two different standards, one of which must have a photon energy between 100 and 500 keV, must be assayed. Accuracy testing is performed as follows:

1. Assay each standard in the dose calibrator three times at the appropriate radionuclide setting. Measure the background at each setting.
2. For each standard, average the three readings and subtract the background to obtain the net activity.
3. Correct the known reference activity for decay and determine the ±10% range of the decay-corrected value.
4. Average measured activities should be within ±10% of the decay-corrected reference activity.

According to the NRC, if the accuracy error is greater than 10%, the dose calibrator should be repaired or replaced.

Geometric Variation

Evaluation of geometric variation determines the effect of sample volume and configuration on the measurement of a sample's activity. For example, 20 mCi (0.74 GBq) contained in a 1-ml volume in a syringe and 20 mCi (0.74 GBq) contained in a 10-ml volume in a glass vial may yield significantly different measurements when assayed in the same dose calibrator. To ascertain the error in measuring activity of varying volumes or shapes, the following procedure may be used.

1. Assay 1–2 mCi (37–74 MBq) ^{99m}Tc in a minimal volume (1–2 drops) in a 20–30-ml vial. Obtain the background reading.
2. Increase the volume in the vial stepwise by adding water. The volumes should be those commonly assayed.
3. Assay the vial after each addition of water and obtain a background reading.
4. Correct each measurement for background and calculate a correction factor for each volume.

$$\%\ \text{correction factor} = \frac{\text{true activity}}{\text{measured activity}}.$$

5. Plot the correction factors against the volumes on linear graph paper.
6. After assaying a vial of activity in the dose calibrator, calculate the true activity using the appropriate correction factor:

$$\text{true activity} = \text{measured activity} \times \text{correction factor}.$$

7. A similar procedure can be used for various size syringes.

According to the NRC, correction factors should be calculated for any geometric variations causing measurements to vary by more than 10% from the true activity.

SCINTILLATION SPECTROMETER

A scintillation spectrometer is an instrument, such as an uptake probe or scintillation well counting system, that uses pulse-height analysis to determine which pulses will be counted. Table 4-6 contains a list of quality control tests and the frequency with which they should be performed on scintillation spectrometers.

Calibration

Calibration of a scintillation spectrometer involves determining the appropriate operating high voltage and amplifier gain.

Operating Voltage. The operating voltage is the high voltage applied to the dynodes of the photomultiplier tube (PMT). The high voltage can be adjusted so that the arbitrary units on the pulse-height analyzer dials, upper and lower level discriminators (ULD and LLD), correspond to meaningful energy (voltage) units. Typically, the dials are divided into 1000 units. A useful calibration is to have each unit equal to 1 keV; then the range of the dial is 0–1000 keV. The operating voltage is determined in the following manner.

1. Use a monoenergetic gamma source of known energy, for example, ^{137}Cs.
2. Set a narrow window around the photopeak energy by adjusting the ULD and LLD of the pulse-height analyzer. For ^{137}Cs, the lower and upper level discriminators would be set at 652 and 672 units, respectively, for a window of 3%.
3. Beginning with the lowest voltage setting, count the source for 1 min at each voltage setting, increasing the voltage until the maximum count rate is observed.

Table 4.6
Scintillation Spectrometer Quality Control

Test	Testing frequency
Background measurement	Daily
Calibration	Daily
Sensitivity	Daily
Energy resolution	Quarterly
Chi-square test	Quarterly

These tests should also be performed after adjustment or repair of the instrument.

4. Plot counts per minute versus energy (voltage) on linear graph paper. The voltage setting at which the highest count rate is obtained is the operating voltage. The units on the pulse-height analyzer dials are now calibrated for 0–1000 keV. The window can be moved up or down to accept pulses from the photopeaks of other radionuclides.
5. Note gain settings. Calibration results are valid only on that gain setting.

The effect of changing voltages on a gamma ray spectrum is shown in Figure 4-6. Increasing the voltage moves the entire gamma spectrum to the right. When the photopeak moves into the preset window, the maximum counting rate is observed.

Amplifier Gain. In the previous discussion, the spectrometer was calibrated to accept pulse heights in the 0–1000 keV range. However, the calibration of the spectrometer is not linear in the low voltage range where lower energy radionuclides, such as ^{125}I, are counted. Nonlinearity means that the photopeak will not be found at the expected voltage. For ^{125}I, the photopeak will not be

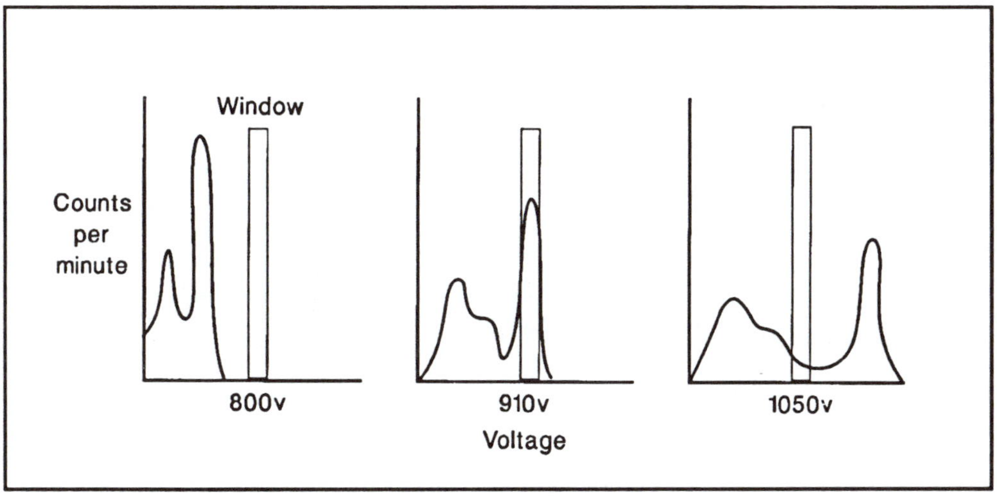

Figure 4.6 Effect of changing voltage on the gamma-ray spectrum. At the lower voltages, the entire spectrum lies below the window, so only the background is being counted. As the voltage increases, the spectrum is shifted to the right, which moves the photopeak into the preset window. Increasing the voltage moves Compton scatter into the counting window.

found at the voltage corresponding to 35 keV but rather at some slightly higher or lower voltage. In addition, calibrating the instrument in this manner eliminates the possibility of counting radionuclides with energies above 1000 keV, such as ^{60}Co (1.17 MeV, 1.33 MeV). Adjusting the amplifier gain, however, will permit counting of very high or very low radionuclide energies. When the amplifier gain is used to alter pulse height and shift the gamma spectrum, one unit on the ULD and LLD dials is no longer equivalent to 1 keV.

Depending on the instrument, one of two types of gain control may be used to adjust amplifier gain: true gain and inverse gain. With true gain control, an increase in gain produces an increase in pulse height with a corresponding decrease in the energy range. For example, a true gain instrument is calibrated on a gain setting of 8 so that the energy range is 0–1000 keV over 1000 dial divisions (Fig. 4-7). If the gain is doubled, the energy range is decreased and the gamma spectrum is shifted to the right. If the gain is halved, then the energy range is increased and the spectrum shifts to the left. Inverse gain operates in the opposite manner. Thus, with this type of amplifier gain, an increase in gain produces a corresponding decrease in pulse height but a corresponding increase in the energy range (Fig. 4-8). To determine which type of gain control an instrument uses, consult the operator's manual.

Energy Resolution

If the conversion of light photons in a sodium iodide detector to an electrical pulse were perfect, the photopeak in a gamma spectrum would look like a narrow line. Instead, pulse heights of varying amplitudes, representing a range of energies around the photopeak energy, form the familiar bell-shaped peak. The width of the photopeak is an indicator of the accuracy of the conversion from light to electrical energy, or the energy resolution of the instrument.

A ^{137}Cs source is typically used to measure energy resolution in the following way:

1. Using the proper operating voltage and a narrow window, measure the counts for a preset time at 10-keV increments around the photopeak.
2. Plot counts per 10 keV interval versus the midpoint of the counting interval (Fig. 4-9).
3. Calculate the full width at half maximum (FWHM) as follows: (a) divide the maximum photopeak count by 2, (b)

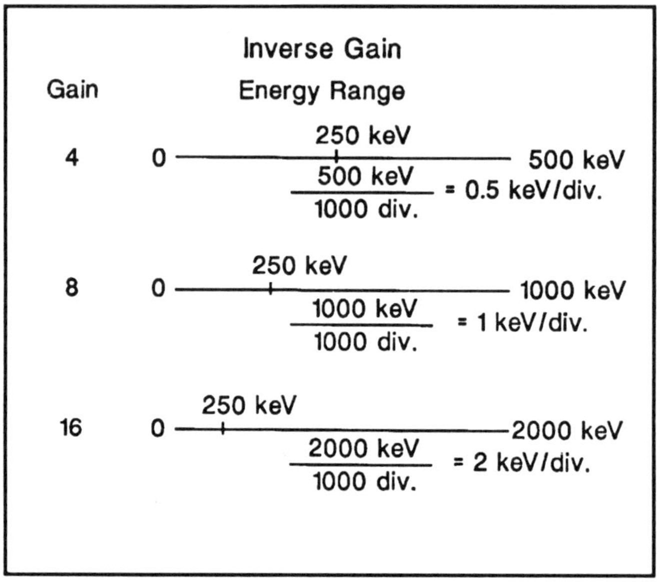

Figure 4.8 Inverse gain control.

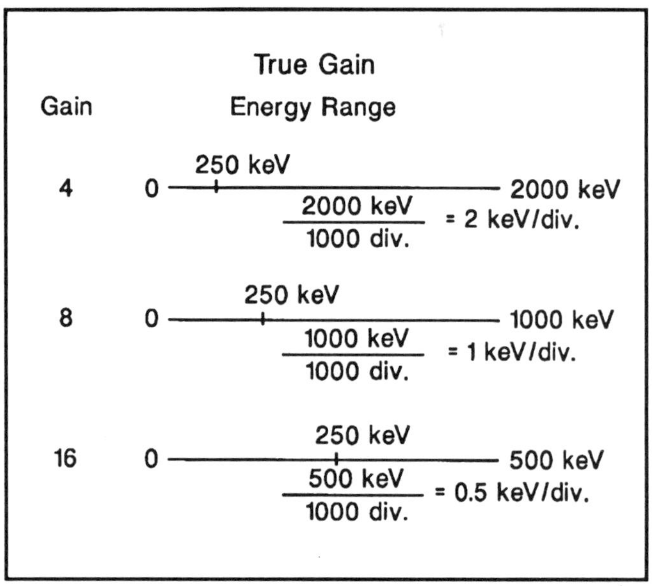

Figure 4.7 True gain control.

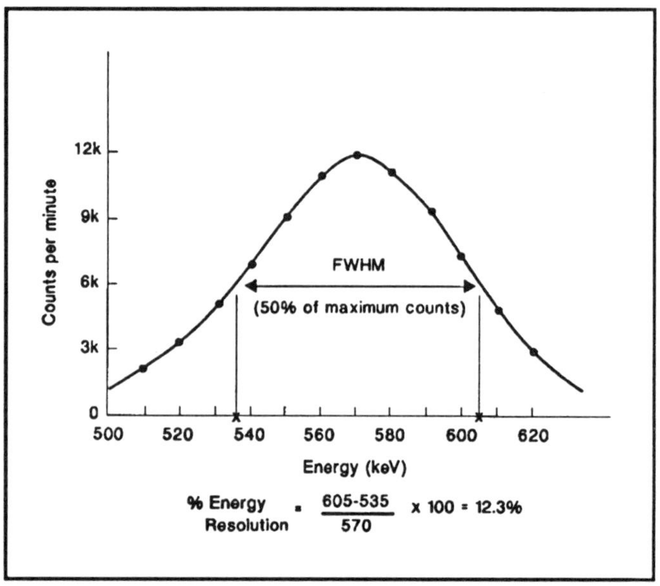

Figure 4.9 Energy resolution determination.

draw a line across the photopeak at the 50% count level determined in step a, (c) drop perpendicular lines to the x-axis where the line in step b intersects the two edges of the photopeak. The distance between the two perpendicular lines (in energy units) is the FWHM.

4. Calculate the % energy resolution as follows:

$$\%\text{ energy resolution} = \frac{\text{FWHM (keV)}}{\text{midpoint of photopeak (kev)}} \times 100.$$

A typical range for ^{137}Cs is 8%–12%. The energy resolution will degrade, that is, the value will become larger as the crystal ages or if a problem develops with the amplifier or photomultiplier tube.

Chi Square Test

The chi square test is a method to check for random errors greater than those that would be predicted. Random errors affect the reproducibility (or precision) of measurements. These are always present in radiation counting because of the random nature of radioactive decay. If a source is counted ten times for 1 min, each measurement will be different even though the same activity is counted each time. The question then becomes whether the variations in the measurement are due to the randomness of radioactive decay or to a malfunction of the counting instrument. To answer that question, a chi square test is conducted as follows:

1. Using a long-lived standard (^{137}Cs or ^{57}Co), collect a series of measurements (20–50), each for a preset time (Fig. 4-10).
2. Compute the mean (average) value.

$$\overline{N} = \frac{\Sigma N_i}{n},$$

where N_i = an individual measurement and n= number of measurements.

3. Calculate the chi square (χ^2) value as follows:

$$\chi^2 = \frac{\Sigma(N_i - \overline{N})^2}{\overline{N}}.$$

4. Using the χ^2 table (Appendix E), find the probability, p, for the number of measurements and calculated χ^2 value. The p value denotes the probability that random variations observed in a series would equal or exceed the calculated χ^2 value.

Acceptable p values are between 0.1 and 0.9. Values greater than 0.9 or less than 0.1 indicate that the variations in the measurements do not match the expected and the instrument should be checked.

N_i	$(N_i - \overline{N})^2$
10150	17956
9988	784
9899	13689
10060	1936
9954	3844
10099	6889
9999	289
10005	121
10027	121
9979	1369
$\overline{N}$ = 10016	Sum = 46,998

$$\chi^2 = \frac{46{,}998}{10{,}016} = 4.692$$

Using the table in Appendix E, for 9 degrees of freedom (n-1), 4.692 falls between an acceptable probability of 0.90 and 0.50, indicating that the variations in counts are probably due to the randomness of radioactive decay rather than instrument malfunction.

Figure 4.10 Chi square calculation.

SURVEY METER

Table 4-7 lists the quality control steps that should be performed on survey meters and the testing frequency required by the NRC. A battery check should be performed immediately before each use, if the instrument has that option. Daily reference checks are performed by measuring a long-lived source, using constant geometry,

TABLE 4-7
Survey Meter Quality Control (NRC)

Test	Testing frequency
Reference check source	Before each use
Calibration	Before initial use and annually

These tests should also be performed following adjustment or repair of the instrument.

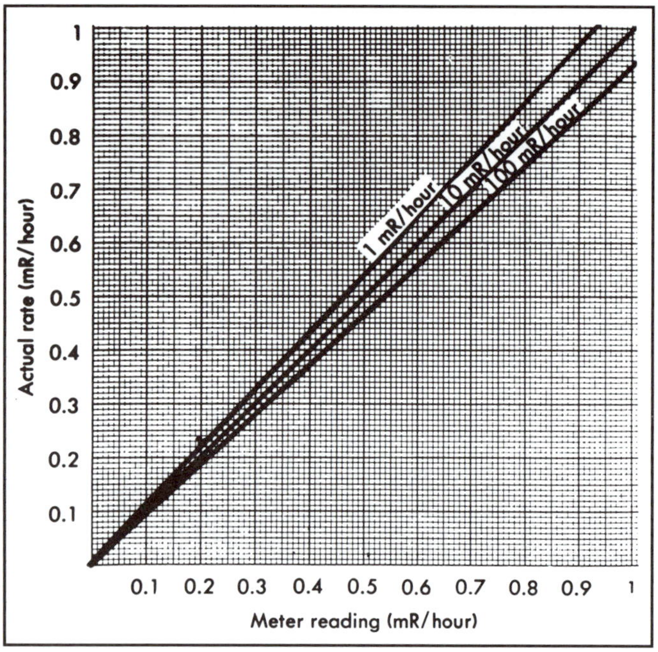

Figure 4.11 Survey meter calibration graph. Convert meter reading (abscissa) to actual dose rate by reading upward to intercept point and then across to ordinate. Multiple ranges may be plotted on the same graph. Reprinted with permission from: Bernier DR, Christian PE, Langan JK, Wells LD, eds. *Nuclear medicine technology and techniques.* St. Louis: CV Mosby; 1989:212.

before each use to verify instrument calibration. Acceptable limits are readings within ±20% of the calibrated exposure rate, which should be posted on the survey instrument (Fig. 4-11). Records of daily reference checks do not need to be kept; however, the NRC does require that survey meter calibration records be maintained for three years.

REFERENCES

1. Bernier DR, Christian PE, Langan JK, eds. *Nuclear medicine technology and techniques,* 3rd ed. St. Louis: Mosby Year-Book; 1994:69–80, 93–94.
2. *Code of Federal Regulations.* Title 10, Subparts C 35.50–35.51. Washington, DC: Nuclear Regulatory Commission; January 1, 1995.
3. Early PJ, Sodee DB. *Principles and practice of nuclear medicine,* 2nd ed. St. Louis: Mosby Year-Book; 1995:150–175, 211–215, 257–290.
4. Graham LS. Quality assurance procedures. In: Simmons GH, ed. *The scintillation camera.* Reston, VA: Society of Nuclear Medicine; 1988:79–98.
5. Halama JR, Henkin RE. *Du Pont guide to instrumentation quality control.* North Billerica, MA: DuPont Company; 1986.
6. Hibbard WM, Lance SP, eds. *Laboratory manual for nuclear medicine technology.* Reston, VA: Society of Nuclear Medicine; 1984.

5 Introduction to SPECT

Robert L. Gladding and Ann M. Steves

Single-photon emission computed tomography (SPECT) has gained widespread acceptance over the last several years and has assumed an important role in routine clinical imaging. This chapter will emphasize the clinical aspects of SPECT. A detailed discussion of the physics principles and image processing related to SPECT is beyond the scope of this review book. The reader is referred to other texts cited at the end of this chapter for such information.

OVERVIEW

SPECT is an imaging technique that permits viewing a thin slice of an organ at one time rather than the entire organ. To accomplish this, a scintillation camera with a rotating detector head is used (Fig. 5-1). The imaging table is designed to permit rotation of the detector head around the patient through 360°. Images are collected at intervals around the patient. The acquisition arc is typically 360°, although 180° acquisitions are common for myocardial imaging. Each image, referred to as a projection, is stored in a computer for later processing. Image processing includes reconstruction of the acquired projections into transaxial, coronal and sagittal slices of the organ of interest.

Croft likens the process to drawing the floor plan of a house by looking in through the windows from the outside (*2*). By walking around the house and looking in each window, a detailed floor plan can be derived. Similarly, each projection acquired serves as a window into an area of the organ being imaged.

In conventional planar imaging, multiple views are acquired to differentiate overlying structures. Deep-seated lesions may be impossible to visualize, even with multiple projections. SPECT helps overcome such problems because contrast resolution, the ability to detect small differences in radiopharmaceutical concentration, is greatly improved with tomographic imaging. This is particularly helpful when imaging distributions of tracers such as ^{201}Tl within the myocardium.

Clinical Applications of SPECT

There are SPECT applications for almost all organ systems. Regional cerebral blood flow studies would be impossible to obtain without the use of tomographic imaging. Small defects in myocardial perfusion studies that could be missed or misread due to attenuation may be easily visualized by generating slices of the left ventricle. Small lesions not visualized on planar views of the lumber spine are clearly delineated with SPECT. Accurate location of a lesion in a specific area of a vertebral body can give the physician a much better idea as to whether an abnormality is due to metastatic disease or is simply a degenerative change. Soft-tissue imaging, such as liver/spleen or lung perfusion, is also improved when SPECT is used.

CROSS-SECTIONAL ANATOMY

Tomographic images can be displayed in the transaxial (transverse), sagittal or coronal planes. The anatomical planes are imaginary flat surfaces used as points of reference to identify the positions of parts of the body (Fig. 5-2). Since tomographic images are acquired by rotating the camera about the long-axis of the patient's body, the initial tomograms are transaxial images, which are derived from the transaxial plane perpendicular to the long-axis of the body. The sagittal and coronal images are generated from the initial transaxial slices.

Some attempt has been made to standardize the display of cross-sectional images. The conventional transaxial cross-section is displayed as if the viewer were standing at the supine subject's feet and looking up through the body (Fig. 5-3). The anterior surface is at the top of the image and the subject's right side is on the viewer's left. A series of transaxial images is presented from the upper portion of the body or organ to the lower (Fig. 5-4). The coronal cross-section is presented with the superior portion of the body or organ at the top and the subject's right side on the viewer's left, as if the viewer were facing the subject. A coronal series is presented from the anterior to the posterior. Sagittal images may be displayed as if the subject were upright or supine. If upright, the superior portion will be at the top of the image and the anterior surface on the viewer's right. If supine, the superior portion will be on the viewer's left and the anterior surface will be at the top of the image. A series of sagittal images is displayed from the right side of the body to the left.

The heart is not aligned along the natural planes of the body. For this reason, the planes of the heart are named differently (Fig. 5-5). From the transaxial cross-section, oblique cross-sections of the myocardium are generated. To obtain the oblique cross-sections, the heart is reoriented during image reconstruction as if the apex of the heart is pointing directly out of the chest. With this orientation in mind, the short-axis is viewed as if standing directly in front of the subject. Cross-sections from the apex of the heart to the base are displayed. The horizontal long-axis is viewed as though

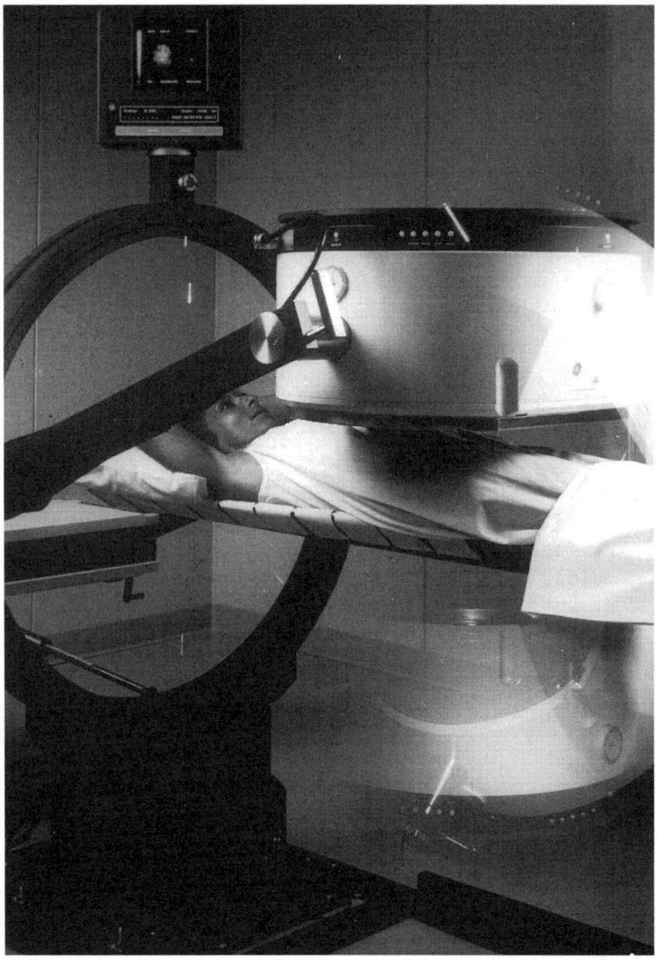

Figure 5.1 Tomographic scintillation camera and imaging bed. Courtesy of GE Medical Systems, Milwaukee, WI.

standing at the supine subject's feet and looking up. Cross-sections from the superior wall to the inferior wall of the heart are presented. The vertical long-axis is analogous to a sagittal projection, in which the subject is viewed from the right side and cross-sections from the septum to the lateral wall are displayed.

ACQUISITION

As with any nuclear medicine procedure, certain technical parameters must be selected before data collection begins.

Matrix Selection

For a standard, large field of view (400 mm diameter) scintillation camera, a 64x64 acquisition matrix is recommended. A matrix of this size provides the optimum pixel size based on the resolution capabilities of the scintillation camera. Larger matrix sizes require more computer storage space and data processing time.

Projections per Rotation

For a given acquisition time, increasing the number of images or projections collected as the camera rotates around the patient reduces the amount of "star" artifact visualized in the reconstructed images (Fig. 5-6). The minimum recommended number of projections for a 360° acquisition is 60.

Acquisition Time

The time required to complete data collection depends on the counting rate, the desired counting statistics and the patient's ability to remain still. The total acquisition time is equal to the number of projections multiplied by the time required for each projection.

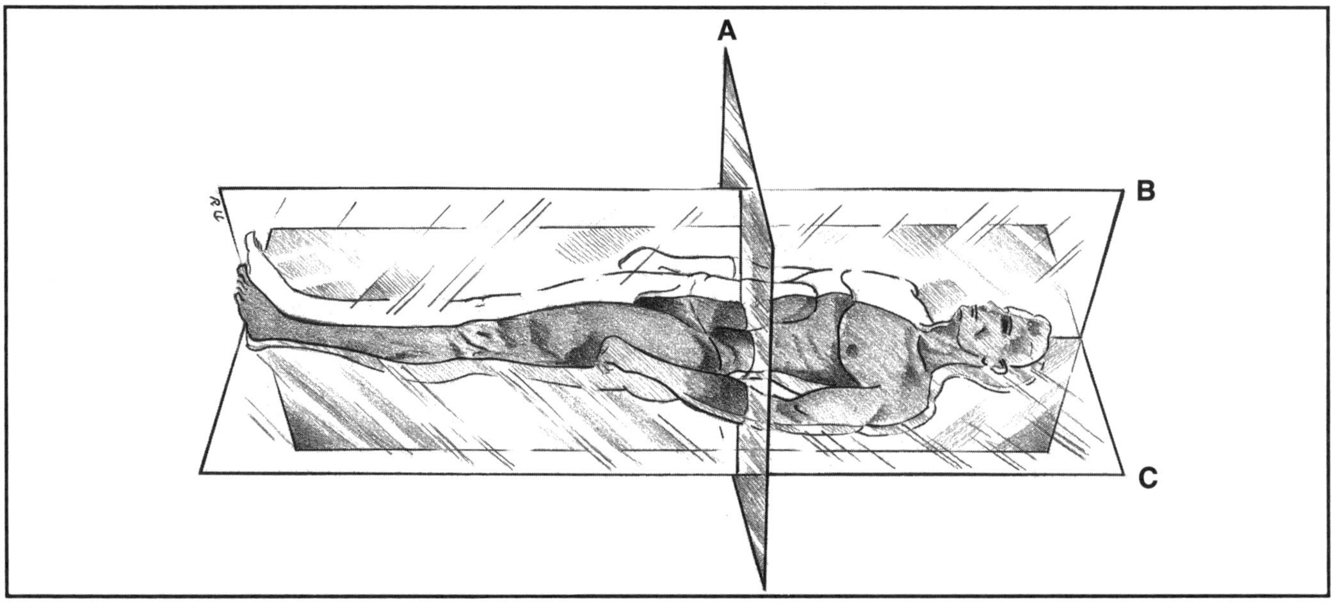

Figure 5.2 Tomographic planes of the body: (A) transverse, (B) sagittal and (C) coronal. Reprinted with permission from: English RJ, Brown SE. *SPECT: a primer*, 2nd ed. Reston, VA: Society of Nuclear Medicine; 1990:95.

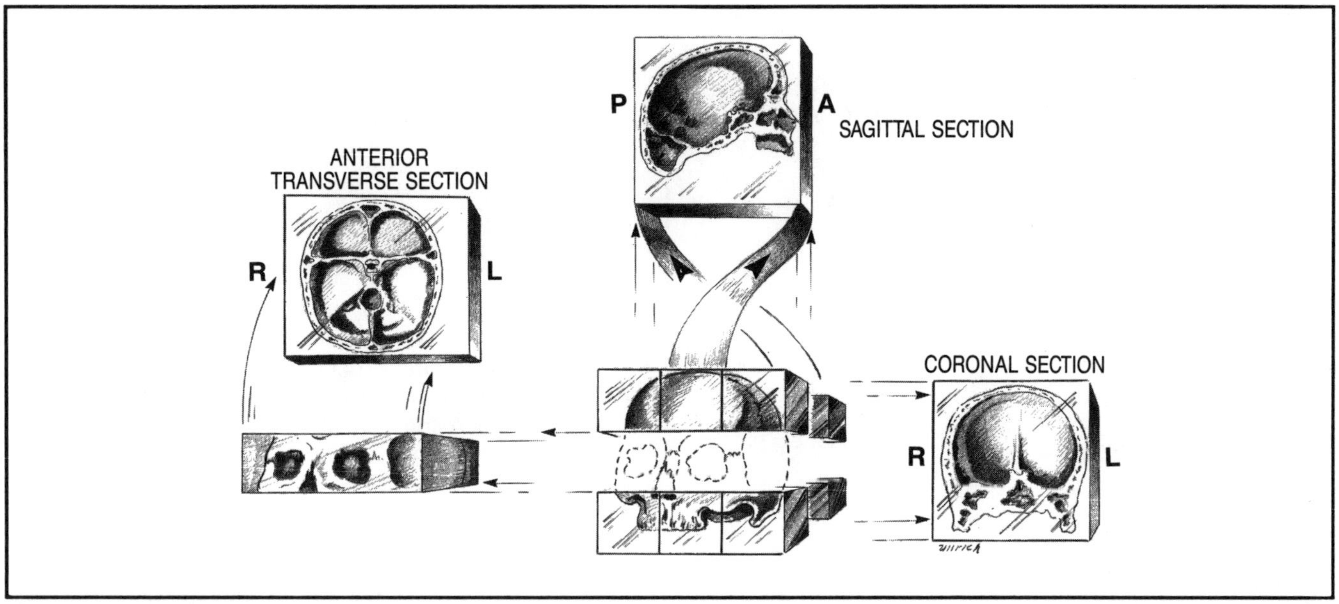

Figure 5.3 Conventional orientation of cross-sections. Reprinted with permission from: English RJ, Brown SE. *SPECT: a primer,* 2nd ed. Reston, VA: Society of Nuclear Medicine; 1990:97.

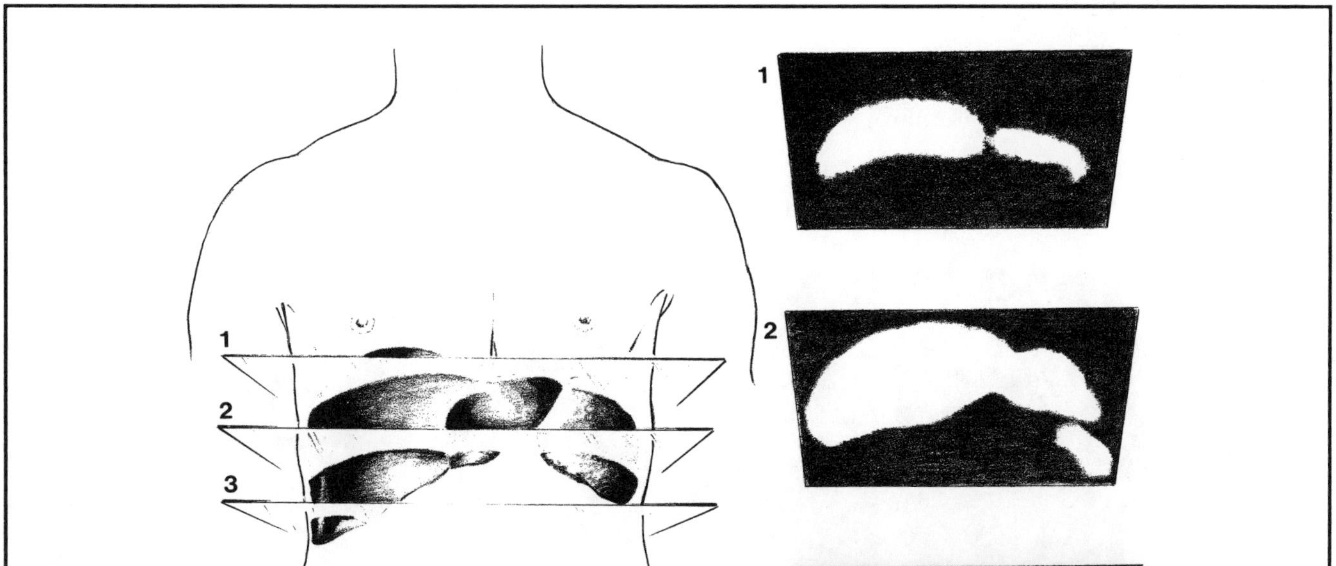

Figure 5.4 Transverse sections of the liver. Reprinted with permission from: English RJ, Brown SE. *SPECT: a primer,* 2nd ed. Reston, VA: Society of Nuclear Medicine; 1990:101.

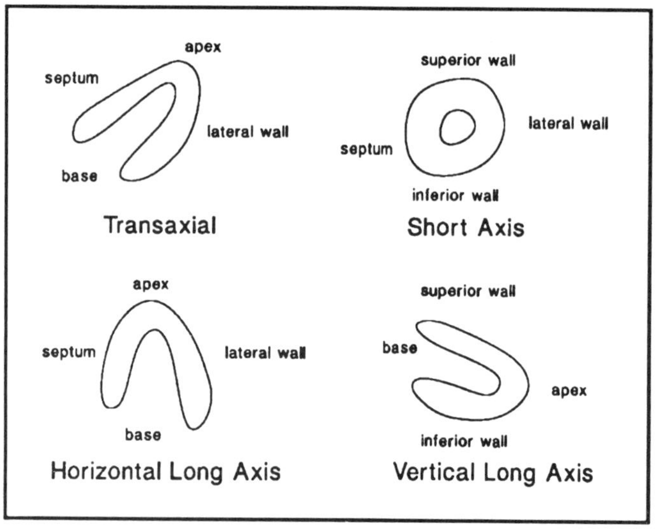

Figure 5.5 Orientation of cross-cardiac sections.

For example, a SPECT study of the spine is to be performed. How long will it take to acquire a 3-million count, 360°, 64-projection tomographic study, if a 500,000 count posterior planar image can be acquired in 3 min?

If 500,000 counts can be acquired in 3 min, the counting rate is:

$$\text{count rate} = \frac{500{,}000 \text{ counts}}{3 \text{ min}}$$
$$= 166{,}666 \text{ cpm}$$
$$\text{total acquisition time} = \frac{\text{total counts}}{\text{count rate}}$$
$$= \frac{3 \text{ million counts}}{166{,}666 \text{ cpm}}$$
$$= 18 \text{ min.}$$

In practice, the total time may be slightly longer than calculated, since the movement of the camera from one projection to the next takes additional time.

Dividing the total counts and total time by the number of projections yields the time per projection and the approximate number of counts in each projection:

$$\frac{\text{time}}{\text{projection}} = \frac{18 \text{ min}}{64 \text{ projections}} = 0.28 \text{ min}$$
$$\frac{\text{counts}}{\text{projection}} = \frac{3 \text{ million counts}}{64 \text{ projections}} = 46{,}875 \text{ counts.}$$

The patient's ability to remain still is not factored into the above equations. It is, nevertheless, an important determinant of a technically satisfactory study. Although an optimum acquisition time means better resolution, a patient who becomes restless or agitated and begins moving will negate any possibility of obtaining high-quality images. With some uncooperative patients, a shorter, lower count study may yield more information than a longer "by the book" acquisition time. Other factors that need to be considered in determining the acquisition time are the patient's weight, the amount of activity administered, the time post-tracer administration and the photon abundance of the radionuclide being imaged.

Radius of Rotation

As in planar imaging, the surface of the patient should be as close to the face of the collimator as possible. Since, however, a noncircular object (the patient's body) is being placed in a circular field, minimizing the patient-detector distance is not always easy. Elliptical or body contouring orbits can help minimize this distance (Fig. 5-7).

Detector Motion

Two types of detector movement can be used to move the detector around the patient. In the "step and shoot" mode, the detector moves to successive preset angles. At each stop, data are collected for a preset time, then the detector moves to the next angle to acquire data. The detector's movement

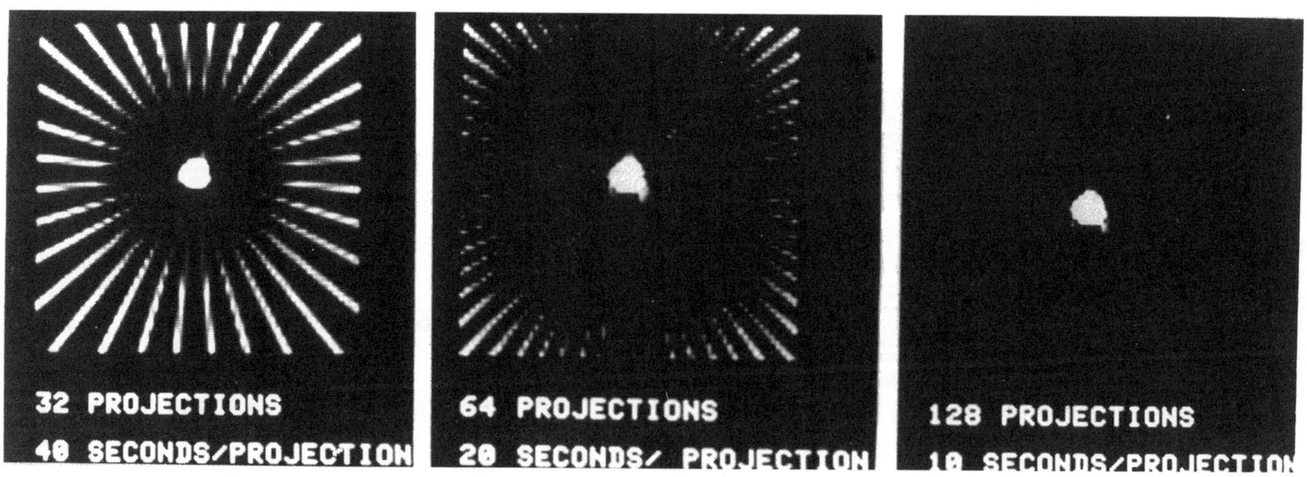

Figure 5.6 Transaxial slice of the line source illustrates reduction of the "star" artifact with an increase in the acquired number of projections. Reprinted with permission from: English RJ, Brown SE. *SPECT: a primer,* 2nd ed. Reston, VA: Society of Nuclear Medicine; 1990:50.

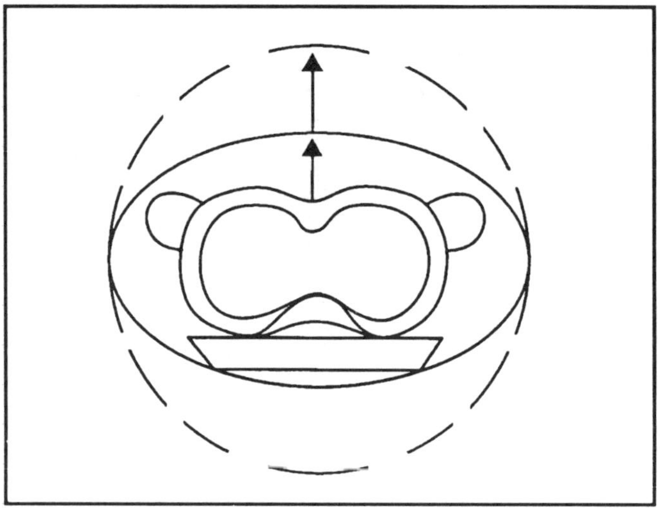

Figure 5.7 Comparison of distance between patient and detector with circular and elliptical orbs.

is controlled by computer software. Moving the detector from one position to the next adds a small amount of time to the total acquisition time. In the continuous rotation mode, data are acquired continuously as the detector rotates through the entire acquisition arc without stopping. Since the data are collected while the detector is in motion, there is a small amount of blurring.

Collimator Selection

Selecting a collimator for tomographic imaging involves the same considerations and compromises as for planar imaging. Because each planar projection is acquired for only a short period of time, it is important to obtain as many counts as possible. Therefore, for the majority of SPECT studies using ^{99m}Tc-labeled agents, a general all-purpose, parallel-hole collimator is indicated. A high-resolution collimator will result in fewer counts.

Specially designed collimators for specific clinical applications are also available. A slant-hole collimator is preferred for brain imaging. By tilting the brain to 30° and angling the detector 30°, all collimator septa will be parallel to the area of interest. Consequently, the detector head can now be placed much closer to the area of interest (the brain) while avoiding contact with the patient's shoulders. When imaging higher energy radionuclides, such as ^{67}Ga, a medium- or high-energy collimator should be used.

Whatever collimator is used, it is imperative that the distance between the face of the collimator and the patient be minimized. In SPECT imaging, this is sometimes more difficult to achieve than in planar imaging. Selecting the most appropriate orbit, circular or elliptical, for the imaging application can help minimize the detector-patient distance. For example, a circular orbit is the best choice for brain imaging, while an elliptical orbit is better for liver or spine imaging.

Clinical Considerations

Minimizing patient motion is extremely important whether planar or tomographic imaging is performed. Planar acquisitions, however, are typically of several minutes duration, while tomographic acquisitions can take from 20 to 30 min. Repeating tomographic studies may not be feasible for patients who are unable to lie still for extended periods. Therefore, it is essential to explain the procedure in advance to the patient to enhance patient cooperation and to obtain a technically satisfactory tomographic study. The technologist should explain the importance of lying still and describe what that means. Perhaps the best way to explain is to let the patient know what he or she may or may not do. For example, suggest that the patient breathe normally and attempt to relax. Noisy distractions should be kept to a minimum.

It is imperative that the technologist position the patient to maximize comfort. Lower back strain may be relieved by elevating and bending the knees with a pillow or support. When head and chin straps are used, they should be snug, but not tight. Better results are usually obtained when straps are used as a reminder to the patient rather than a physical restraint. An efficient set-up reduces the length of time that a patient must lie in one position. Turning off overhead lights and providing a blanket also can enhance patient comfort.

It is crucial that the detector head be leveled (made parallel to the axis of rotation) before data acquisition begins (Fig. 5-8). Reconstruction of transaxial images assumes that

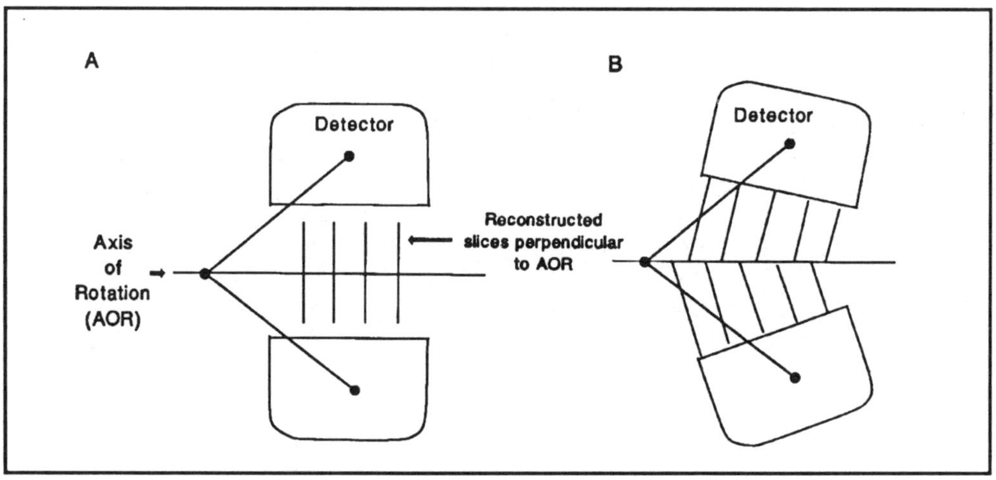

Figure 5.8 Effect of detector head tilt. With the detector head parallel to the axis of rotation, AOR (A), the holes of the parallel-hole collimator will gather counts from the same slice all the way through the patient. When the detector is not parallel to the AOR (B), data from several adjoining slices will be superimposed, which can compromise resolution.

the reconstructed slices are perpendicular to the axis of rotation. Any tilt of the detector head will cause counts to be misplaced in the reconstructed images.

While imaging is in progress, the technologist should remain in the imaging room to encourage the patient to lie still, to observe the motion of the detector and to move potential obstacles (such as catheters and intravenous and oxygen lines) from the detector's path. The patient should be made aware that the "moving machine" is being monitored and controlled by the technologist.

When imaging the head, a headholder will reduce movement and will position the patient to allow rotation of the detector about the head. The patient should be advised not to talk, again to minimize any motion of the head. A specially designed detector head permits closer positioning of the detector to the patient's head by eliminating interference with the shoulders as the detector rotates about the patient.

Imaging the chest or abdomen necessitates placing the patient's arms out of the field of view. This is particularly difficult for the patient when the chest is being imaged, as the arms must be held over the head for an extended period of time. Again, talking and coughing may introduce motion artifacts into the clinical images.

Radionuclide concentrations such as an infiltration site or a full bladder also produce artifacts that may interfere with image interpretation. Sites of tracer infiltration usually can be removed from the field of view with careful placement of the patient's arms.

Multihead Detectors

Many nuclear medicine departments are purchasing SPECT camera systems with multiple detector heads. There are many advantages to such systems, including a shorter radius of rotation, increased sensitivity and resolution, shorter acquisition times and increased patient comfort. Some multidetector systems are dedicated to neuro imaging, but the majority are capable of imaging all areas of the body.

IMAGE RECONSTRUCTION AND PROCESSING

After acquisition, images are generated from the data stored in the computer. Proper reconstruction techniques are imperative if accurate information is to be derived from the raw data. Although techniques vary among different computer systems and software, certain basic functions are performed.

Filtering. A variety of filters are available that, when applied to the raw data, either enhance edges or smooth the image to reduce "noise."

Attenuation Correction. To correct for photon absorption in overlying body tissue, attenuation correction methods are sometimes used.

Slice Generation. The two-dimensional projections that are acquired as the detector rotates about the patient are reconstructed into three planes. First, images of the transaxial plane are generated. Next, coronal and sagittal images are derived from the transaxials. For the heart, the short-axis and vertical and horizontal long axes are derived from the transaxials. The image reconstruction process is called filtered backprojection. For interpretation, the images are displayed as described in the cross-sectional anatomy section of this chapter.

QUALITY CONTROL

Quality control for tomographic cameras should first include those procedures used to test conventional scintillation cameras. Daily uniformity checks and weekly resolution and linearity tests are as important for tomographic cameras as they are for planar imaging instruments. Poor performance as a planar imaging device will not be enhanced when tomographic imaging is attempted.

Quality control tests specific to tomographic cameras include center of rotation (COR) and uniformity corrections. Uniformity correction should not be confused with daily uniformity checks to assess photomultiplier tube function.

Center of Rotation Correction

Center of rotation correction must be performed daily or at least on the days that the scintillation camera is used to perform tomography. COR correction is performed to ensure that the axis of rotation, the point about which the detector rotates, falls in the center of the computer matrix for each projection acquired. For example, in a 64x64 matrix, the center coordinates would be located at pixels 32.5 and 32.5 (Fig. 5-9). The rotation arc of the detector is not a perfect cir-

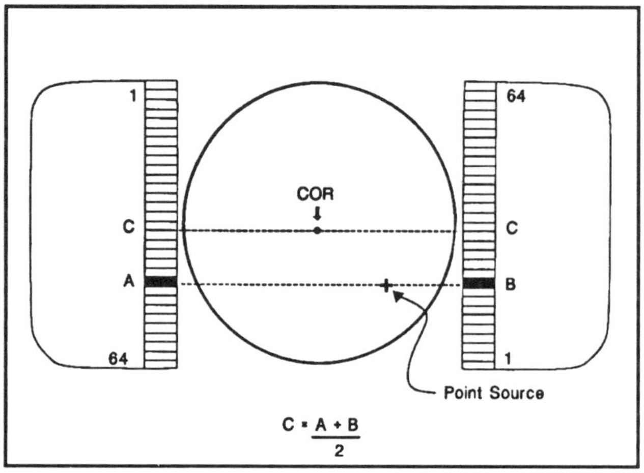

Figure 5.9 COR is calculated by identifying the pixel with the maximum number of counts for each opposing projection in a pair. A and B are the pixel numbers containing the maximum number of counts; C is the COR value for that pair of projections. The software then stores the COR correction factors to be applied during acquisition.

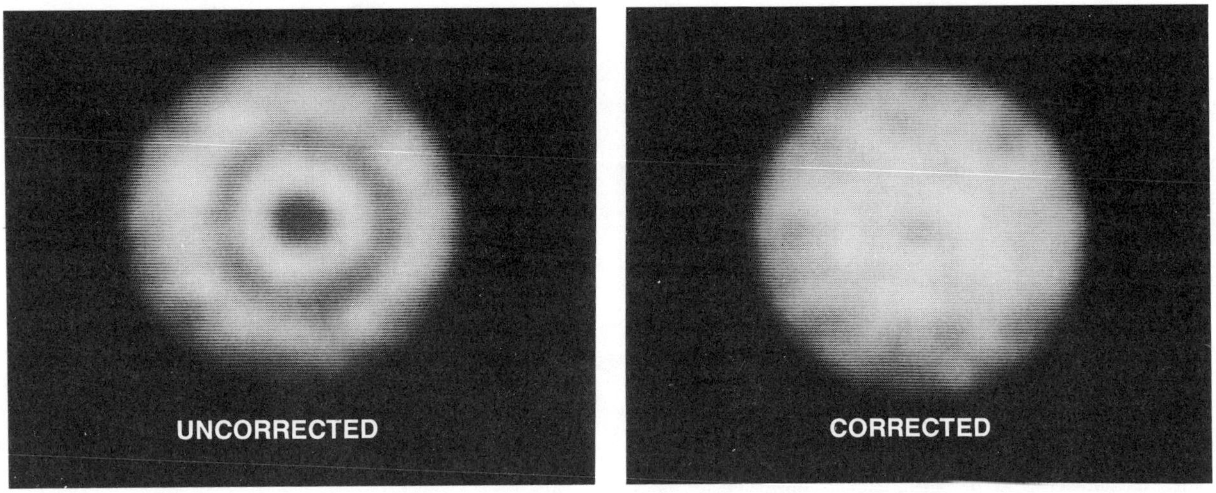

Figure 5.10 Cylindrical phantom with uniform radionuclide distribution, uncorrected and corrected with a 30-million count flood. Reprinted with permission from: English RJ, Brown SE. *SPECT: a primer,* 2nd ed. Reston, VA: Society of Nuclear Medicine; 1990:32.

cle or ellipse. Hence, the axis of rotation may not fall in the center of the computer matrix and a correction factor must be applied. Failure to account for misalignment of the axis of rotation with the center of the matrix degrades image quality because counts are incorrectly placed in the reconstructed images.

COR should be determined for each collimator used for SPECT imaging. The procedure involves acquiring an even number of point source images (projections) over 360°. Using the manufacturer supplied software, the COR is calculated for each set of 180° opposing projections (Fig. 5-9). The average of these values is stored and applied during later tomographic acquisitions. COR values should be recorded and compared to preceding measurements. Variations of no more than half a pixel are considered acceptable.

Uniformity Correction

In planar imaging, nonuniformities across the field of view are corrected with electronic circuitry. Tomographic imaging, however, tolerates a much smaller variance in field uniformity. Even small nonuniformities introduce ring artifacts into the reconstructed images (Fig. 5-10).

To reduce nonuniformity artifacts in reconstructed images, the planar projections are corrected with a 30-million count flood source image. For a 64x64 matrix on a standard size field of view camera, a 30-million count flood yields a standard deviation of only 1% across the field of view (Fig. 5-11). A uniformity correction performed with such a high count density flood image results in fewer artifacts in the reconstructed SPECT images.

After the flood correction image is stored in the computer, the software calculates an average pixel value for the flood matrix. A correction factor for each pixel is then calculated using the formula:

$$F_i = \frac{\text{average flood counts}}{C_i},$$

where F_i equals the correction factor for the ith pixel and C_i equals the counts in the ith pixel.

Each projection image is multiplied by the correction factor matrix to obtain a uniformity corrected image (Fig. 5-12). Since a particular correction matrix should be applied only to data acquired under the same conditions, a uniformity correction matrix should be acquired for each combination of collimator, matrix size and zoom factor used for tomographic imaging. It is recommended that these be collected weekly.

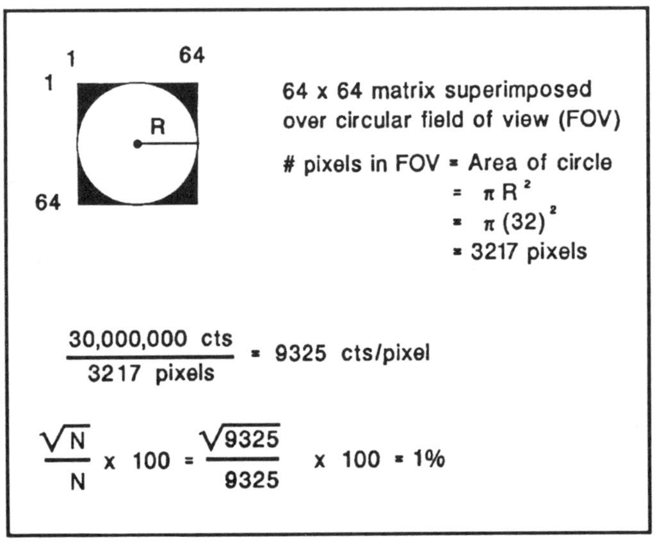

Figure 5.11 Correction of flood statistics.

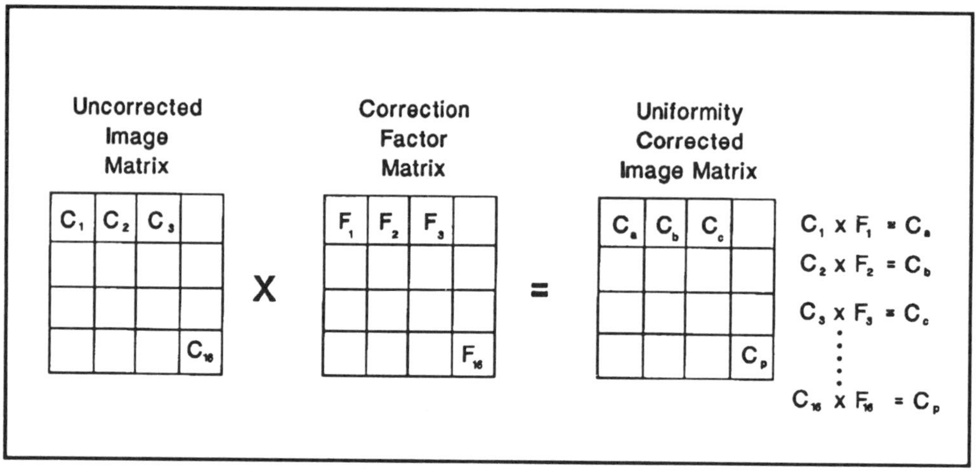

Figure 5.12 Method used to correct images for uniformity.

REFERENCES

1. Brust KD, Graham MM. Aspects of patient imaging with SPECT. *J Nucl Med Technol* 1987; 15:133–137.
2. Croft BY. *Single-photon emission computed tomography.* Chicago: Year Book Publishers, Inc.; 1986:11–20, 68–80, 123–142, 181–200.
3. DePuey EG. *Artifacts in SPECT ^{201}Tl and gated blood-pool imaging* (audiovisual). Reston, VA: Society of Nuclear Medicine; 1986.
4. Eisner RL. Principles of instrumentation in SPECT. *J Nucl Med Technol* 1985; 13:23–31.
5. English RJ, Brown SE. *Single-photon emission computed tomography: a primer.* 2nd ed. Reston, VA: Society of Nuclear Medicine; 1990:25–67, 93–119.
6. Feldkamp MJ. SPECT quality improvement. *J Nucl Med Technol* 1994; 22:35–38.
7. Ficken V, McCartney W. SPECT quality control: a program recommended by the American College of Nuclear Physicians and the ACNP Corporate Committee. *J Nucl Med Technol* 1994; 22:205–208.
8. Folks R, Banks L, Plankey M, et al. Cardiovascular SPECT. *J Nucl Med Technol* 1985; 13:150–161.
9. Greer KL, Coleman RE, Jaszczak RJ. SPECT: a practical guide for users. *J Nucl Med Technol* 1983: 11:61–65.
10. Greer KL, Jaszczak RJ, Harris CC, et al. Quality control in SPECT. *J Nucl Med Technol* 1985; 13:76–85.
11. Halama JR, Henkin RE. Quality assurance in SPECT imaging. *Appl Radiol* 1987; 16:41–50.
12. Harkness BA, Rogers WL, Clinthorne NH, et al. SPECT: quality control procedures and artifact identification. *J Nucl Med Technol* 1983; 11:55–60.
13. Lee K. *Computers in nuclear medicine: a practical approach.* Reston, VA: Society of Nuclear Medicine; 1991:189–228.
14. Rowell K, ed. *Clinical computers in nuclear medicine.* Reston, VA: Society of Nuclear Medicine; 1992.

Additional Physics-Related References

15. Brooks RA, DiChiro GD. Theory of image reconstruction in computed tomography. *Radiology* 1986; 14:561–572.
16. Galt JR, Hise HL, Garcia EV, et al. Filtering in frequency space. *J Nucl Med Technol* 1986; 14:152–162.
17. Garcia EV. Digital processing in nuclear medicine imaging. *J Nucl Med Technol* 1986; 14:21–30.
18. Heller SL, Goodwin P. Instrumentation: basic principles and recent innovations. *Semin Nucl Med* 1987; 17:184–199.

6 Film Processing

Ann M. Steves

Film processing is the last step in producing a nuclear medicine image. It is as important to include the automatic film processor in the overall quality assurance program as it is to include dose calibrators, scintillation cameras and other equipment related to the practice of nuclear medicine technology.

FILM PROCESSORS

The film processing cycle consists of four steps (Fig. 6-1). After a film has been introduced into the automatic film processor, it is cycled through each of the four steps for the appropriate amount of time. Although the entire process often is referred to as developing the film, image development actually occurs in Step 1 when the silver halide crystals in the film's emulsion that have been exposed to light are reduced to metallic silver. During the film's travel through the fixer, the unexposed or undeveloped silver halide crystals are removed and the reducing action of the developer is neutralized to stop the developing process. The film is then washed to remove the chemicals from Steps 1 and 2. Finally, the film travels through a hot air blower to dry it. Depending on the automatic film processor, the complete four-step cycle is completed in 1–2 min.

It is important that the film processing chemicals, the developer and fixer, be mixed according to the manufacturer's instructions to achieve the proper pH and concentration for optimum film development. The temperature of the developer must be maintained within ±2° of the recommended temperature. The length of the developing time is affected by the temperature of the developer solution. As the temperature increases, the amount of developing time required decreases and vice versa. Since a film remains in the developer for a fixed amount of time as it travels through the automatic processor, temperature changes can lead to films that are too dark or too light. The rate at which chemicals in the developer and fixer tanks are replenished is also important. Replenishment rates should be adjusted according to the number and size of the films run each day. Too little replenishment may lead to underdeveloped films, while over-replenishment wastes chemicals.

ROUTINE MAINTENANCE

To maintain consistent processor performance and to identify potential problems, the following routine maintenance is recommended.

Daily

1. Check to ensure that the water has been turned on and that the water temperature is 5–10° F lower than the developer temperature.
2. Make sure that the developer and fixer solution levels are adequate.
3. Check developer temperature and adjust if necessary.
4. Run several unprocessed films to clean the rollers and to check for artifacts such as scratches and static electricity.
5. Rinse crossover racks at the end of the day and leave the processor top ajar for ventilation.

Weekly

1. Adjust the developer and fixer replenishment rates to match the number and size of films processed.
2. Using a stopwatch, time the transit of a film through the processor. The time should be consistent from week to week.
3. Check the tanks and rollers for chemical build-up and algae.

Monthly

1. Clean tanks and rollers thoroughly.
2. Fill the processor tanks with fresh developer and fixer solutions.
3. Check rollers and gears for wear.

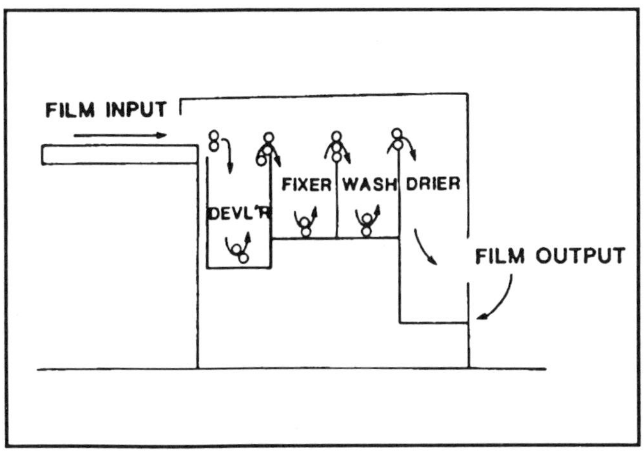

Figure 6.1 Schematic diagram of an automatic film processor. Reprinted with permission from: Cyr L, Dick D, Huda W, O'Connor S. Film processors in nuclear medicine. *J Nucl Med Technol* 1986;14:66.

Table 6-1
Troubleshooting Suggestions

Problem	Solution	Test film conditions		
		Fogged	Light	Dark
Improper developer temperature	Readjust to manufacturer's specifications		X	X
Developer diluted	Check for water overflow into developer tank		X	
Developer replenishment rate faulty	Readjust to manufacturer's specifications		X	X
Developer replenishment chemistry improperly mixed	Change all developer chemicals; follow directions exactly		X	X
Safelight faulty	Check specifications for bulb size and filter type	X		
Light leaks	Check processor and darkroom carefully; if processor speed is adjustable, check cycle time	X		
Chemistry contamination	Check overflow, foreign matter in tanks	X		X

Reprinted with permission from: *Du Pont guide to film quality control for nuclear medicine.* N. Billerica, MA: Du Pont Co.; 1987.

TROUBLESHOOTING

Table 6-1 lists common film processor problems and how these conditions appear on film.

REFERENCES

1. Cyr L, Dick D, Huda W et al. Film processors in nuclear medicine. *J Nucl Med Technol* 1986; 14:66–692.
2. *Du Pont guide to film quality control for nuclear medicine.* N. Billerica, MA: E.I. du Pont de Nemours & Co.; 1987.

7 Cardiovascular System

Timothy D. Baker

In the past twenty years, nuclear imaging of the cardiovascular system has changed from a sporadically used tool in the university setting to a major component of the day-to-day work in most nuclear medicine departments. Because of the advent of faster computers and new radiopharmaceuticals, nuclear cardiology can assess everything from myocardial viability to congenital blood flow abnormalities. An understanding of all aspects of nuclear cardiology is now essential in the education of nuclear medicine technologists.

CARDIAC ANATOMY AND PHYSIOLOGY

The heart is a muscular organ that rests in the center of the chest in an area called the mediastinum. Two-thirds of the heart lie left of the midline next to the base of the left lung. The heart is angled away from the midline with the apex being approximately 30–50° from the sternum (Fig. 7-1).

The heart is divided into four chambers. The upper chambers, the atria, allow blood to enter the main pumping chambers, the left and right ventricles (Fig. 7-2). The right atrium and ventricle are separated by the tricuspid valve. The right ventricle pumps blood to the lungs for oxygenation through the pulmonary artery. The newly oxygenated blood returns to the heart by way of the pulmonary vein and enters the heart at the left atrium. The blood then passes across the mitral valve into the left ventricle, at which point it is introduced into the systemic circulation by passing through the aortic valve and into the aorta.

Coronary Circulation

Circulation into the heart muscle itself is called coronary circulation. Coronary circulation begins at the base of the aorta with the right and left coronary arteries. The right coronary artery (RCA) exits the aorta and usually follows the right posterior sulcus and branches posteriorly toward the apex. The RCA supplies the posterior and diaphragmatic areas of the myocardium. In some patients, the RCA also supplies the apex. The left coronary artery (LCA) exits the aorta at the level of the left coronary sinus. The LCA branches into the left anterior descending artery (LAD) and the left circumflex artery (LCX). The LAD usually traverses down the anterior surface of the heart to provide blood to the septal and anterior walls of the myocardium. In most patients, the LAD will also provide blood to the apex. The circumflex and its branches service the lateral free wall (Fig. 7-3).

Cardiac Electrical Conduction System

A cardiac cycle is the period from the end of one heart contraction (systole) to the end of the next. In between the two contractions is a period of relaxation or diastole. Each cardiac cycle is initiated by electrical stimulation in the heart that prepares it to contract.

The electrical impulse that initiates contraction begins in the sinoatrial (SA) node, a small mass of specialized tissue located in the right atrium near the entrance of the superior vena cava (Fig. 7-4). The SA node is the pacemaker for the heart and generates regular impulses at the rate of 60–100 impulses per minute. The impulses from the SA node are directed to the atrioventricular (AV) node where the impulse transmission is slowed. The AV node serves as a gatekeeper for the ventricles and as such allows only 40–60 impulses per minute to pass on to the ventricles. From the AV node, impulses travel through the Bundle of His to the right and left bundle branches that carry the impulses to the tips of both ventricles. The terminal branches for the two bundle branches, the Purkinje fibers, carry the impulses to the individual myocardial cells, which results in simultaneous contraction of all parts of both ventricles.

The electrocardiogram (ECG) is a graphical representation of the electrical activity of the heart. A normal ECG pattern is composed of a P-wave, a QRS complex and a T-wave (Fig. 7-5). Each of these is related to an event in the cardiac cycle. The P-wave represents atrial depolarization or activation of the atria. Atrial depolarization is initiated by the SA node and immediately precedes contraction of the atria. The slowing of impulse transmission at the AV node is indicated by the interval between the P-wave and the QRS complex. Also, during this interval, the blood flows from the atria into the ventricles. The QRS complex denotes depolarization of the ventricles. As these chambers contract, the blood flows from the ventricles into the pulmonary arteries and aorta. The ST-segment or interval represents a rest period between depolarization and repolarization (relaxation) of the ventricles. Repolarization of the ventricles is delineated by the T-wave. The contraction and relaxation of the atria and the ventricles are 180° out of phase to one another; that is, the atria are contracting when the ventricles are relaxing and vice versa. Relaxation of the atria is not seen in the ECG because it is obscured by the QRS complex.

In a healthy individual, the normal ECG pattern is repeated 60–100 times per minute, which corresponds to the number of heart beats per minute. The cardiac rhythm is regular and the P-wave, PR interval and QRS complex occur at constant intervals.

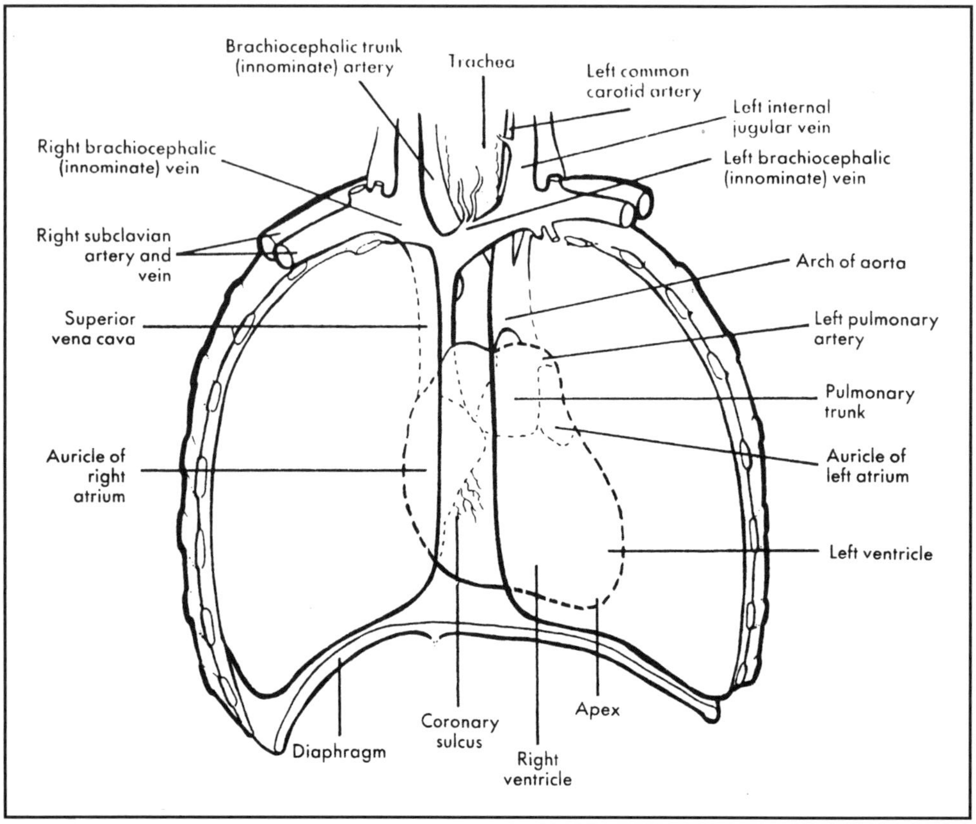

Figure 7.1 Anterior schematic of the anatomy of the heart and great vessels.

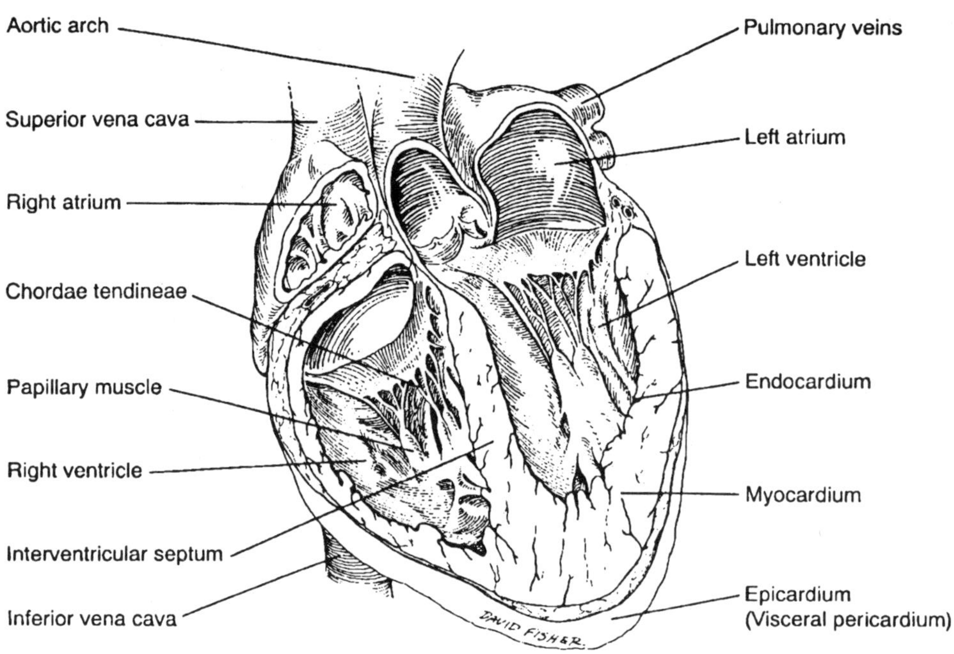

Figure 7.2 The human heart is divided into four chambers with walls of varying thickness.

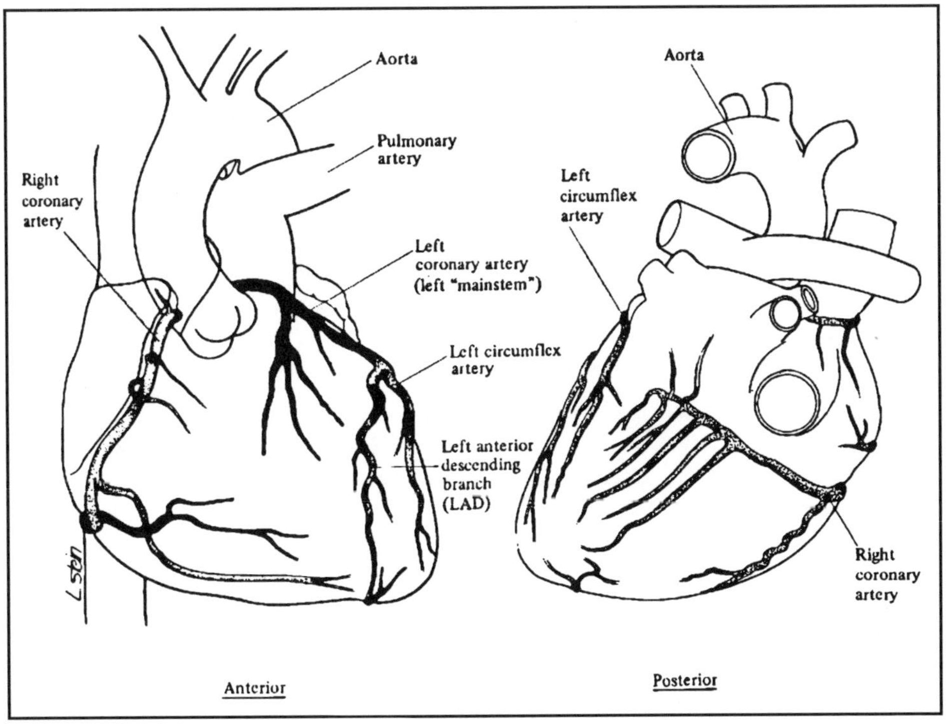

Figure 7.3 Two main vessels arising directly from the aorta–the right and left coronary arteries–supply nutrients and oxygen to the myocardium. The right coronary artery supplies the right atrium and ventricle as well as the inferior part of the left ventricle. The left circumflex artery supplies the posterior wall of the left ventricle and a portion of the inferior and lateral walls. The left anterior descending artery supplies much of the left myocardium and the interventricular septum. Reprinted with permission from: *Introduction to nuclear cardiology: a technologist training manual.* N. Billerica, MA: DuPont EN Medical Products; 1984:11.

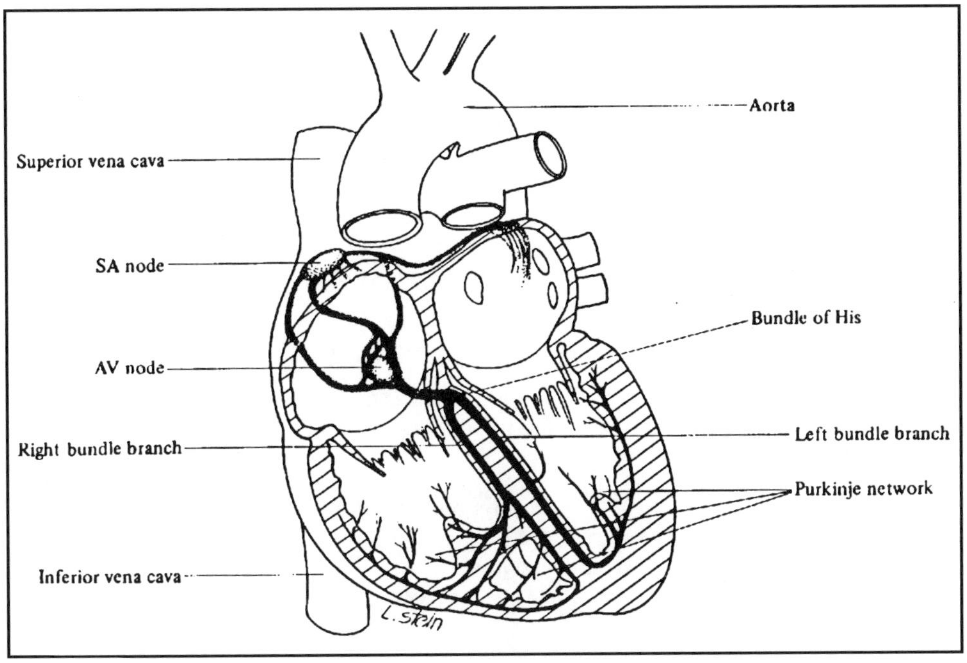

Figure 7.4 The cardiac conducting system is responsible for initiating and transmitting the electrical impulse that causes the heart to contract. Reprinted with permission from: *Introduction to nuclear cardiology: a technologist training manual.* N. Billerica, MA: DuPont NEN Medical Products; 1984:14.

It is in the ST-segment that a lack of blood flow may be demonstrated by a depression of this line below the baseline. This is of particular interest to nuclear medicine practitioners because during a stress study, the patient's ECG may exhibit S-T depression, indicating that the demand or supply of blood to the myocardium has changed.

MYOCARDIAL IMAGING

Myocardial imaging can be used to demonstrate myocardial ischemia or necrosis resulting from myocardial infarction. Infarct-avid or hot spot myocardial imaging is used to visualize areas of acute myocardial infarction and is performed with ^{99m}Tc-pyrophosphate. Myocardial perfusion can be demonstrated with [^{201}Tl]thallous chloride or ^{99m}Tc-sestamibi.

Infarct-Avid Imaging

Myocardial infarction begins with the denial of blood to the myocardium by a blocked coronary artery or by blunt chest trauma that injures part of the heart. As myocardial cells begin to die, tissue necrosis begins. During cell necrosis, the

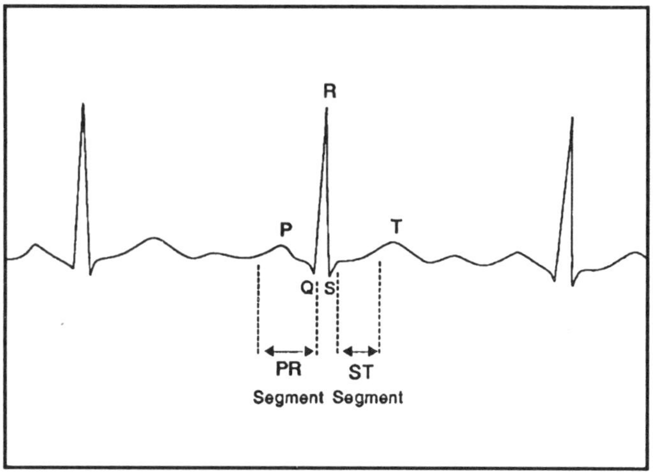

Figure 7.5 Normal ECG pattern.

cellular mitochondria take in phosphates while the cell releases large amounts of macromolecules in the form of proteins. In 1975, it was discovered that bone imaging agents, such as the polyphosphates, accumulate in sites of myocardial injury. The action of the mitochondria and the high binding affinity of polyphosphates to proteins made ^{99m}Tc-pyrophosphate one of the first clinically useful myocardial imaging agents.

Technetium-99m-pyrophosphate imaging is indicated when there is a question about the possibility or extent of myocardial infarction or injury. In most cases, this type of imaging is performed on patients for whom other data such as the ECG or cardiac enzymes are inconclusive. ECG problems such as left bundle branch block or extensive previous infarctions can mask a recent insult. Cardiac enzymes often are not elevated for several days after an event.

Clinical Procedure

Individual department protocols may vary; the following method is a suggested clinical procedure to perform infarct-avid imaging.

1. Collect relevant medical history, including recent injuries or surgeries to the thoracic area; the location, duration and frequency of pain, and serum enzyme levels.
2. Administer 15–25 mCi (370–925 MBq) ^{99m}Tc-pyrophosphate intravenously.
3. As with any bone agent, encourage the patient to drink fluids and to void frequently.
4. Image 2–3 hr following tracer administration. Obtain 1 million counts in each view with a low-energy, high-resolution, parallel-hole collimator.
5. Standard views of the cardiac area include the anterior, 45° left anterior oblique (LAO) and 70° LAO or left lateral projections to evaluate each of the major walls of the left ventricle. For the anterior and LAO images, position the patient so that the sternum is located halfway down the field of view and to the left of the center of the field of view to include the entire left side of the chest. For the steep LAO or lateral view, position the patient so that the sternum is at the left edge of the image.

Image Findings

Since pyrophosphate is a bone imaging agent, bony structures such as the ribs and sternum are normally visualized. No soft-tissue activity should be seen in the area of the heart (Fig. 7-6A).

Increased tracer uptake in the region of the myocardium is abnormal (Fig. 7-6B). When interpreting the images, the physician typically compares the activity in the cardiac areas to bone activity to grade the severity of the infarct.

Technical Considerations

Cellular necrosis begins immediately after an insult. The point at which ^{99m}Tc-pyrophosphate can bind to the products of cellular decay, however, does not occur until some time after the event. Imaging should not take place until 24–72 hr have passed since the initial myocardial event or injury. Imaging before 24–72 hr or beyond 7–10 days may lead to false-negative results and unnecessary radiation exposure to the patient. If the injury is the result of blunt trauma to the chest, fractures of the ribs or sternum may also be present. Since ^{99m}Tc-pyrophosphate is also used as a bone imaging agent, these fractures may be present on the image and obscure visualization of the myocardium. This becomes more of a problem the longer imaging is delayed from the time of injury.

MYOCARDIAL PERFUSION IMAGING

Myocardial perfusion imaging has become a major component of daily imaging procedures performed in most nuclear medicine departments. Because of the high incidence of coronary artery disease (CAD) in the United States, physicians need a low-cost method of screening symptomatic patients without cardiac catheterization. Thallium-201, and, more recently ^{99m}Tc-sestamibi, give the physician a powerful tool for finding CAD in high risk patients. In this section, various methods of physical and pharmacologic stress and radiopharmaceuticals with their associated imaging protocols are discussed.

Treadmill Exercise Testing

In many cases, individuals with CAD do not know they are at risk because the symptoms of CAD do not become obvious until patients exert themselves. Exercise increases the heart rate, which in turn causes the myocardium to demand more blood from the coronary circulation. For CAD patients, the coronary circulation cannot meet the demand placed upon it. Only then do these patients experience chest pain (angina pectoris), neck or jaw pain, arm pain or shortness of breath.

The purpose of treadmill exercise testing is to evaluate the potential CAD patient in a controlled setting by recreating symptoms the patient experiences on exertion. With the aid of a 12-lead ECG, these clinical symptoms can be correlated with electrical data to determine if ischemic changes occur. Nuclear imaging can be added to the test by the administration of a radiopharmaceutical during peak exercise to visualize ischemic areas in the myocardium induced by exercise.

Patient History and Preparation. In treadmill testing, a certain level of exercise must be reached for adequate evalua-

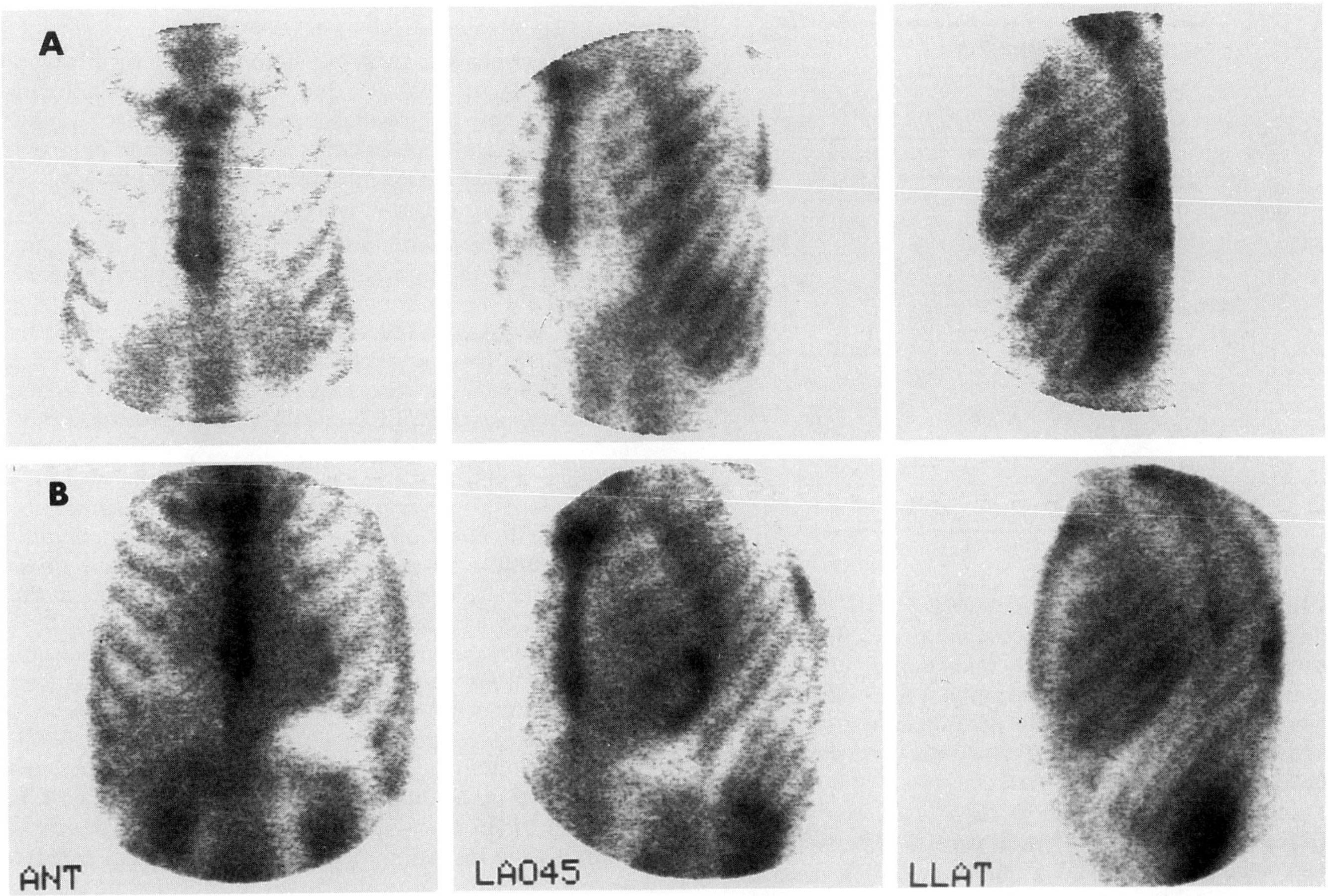

Figure 7.6 Technetium-99m-pyrophosphate images. (A) Normal pyrophosphate images depict radioactivity in only the bony structures of the thorax and in the kidneys. (B) Intense uptake in the area of the heart indicates an abnormal finding. Courtesy of the Department of Veterans Affairs Medical Center, Nashville, TN.

tion of the patient. This level is usually 85% of the patient's maximum heart rate. The nuclear medicine technologist may be required to participate in gathering data related to the patient's history. Usually, this will include questions about the patient's family medical history, lifestyle (smoking, alcohol consumption, exercise, etc.) and recent symptoms. Another part of the history is listing all currently used medications. This is important since many medications, such as beta-blockers for hypertension, adversely affect the patient's ability to reach an adequate level of myocardial demand during treadmill exercise. A physical or pharmacologic limitation that may affect the patient's ability to reach a target heart rate must be brought to the attention of the physician in charge of the stress procedure. Table 7-1 lists some medications that can affect exercise response.

For myocardial perfusion imaging, the technologist must insure that a large-bore intravenous catheter is in place to allow injection of the radiopharmaceutical at peak exercise. It is the technologist's responsibility to make sure that the catheter does not leak near the injection site. This is important because if the radiopharmaceutical is injected into the catheter while it is leaking, there is potential for radioactive contamination of the patient and equipment, as well as for technically suboptimal images.

During the exercise procedure, all radiation safety practices should be observed. For the technologist, this would include the use of gloves, protective clothing and a syringe shield. All other personnel involved in the test should also wear gloves to prevent the possible spread of radioactive contamination in case of a spill or leaking catheter.

For ECG monitoring, electrodes are placed on the patient's chest (Fig. 7-7). Securely attached electrodes will ensure a quality ECG. The areas of the skin should be cleansed with alcohol to remove any skin oils and should be lightly sanded to achieve good electrical contact. The electrodes are then coated with gel and placed directly onto the sandpapered areas. Excess hair may prevent adequate electrical contact and may necessitate dry shaving small areas where the electrodes will be attached. The razor and sandpaper should not be reused on other patients and should be disposed of along with other biohazardous material.

Exercise Protocols. There are two main exercise protocols; the most common is the Bruce protocol. In this protocol, speed and elevation of the treadmill increase every 3 min. These stages, as they are called, represent an increase in the patient's workload, thereby increasing the patient's heart rate. The second method is called the modified Bruce protocol. This is a variation of the Bruce protocol in which the elevation increases slightly every 3 min, but the speed remains at a slow pace. This is generally reserved for patients with very limited exercise capacity.

Table 7.1
Drugs That Can Affect Exercise Response

Drug	Discontinue prior to test
Nitroglycerin	1 hr
Long-acting nitrates	1 day
Tranquilizers/Sedatives	1 day
Antiarrhythmic agents	2 days
Beta blockers	2 days
Diuretics	4 days
Antihypertensives	4–7 days
Digitalis	1–2 wk

Pharmacologic Stress Agents

Because of physical limitations, poor motivation or medications that hinder adequate myocardial demand, many patients cannot perform a treadmill test. These patients will benefit from a fairly new class of drugs known as pharmacologic stress agents. Table 7-2 provides a quick and easy reference for all currently approved pharmacologic stress agents.

Dipyridamole USP (Intravenous Persantine®)

Dipyridamole has been a common oral medication for patients suffering with CAD for many years. Dipyridamole increases the level of exogenous adenosine in the patient's blood, which acts as a powerful vasodilator. This vasodilation creates a "myocardial steal" phenomenon that diverts blood away from the myocardium that is served by coronary arteries that may have significant stenosis. When used in conjunction with myocardial perfusion imaging agents, differences in myocardial perfusion become apparent during imaging.

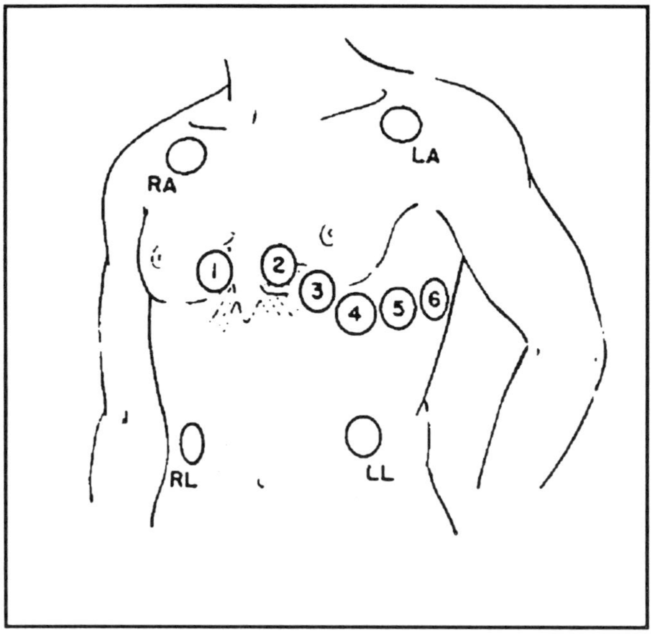

Figure 7.7 Sites of electrode placement for cardiac stress testing. Reprinted with permission from: Bernier DR, Christian PE, Langan JK, Wells LD, eds. *Nuclear medicine technology and techniques,* 2nd ed. St. Louis: CV Mosby; 1989:368.

Patient History and Preparation. A thorough patient history or a full review of the patient's medical record are essential for successful use of dipyridamole in myocardial imaging. First, the technologist must be assured that the patient has been without food or drink for a minimum of 6 hr prior to testing. Stomach contents may not only contribute to nausea during administration of dipyridamole but may also change the availability of blood to the myocardium. Second, the patient must have been without aminophylline or theophylline derivatives for at least 48 hr. These drugs may interfere with the mechanism of dipyridamole. Finally, the technologist must confirm that the patient does not have any drug sensitivities or allergies to dipyridamole, aminophylline or its derivatives.

Since the dosage of intravenous dipyridamole is calculated according to the patient's weight, the most recent measurement should be obtained. This can be done by patient interview, medical record review or directly weighing the patient. In any intravenous dipyridamole stress protocol, a large-bore (20-gauge or greater) catheter should be started to ensure easy pharmaceutical administration. As in treadmill exercise testing, a 12-lead ECG should be set up to monitor the patient's cardiac status during any pharmacologic stress procedure.

Resting Administration Protocol. Resting dipyridamole tests are performed with the patient fully prepped in the supine position. Dipyridamole administration is accomplished by intravenous drip or by injection with a syringe into the port of the intravenous tubing. Dipyridamole is diluted to 50 cc and administered at a rate of 12.5 cc/min or 0.14 mg/kg/min. The patient's dosage, prepared by a licensed pharmacist, is calculated at 0.56 mg/kg of body weight. Dipyridamole administration is completed in 4 min. Since the peak action of dipyridamole occurs about 2 min after the termination of administration, radiopharmaceutical injection is delayed until then. Common side effects of intravenous dipyridamole are chest pain or tightness, dyspnea, headache and in a few cases, nausea and vomiting. In most patients, these symptoms can be relieved with intravenously administered aminophylline, given over 60 sec, or sublingual nitrates. Depending on the radiopharmaceutical, imaging should proceed as with any other stress study.

Exercise Administration Protocol. Although many patients can perform some level of exercise, few patients with CAD can reach an acceptable heart rate. The use of dipyridamole alone in these patients may not be appropriate. Instead, a combination protocol using low-level exercise and dipyridamole infusion has been shown to decrease side effects, increase target-to-background ratios and enhance ECG effects of dipyridamole over

Table 7.2
Protocols for Administration of Dipyridamole, Adenosine and Dobutamine

Patient preparation	For 3 hr prior to test, NPO except water. For at least 12 hr prior to test: If dipyridamole, withhold xanthine derivatives (caffeine, theophylline, etc.). If adenosine, withhold xanthine derivatives (caffeine, theophylline, etc.) and oral dipyridamole. If dobutamine, withhold beta blockers.
Imaging	Standard SPECT or planar myocardial perfusion imaging protocols.
Preparation	Dipyridamole: Patient weight in kg × 0.56 mg/kg drawn up in syringe from 5 mg/ml vials. Adenosine: Ten 2-ml vials (6 mg/ml) diluted in 30 ml normal saline for a concentration of 2.4 mg/ml *or* one 30-ml vial with a concentration of 3 mg/ml. Calculate dose relative to patient weight. Dobutamine: Dilute 120 mg/20 ml dobutamine with 30 ml saline. Calculate dose relative to patient weight.
Standard procedure	1. Confirm physician's lab order; explain procedure; obtain consent. 2. Obtain resting 12-lead ECG and blood pressure. 3. Physician examines and questions the patient regarding relative contraindications. *If any of the exclusion criteria are present, discuss risk/benefit with the referral physician.*
Dipyridamole	1. Start normal saline or D5W i.v. drip. 2. Infuse dipyridamole over 4 min (infusion pump or manual administration). Inject radiopharmaceutical at 8 min. 3. Record ECG and blood pressure at rest and every minute during infusion. 4. Keep aminophylline available: in the event of serious side effects, administer 1–2 min after myocardial perfusion agent is given. 5. Terminate monitoring at 15 min postinfusion if no adverse side effects, ECG changes or hemodynamic changes have occurred. 6. Monitor until patient is stable, if aminophylline was given or changes were noted.
Adenosine	1. Start i.v. drip with normal saline, dual-port extension set and three-way stopcock attached to an infusion pump. 2. Use the most appropriate of the following infusion sequences: Standard 6-min infusion: infuse adenosine at a rate of 140 μg/kg/min for 6 min, with slow radiopharmaceutical injection at the end of the 3 min. Alternate 7-min titrating infusion (typically used for high risk patients): infuse adenosine at a rate of 50 μg/kg/min for 1 min, followed by stepped increases to 75, 100 and 140 μg/kg/min for each consecutive min. Inject radiopharmaceutical at the end of 4 min. Continue infusion at the rate of 140 μg/kg/min for 3 min. 3. Record ECG and blood pressure at rest and every minute during the infusion and for the first 5 min after cessation of infusion. 4. Keep aminophylline available: In the event of serious side effects, administer at the discretion of the physician. 5. Terminate monitoring at 5 min postinfusion, if no adverse side effects, ECG changes or hemodynamic changes have occurred. 6. Monitor until patient is stable, if aminophylline was given or changes were observed.
Dobutamine	1. Start i.v. drip with normal saline, dual-port extension set and three-way stopcock attached to an infusion pump. 2. Infuse dobutamine at a rate of 5 μg/kg/min for 3 min followed by stepped increases to 10, 20, 30 and 40 μg/kg/min for each consecutive 3 min. Inject radiopharmaceutical at the initiation of the maximum dose (13 min or 1 min following initiation of the maximally tolerated dose). Continue infusion at the rate of 40 μg/kg/min for 2 min. 3. Record ECG and blood pressure at rest and every minute during the infusion and for the first 6 min after cessation. 4. Keep esmolol available: In the event of serious side effects, administer at the discretion of the physician. 5. Terminate monitoring at 5 min postinfusion, if no adverse side effects, ECG changes or hemodynamic changes have occurred. 6. Monitor until patient is stable, if esmolol was given or changes were observed.

using dipyridamole alone. Many combination protocols have been proposed utilizing walking, bicycle stress and hand-and-arm exercise during or immediately after dipyridamole infusion. One such protocol enhances dipyridamole effects by using the modified Bruce treadmill protocol. The patient is prepared as for any treadmill myocardial study. A pharmacist prepares dipyridamole to be administered in the usual concentration. Dipyridamole administration begins when the patient begins walking and continues for the full 4 min. The patient continues walking during the second stage; the radiopharmaceutical is injected at the end of the second stage. The patient continues walking for 1 min into the third stage, at which time exercise is terminated. Imaging then proceeds as usual. Aminophylline may be administered after dipyridamole infusion without affecting subsequent images.

Contraindications. There are few contraindications for dipyridamole administration. Patients with drug sensitivities to dipyridamole or aminophylline should be excluded. Patients who have a history of bronchospasm should be excluded because dipyridamole may exacerbate the condition. Dipyridamole should be postponed for those patients who have chronic lung disease and have used aminophylline or its derivatives in the previous 48 hr. Patients who are currently on oral dipyridamole may undergo dipyridamole stress imaging.

Adenosine

The mechanisms of dipyridamole and adenosine are actually the same. Dipyridamole increases the level of exogenous adenosine in the patient's blood. Adenosine, in turn, activates the A2 receptors on the cell membrane of smooth muscle. This creates the vasodilation seen with both stress agents. However, the short plasma half-life of adenosine ($<$ 10 sec), compared to that of dipyridamole (20–30 min), means that the two stress agents have different administration protocols. Adenosine's short plasma half-life also means that its side effects are more transient, but they may also be more severe.

Administration Protocol. The patient interview and preparation is similar to that for the dipyridamole protocol. The patient is placed supine with a patent intravenous catheter. Adenosine is prepared by a pharmacist at a dosage of 240 μg/kg of patient body weight. Adenosine is infused at a rate of 40 μg/kg/min over 6 min. The radiopharmaceutical is administered 3 min into the adenosine infusion. Because of adenosine's transient nature, reversal of side effects with aminophylline is usually not needed, but it may be administered if symptoms persist. Imaging can proceed from this point depending on the radiopharmaceutical.

Contraindications and Side Effects. Contraindications for adenosine stress imaging are the same as for dipyridamole stress imaging. Close attention must be paid to clinical symptoms and ECG data during adenosine administration to note any rapid changes in the patient's condition.

Dobutamine

Both adenosine and dipyridamole act by increasing the flow of blood to the myocardium by vasodilation. Dobutamine is the only approved pharmacologic stress agent that works by increasing the demand for blood by the myocardium. Dobutamine is a positive inotropic agent (a substance that affects the force of myocardial contractions) that stimulates the myocardium's beta-1 receptors. This stimulation increases the force and frequency of the contraction. Essentially, dobutamine mimics the effect of exercise on the heart.

Patient Preparation. The patient preparation for dobutamine imaging is similar to that for the treadmill exercise test. A large-bore intravenous catheter is established in a peripheral vein. Patients should refrain from the use of beta blockers for at least 24 hr because they bind to the beta sites of the myocardium and inhibit the effect of dobutamine.

Administration Protocol. Dobutamine administration is broken down into stages very similar to that of a treadmill test. Intravenous infusion begins at a rate of 5 μg/kg/min for 3 min. Stepped increases follow at 5-min intervals to infusion rates of 10, 20, 30 and 40 μg/kg/min. At the beginning of the last stage, the radiopharmaceutical is injected. The duration for this 40 μg/kg/min infusion lasts only 2 min because of the high dosage. ECG data should be obtained at rest before infusion and every 5 min after the beginning of infusion. A 5-min postinfusion ECG should also be obtained. Vital signs should be taken at rest and every minute during infusion until the 5-min postinfusion ECG. Propranolol should be kept available to reverse any side effects. The patient should remain supine until all ECG and clinical data are obtained and imaging is about to begin.

Contraindications and Side Effects. Beta blockers are the primary contraindication for dobutamine stress testing. These antihypertensives should be discontinued for 24 hr prior to testing. Dobutamine side effects are similar to those of treadmill testing and patients may experience chest pain, dyspnea, ECG changes or nausea. Dobutamine should be discontinued if these symptoms become too severe and propranolol should be administered to reverse the side effects.

Thallium-201-Thallous Chloride

For many years, researchers worked to find an acceptable method of assessing myocardial perfusion using radionuclides. Many different nuclides were tested before ^{201}Tl was first used in the 1970s. Thallium is an analog of the element potassium (K), which is used by the myocardium during contractions. Thallium does not collect in the myocardium permanently but is constantly being pumped in and out of the myocardial cells. This phenomenon makes ^{201}Tl an ideal agent for assessing the extent of CAD and for determining the viability of the affected myocardium. Because of the number of individuals suffering from CAD in the U.S. and the availability of ^{201}Tl, this procedure has become a staple of the average nuclear medicine department.

For coronary blockages, because of the restriction of blood flow, ^{201}Tl cannot enter the myocardium to the same extent as when blood flow is unrestricted. This condition is intensified during exercise, when the myocardium's demand for oxygen is greater. The partially blocked coronary artery, however, cannot respond normally by dilating to increase blood flow to meet oxygen demand. Since the amount of ^{201}Tl uptake is based on the amount of blood flow to that area of the myocardium, ischemic regions will concentrate less ^{201}Tl and appear as areas of decreased radioactivity on the images. When the patient is at rest and the myocardium's need for extra oxygen has lessened, blood flow in the diseased artery may be adequate for the resting state. Since ^{201}Tl is constantly being pumped in and out of myocardial cells into the circulation, ^{201}Tl redistribution into previously ischemic areas can occur and is visualized on resting ^{201}Tl images, 24-hr delayed images or reinjection images. Defects visualized on the stress images appear to fill-in with tracer on rest images. Infarcted areas will not accumulate tracer during rest or at stress imaging because the myocardial cells in these areas are no longer functional. Such data provide a highly accurate picture of the amount of viable or salvageable myocardium.

Stress/Rest Image Acquisition. Exercise and pharmacologic stress protocols were previously discussed. With the advent of faster computers and cameras capable of tomographic imaging, many patients can be evaluated more extensively than ever before using ^{201}Tl. The choice between planar imaging or tomographic imaging may depend on a patient's ability to remain still during data acquisition.

Planar Imaging. Imaging should begin within 10 min of ^{201}Tl administration to ensure that ^{201}Tl redistribution has not begun. The patient should be placed in a supine position on the imaging table that will allow *exact* duplication of the angles of imaging. Some facilities acquire three standard images: anterior, 45° LAO and 70° LAO. This method saves time and makes angle reproduction easier on delayed imaging. It does not, however, ensure that the same part of the myocardium is being evaluated from patient to patient since the apical angle in the mediastinum may vary. Another positioning method involves first finding the best septal resolution LAO angle. From this angle, subtract 45° for the anterior angle and add 25° for the steep LAO angle. For example, the best septal resolution for a particular patient may occur at 35° LAO. The anterior view would actually be 10° RAO and the steep LAO would be at 60°. This method takes more time and makes angle reproduction trickier, but it helps ensure that image interpretation by the physician is not dependent on patient anatomy.

The imaging time may vary from 300 to 400 sec per image. The computer matrix is a 64x64x8 for most programs, although some will allow processing with a 128x128x8 matrix. In addition to the angle information (including any caudal angles), the time should also be recorded since most processing programs use the elapsed time to calculate any abnormal washout of ^{201}Tl. A low-energy, all-purpose collimator is used. Due to the low count rates associated with ^{201}Tl imaging, a high-resolution collimator should not be used since longer imaging times increase the possibility of ^{201}Tl redistribution during acquisition.

After the stress images are acquired, the patient should be instructed to return for delayed imaging in 3–4 hr. The patient may be instructed not to eat during this time, or may be permitted a light snack, avoiding caffeine, sugar and carbohydrates. In delayed imaging, the angles and patient position relative to the camera must be reproduced exactly. This will ensure that any changes visualized on the delayed images are not due to positioning errors but rather reflect physiologic changes in the patient.

Image processing usually consists of a comparison of the early and delayed images. Normal myocardial perfusion images display uniform tracer distribution throughout the left ventricle (Fig. 7-8). The right ventricle is either visualized poorly or not at all. Since only healthy myocardial tissue extracts ^{201}Tl from the blood, areas of decreased perfusion or infarcted tissue will be visualized as cold defects (Fig. 7-9). Computer analysis of each section of the myocardium may be performed as well as calculation of the percent washout of ^{201}Tl and heart-to-lung ratios.

SPECT Imaging. Patient preparation for SPECT ^{201}Tl stress/rest imaging is the same as for planar imaging up to the point of patient positioning. In SPECT imaging, the patient is placed supine on a tomographic imaging table with the left arm above the head to avoid attenuation in the area of the heart. The patient is positioned so that the long axis of the body will be in the camera's center of rotation. The heart should be placed at the widest point of the field of view. These steps will help ensure that the heart remains in the field of view throughout the detector's rotation. The camera is then placed in the 45° RAO position to begin the acquisition. Images may be acquired over 180° or 360°. The matrix should be set at 64x64x8. A 128x128x8 matrix should not be used because this would reduce the counts/pixel by a factor of four and decrease the quality of the reconstructed images. The imaging time is comparable to that of planar imaging. After the stress images are obtained, the patient is given the same instructions as for planar imaging. The same imaging procedure is repeated at rest.

Processing details of tomographic myocardial images may vary. The reconstructed slices, short-axis, vertical and horizontal long axes, are typically paired stress to rest for visual comparison.

Rest Imaging Protocols. Resting ^{201}Tl studies are sometimes performed to assess the patient who may have suffered an acute myocardial infarction. Since ^{201}Tl localizes only in areas of viable myocardium, any defect seen at rest can be representative of necrotic or scarred tissue. The patient preparation is similar to that for exercise testing in that the patient should be NPO for at least 4 hr. Medications do not usually interfere with rest studies and the restriction of medications is not usually an issue with these patients because of their poor condition. Two to 4 mCi (74–148 MBq) of ^{201}Tl are injected intravenously and imaging proceeds as usual.

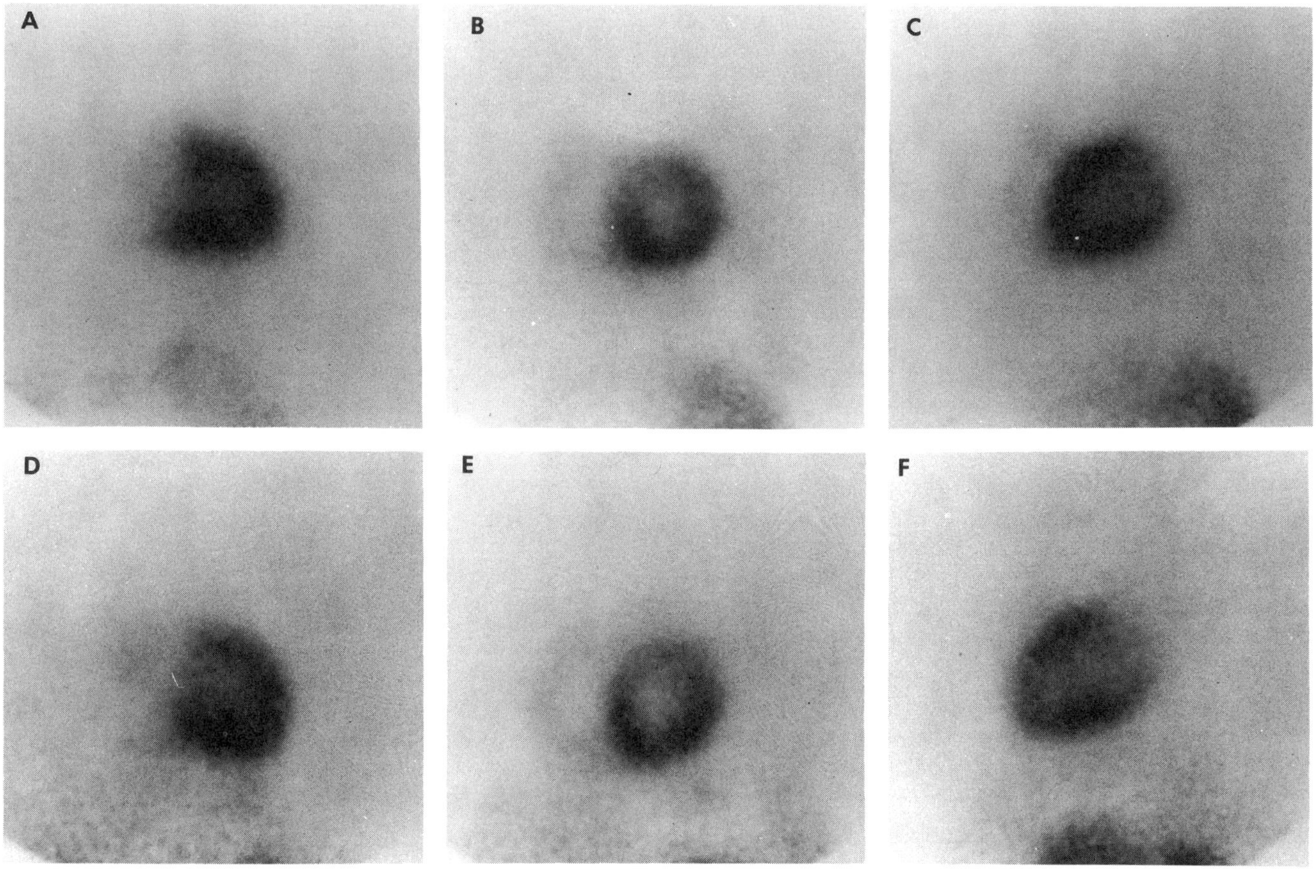

Figure 7.8 Normal planar thallium images in the anterior, 40° LAO and 70° LAO projections. Stress images (A-C) and delayed images (D-F) demonstrate essentially the same tracer distribution with no defects. Courtesy of the Department of Veterans Affairs Medical Center, Buffalo, NY.

Thallium reinjection at rest has been shown to increase the sensitivity of ^{201}Tl imaging for the detection of viable myocardium. This procedure can be performed at the 3–4-hr mark after delayed imaging or even 24 hr later. In this procedure, the patient receives an intravenous injection of 1–2 mCi (37–74 MBq) ^{201}Tl at rest. This dose provides an abundance of available ^{201}Tl for the myocardium. Imaging begins 45–60 min after ^{201}Tl administration. Planar or SPECT images are then obtained just as they were for earlier image sets. These reinjection images are then compared to stress and rest images to identify any areas of ^{201}Tl redistribution. A lack of ^{201}Tl in a part of the myocardium after reinjection means there is a high probability of nonviable tissue.

Contraindications Thallium activity is kept low due to the radiation dose to the patient. Because of thallium's low energy, many of the emissions are absorbed by the body. Clinically, the only contraindications for ^{201}Tl imaging are those associated with the type of stress used during the examination. Obese patients or women with large breasts may be better imaged with ^{99m}Tc-sestamibi because of attenuation defects found with ^{201}Tl.

Technetium-99m-Sestamibi

In the 1980s, researchers worked to find a myocardial perfusion agent with better imaging characteristics than ^{201}Tl. Much of this research centered on finding a ^{99m}Tc-based radiopharmaceutical that would yield high myocardial count rates while delivering a modest radiation dose to the patient. Technetium-99m-sestamibi, marketed under the name Cardiolite®, avidly collects in perfused myocardial cells, although the mechanisms for this action are not well understood. Technetium-99m-sestamibi has changed the way many nuclear medicine departments evaluate patients with CAD. Unlike ^{201}Tl, ^{99m}Tc-sestamibi has little or no redistribution over time, which provides significant flexibility in terms of imaging and camera utilization. This flexibility is somewhat offset by the fact that myocardial ischemia cannot be measured with a single injection of radiopharmaceutical.

Patient Preparation. The patient history should be obtained and the procedure should be fully explained to the patient. The preparation of the patient undergoing ^{99m}Tc-sestamibi resting studies is much the same as for rest ^{201}Tl studies. The patient should be NPO for at least 4 hr before tracer administration and medications are not usually with held. For stress studies, the preparation is more a function of the type of stress used. Refer to earlier sections for these preparations.

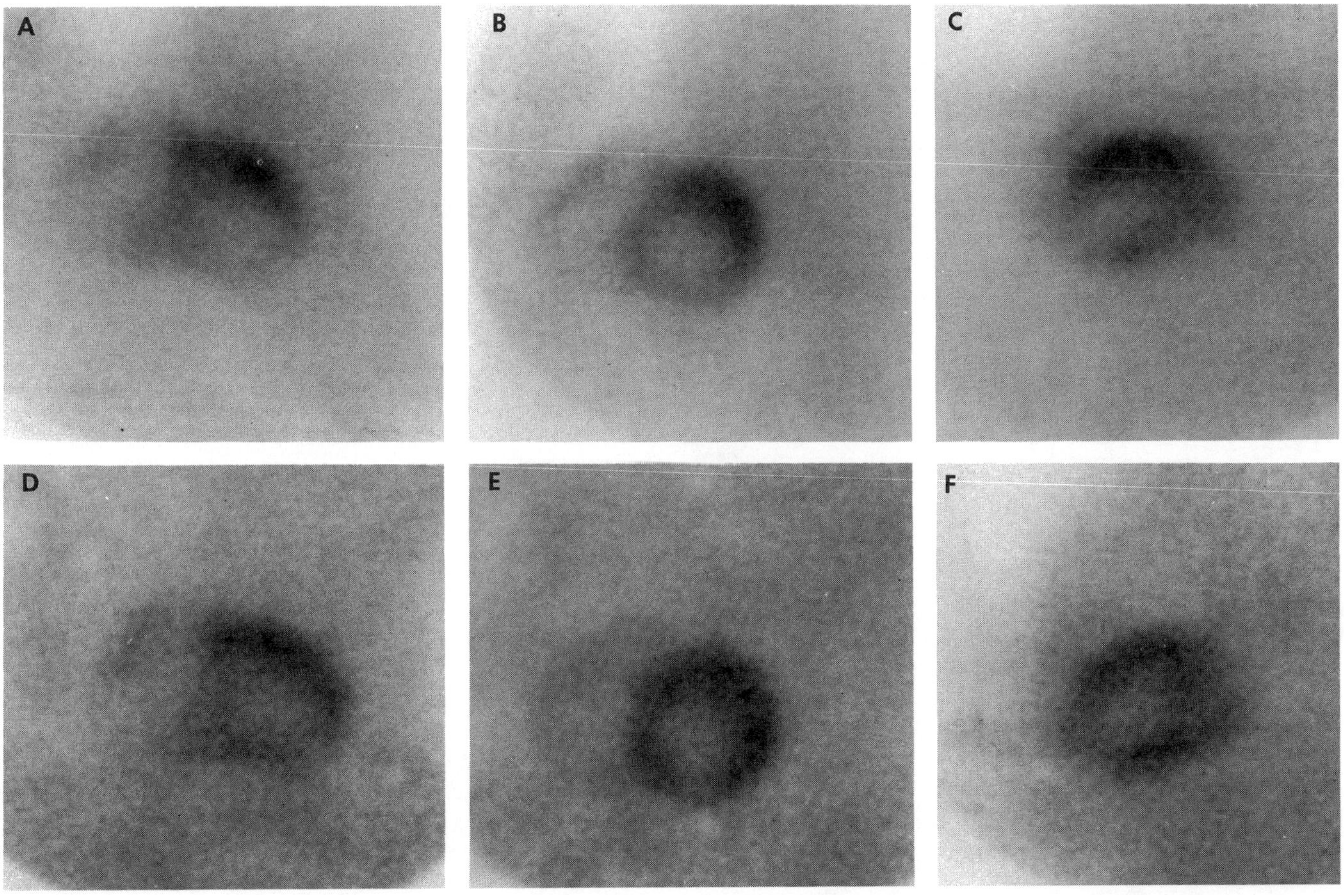

Figure 7.9 Abnormal planar thallium images in the anterior, 40° LAO and 70° LAO projections. Stress images (A-C) show perfusion defects in the inferior, septal and apical areas of the left ventricle. Delayed images (D-F) demonstrate tracer redistribution in these areas, a pattern consistent with exercise-induced ischemia. Courtesy of the Department of Veterans Affairs Medical Center, Buffalo, NY.

Rest Protocol. As with ^{201}Tl studies, ^{99m}Tc-sestamibi rest imaging is performed to assess the extent and severity of acute myocardial infarction. After the patient's preparation is completed, 20–30 mCi (740–1110 MBq) ^{99m}Tc-sestamibi are injected intravenously. If desired, a first-pass wall motion study may be obtained during injection. Unlike ^{201}Tl, ^{99m}Tc-sestamibi imaging does not begin immediately. Initial hepatic and lung background levels are high enough to obscure the myocardium. Instead, imaging occurs anytime between 1–3 hr later. In addition, the patient also may be allowed to have a light fatty meal 45–60 min after tracer administration. This not only makes for a more compliant patient, but it also stimulates gallbladder contraction. Much of the activity not collected in the myocardium will be collected in the hepatobiliary system. When the gallbladder contracts, this activity will be spread throughout the small bowel, thereby helping to eliminate singular areas of intense activity.

Planar imaging is performed with the patient supine. The camera should be peaked for the 140-keV photopeak of ^{99m}Tc. High-resolution collimation is used in stead of LEAP collimation because of the high photon flux. This allows the use of a 128x128x16 matrix for computer acquisition and will give images of greater detail. Images are acquired in the anterior, 45° LAO and 70° LAO projections to evaluate the walls served by the three main coronary arteries. Imaging time should be between 300–400 sec per image and shielding should be used to block any gastrointestinal activity that may interfere with image interpretation. If the rest study is performed in conjunction with a stress study, care should be taken to reproduce the angles exactly.

SPECT imaging is performed with the patient supine on an appropriate tomographic imaging table. Patient positioning is similar to that for SPECT ^{201}Tl imaging. Again, a high-resolution collimator is used. Care should be taken to use the center of rotation correction for this collimator. A 128x128x8 matrix can be used, but a 64x64x16 matrix will give a higher density image with less noise on reconstruction. Imaging is performed in the same manner as ^{201}Tl imaging, with a 180° or 360° rotation. Imaging time per projection can be reduced to 10–20 sec because of the high photon flux. If a rest SPECT study is done in conjunction with a stress study, care must be taken to ensure that patient positioning is duplicated in both sets of images. Reconstruction of the SPECT images may be performed using a variety of filters. The reconstructed slices are then backprojected through a ramp filter before final presentation.

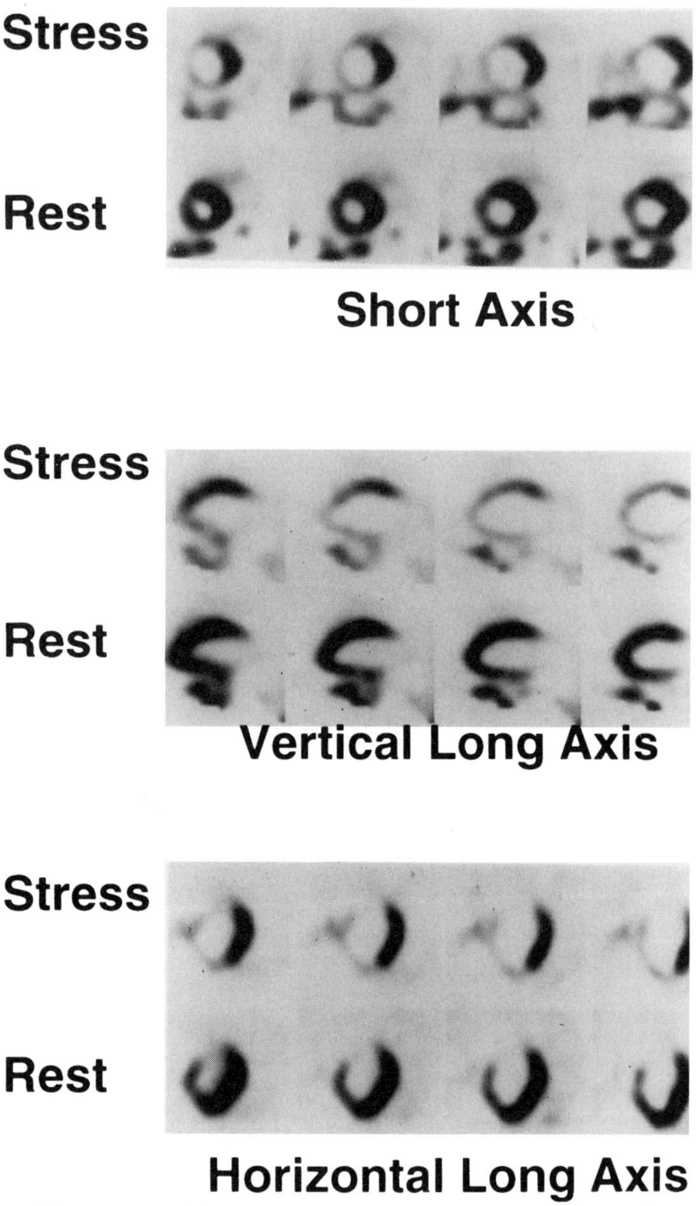

Figure 7.10 Selected slices from an abnormal myocardial perfusion study performed with ^{99m}Tc-sestamibi. Courtesy of Walker Baptist Medical Center, Jasper, AL.

Stress Protocols. Because ^{99m}Tc-sestamibi remains fixed in the myocardium, many different protocols have been developed to evaluate CAD patients. These can be roughly subdivided into one-day and two-day protocols. The one-day protocols can be further subdivided into stress-rest and rest-stress protocols.

Two-Day Stress Protocol. The two-day protocol, first devised for ^{99m}Tc-sestamibi evaluation of CAD, uses two separate injections, if needed, on two separate days to obtain rest and stress information. The patient is first prepared for the stress study just as for any other stress study using radiopharmaceuticals. Twenty to 30 mCi (740–1110 MBq) ^{99m}Tc sestamibi are administered at the appropriate time during the stress procedure. Planar or SPECT imaging is then performed 60–90 min following tracer administration.

If a defect is present on the initial stress images or if ECG or clinical changes occur during the stress procedure, the physician may ask that a rest study be performed. The rest study is then performed on the next available day, at which time 20–30 mCi (740–1110 MBq) ^{99m}Tc-sestamibi are injected intravenously at rest. Images are acquired as in the stress study. The rest images are then compared to the stress images to confirm stress-induced ischemia or infarction. For those patients with normal stress studies, no further imaging is required, thus saving time and money. However, this protocol is sometimes logistically difficult to perform since it may require two separate visits by the patient. This is especially true in the case of outpatient procedures.

One-Day Stress-Rest Protocol. This protocol is patterned after the stress-rest ^{201}Tl protocol. This study is performed with the same stress protocol as in other stress studies using radiopharmaceuticals. Five to 10 mCi (185–370 MBq) ^{99m}Tc-sestamibi are administered intravenously 1 min before the termination of exercise or in conjunction with a pharmacologic stress agent at the appropriate time. Imaging is performed 45–90 min after tracer administration as previously described. After 4 hr, with the patient at rest, a second injection of 25–30 mCi (925–1110 MBq) ^{99m}Tc-sestamibi is administered. Imaging occurs at 60–90 min postinjection. These images are then compared to the stress images (Fig. 7-10). Although this protocol requires only one visit to the imaging lab, the time between initial stress and conclusion of the rest images may be as long as 6 hr.

One-Day Rest-Stress Protocol. This protocol is much the same as the stress-rest protocol except that the sequence is reversed. The rest images are obtained 45–90 min after intravenous administration of 5–10 mCi (185–370 MBq) ^{99m}Tc-sestamibi. The patient is then stressed 3–4 hr later when 25–30 mCi (925–1110 MBq) of the tracer are injected at the appropriate time. Imaging occurs 60–90 min later, taking care to reproduce the views as closely as possible. Image reconstruction is performed on each image set and the two sets of images are then compared for perfusion differences. The difference in activity administered for the stress images will offset any ^{99m}Tc remaining from the initial rest study and will be sufficient to demonstrate ischemic myocardium.

Dual-Isotope Protocols. Recently there has been marked interest in using ^{201}Tl and ^{99m}Tc-sestamibi to assess patients with CAD. The purpose of this approach is to eliminate the problems associated with the one-day and two-day ^{99m}Tc sestamibi protocols. This combination protocol has shown a high sensitivity for the detection of coronary stenosis with a much shorter time in the department for the patient as compared to that for single tracer studies using ^{201}Tl or ^{99m}Tc-sestamibi. This method begins with the intravenous administration of 3.0 mCi (111 MBq) ^{201}Tl with the patient at rest. Planar or SPECT imaging proceeds 10–30 min later. Immediately after rest imaging, the patient is prepared for stress testing. The patient then undergoes stress testing and 20–30 mCi (740–1110 MBq) ^{99m}Tc-sestamibi are administered at the ing the exam. Imaging occurs 60–90 min postinjection using the identical imaging procedure as for rest ^{201}Tl images. Both sets of images are obtained with high-resolution collimation. To ensure adequate count density, the ^{201}Tl data will need to be acquired for a longer period than the ^{99m}Tc-sestamibi data. A 64x64x8 matrix is used during the rest acquisition and a 64x64x16 matrix is used for the stress acquisition. Reconstruction is performed for each image set. The image slices are then compared to detect ischemic areas (Fig. 7-11). Because of the difference in energy of the two radionuclides and the order in which the studies are performed, there is no significant overlap of their photopeaks.

Contraindications and Side Effects. There are no known contraindications for the administration of ^{99m}Tc-sestamibi. The most common side effect associated with ^{99m}Tc-sestamibi is a transient metallic taste. Most side effects experienced by patients are those associated with stress testing.

FUNCTIONAL IMAGING OF THE HEART

The primary function of the heart is to act as a mechanical pump to distribute blood throughout the body. Two techniques are used to assess cardiac function: the gated equilibrium method or the first-pass method.

Gated Equilibrium Left Ventricular Analysis

The most common cardiac function test performed in most nuclear medicine departments is gated left ventricular analysis. This test, also known as a MUGA study (multigated analysis) or radionuclide ventriculogram (RNV), measures the parameter of cardiac function known as ejection fraction and may be performed at rest or during stress. The test is an accurate measurement of cardiac function and can be repeated often to measure the patient's progress during the course of cardiac drug therapy or to measure the effects of chemotherapy on a cancer patient's heart. Data are acquired by dividing the cardiac cycle into 16, 24 or 32 segments, based on the software available (Fig. 7-12). During each cardiac cycle, data are continually added together with previous cycles. Over the course of a few hundred beats, the cumulative information gathered gives an accurate picture of cardiac wall motion. Since the cardiac cycle is now divided into discrete frames, diastolic and systolic frames can be identified based on the number of counts in the left ventricle. Ejection fraction and wall motion analysis are obtained from this information.

Patient Preparation. A three-lead ECG is put in place to signal the computer to begin accumulating data during the cardiac cycle. In addition, for the stress study, the patient's

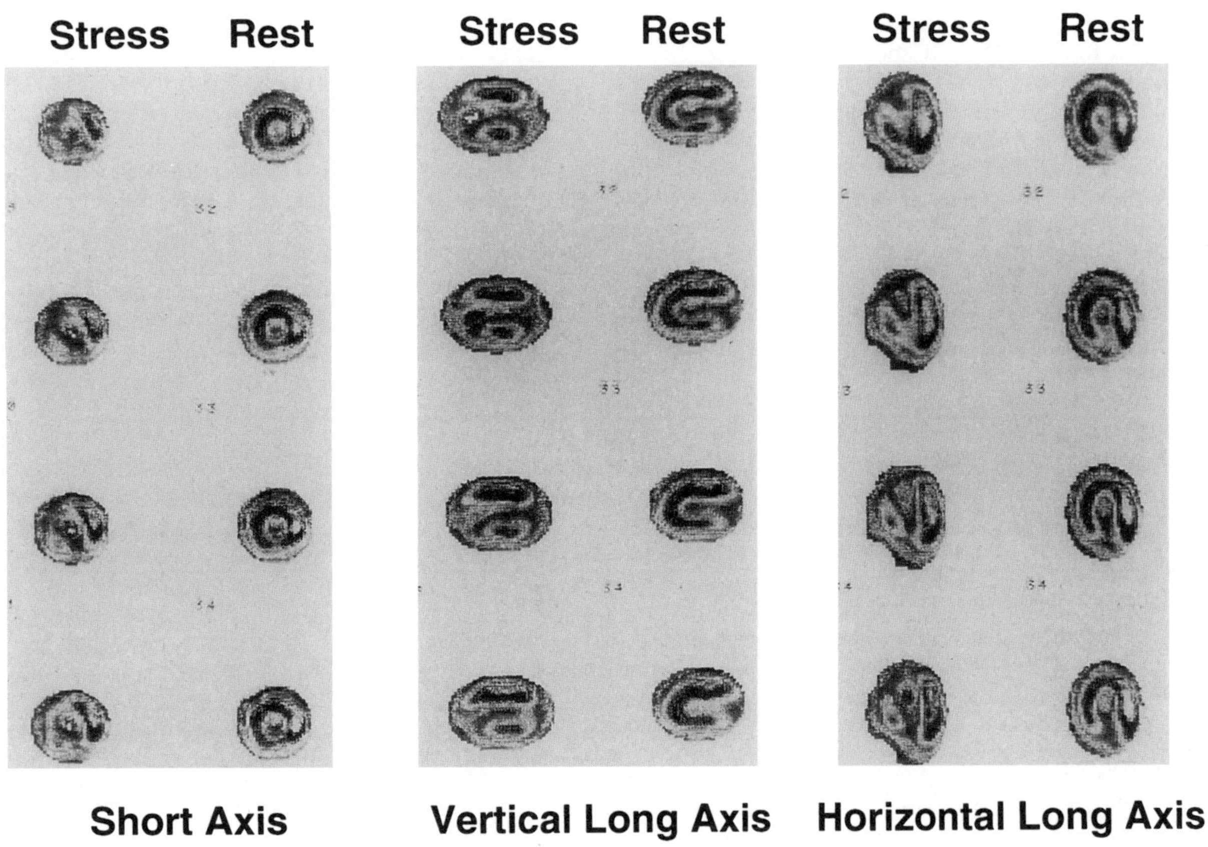

Figure 7.11 Selected slices from a dual-isotope myocardial perfusion study demonstrates stress-induced ischemia in the apex of the left ventricle. Thallium-201-thallous chloride was administered at rest and ^{99m}Tc-sestamibi was administered during exercise. Courtesy of Cardiovascular Associates, Birmingham, AL.

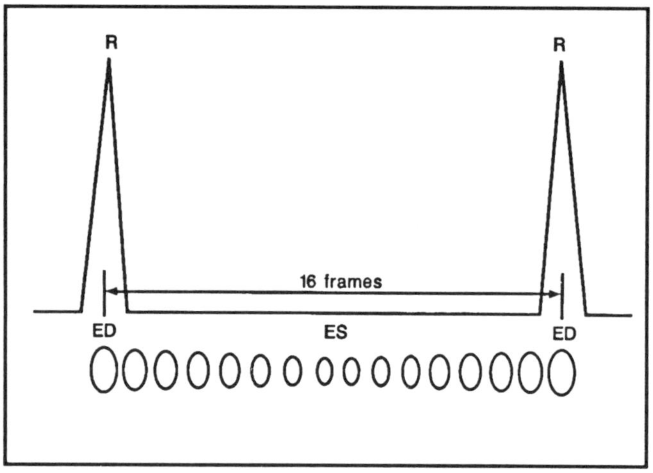

Figure 7.12 Relationship of left ventricular volume and ECG tracing. A representative cardiac cycle (from which left ventricular ejection fraction is calculated) is generated by adding together data from hundreds of cardiac cycles.

thorax is immobilized on a stress table attached to a bicycle ergometer. This system allows the patient to exercise and be imaged simultaneously.

Radiopharmaceuticals. There are two radiopharmaceuticals available for gated equilibrium ventricular function imaging. Human serum albumin (HSA) is a purified product of human blood that can be labeled with ^{99m}Tc. Technetium-99m-HSA gives high-resolution images of the blood pool inside the ventricles. Because HSA is a protein, liver uptake can be a problem if imaging is not started within a few minutes of tracer administration. Technetium-99m-labeled red blood cells (RBCs) is the most common radiopharmaceutical used in gated left ventricular imaging because of its convenience and low cost.

One of three methods, the in vitro, in vivo and modified in vivo, may be used to label the patient's own RBCs. The in vitro method involves withdrawing 2–10 cc of blood from the patient and combining the blood with a reducing agent such as stannous pyrophosphate in the presence of an anticoagulant. Technetium-99m-pertechnetate is then added and incubated with the blood for 20–30 min. During this time, the pertechnetate ion is reduced so that it can be transported across the RBC membrane and attach to hemoglobin. The actual incorporation of the pertechnetate ion into hemoglobin is not well understood, but this method yields a very high labeling efficiency. The newly labeled blood is then reinjected back into the patient for imaging. This label is extremely stable and imaging can be performed up to 4 hr later.

The in vivo method starts with an intravenous injection of 3–10 mg stannous pyrophosphate. This material is allowed to circulate for 15–20 min while the patient is prepared for imaging. The patient is then given an intravenous injection of 20–30 mCi (740–1110 MBq) [^{99m}Tc]pertechnetate. Although the labeling efficiency of the in vivo method is lower than that obtained with the in vitro method, the tagging efficiency is adequate to permit imaging for up to several hours after RBC tagging. To increase the labeling efficiency of the in vivo method, a modified in vivo technique was developed. Table 7-3 compares the two in vivo labeling techniques.

Stress Imaging. Imaging cardiac function under stress is based on the premise that ischemic myocardium does not contract as well as normal myocardium. Following patient preparation and radiopharmaceutical administration, the patient is placed supine on an imaging table interfaced with a bicycle ergometer and the patient's thorax is immobilized. The bicycle ergometer is a method of creating a cardiac workload at a controlled rate much like a treadmill. This method allows the patient to be semi-erect while exercising. The gamma camera is placed at the 45° LAO or best septal resolution LAO to separate the two ventricles. A 64x64x8 acquisition matrix, with the cardiac cycle divided into 16, 24 or 32 segments, depending on the available software, is used. An 8-bit pixel depth is suggested since the limited time for each stage will prevent pixel saturation and an 8-bit

Table 7.3
Technetium-99m Labeling of Red Blood Cells by the In Vivo and Modified In Vivo/In Vitro Methods

In vivo method	In vivo/In vitro method
Step 1. Inject stannous pyrophosphate.	Step 1. Inject (i.v.) stannous pyrophosphate.
Step 2. Wait ~ 20 min, then inject (i.v.) 20–25 mCi [^{99m}Tc]sodium pertechnetate.	Step 2. Wait ~ 20 min.
	Step 3. Withdraw (by venipuncture) ~ 8 ml whole blood into a shielded syringe containing 20–25 mCi [^{99m}Tc]sodium pertechnetate.* Gently mix at room temperature for 10 min.
	Step 4. Reinject contents of syringe.

*Syringe may be heparinized with *very* dilute solution (10 units/ml) or contain ACD (acid-citrate-dextrose) as anticoagulant.

Reprinted with permission from Chilton HM, Witcofski RL. *Nuclear pharmacy.* Philadelphia: Lea & Febiger; 1986:136.

depth will increase the speed of image processing. A 3-min rest study is obtained at baseline before stressing begins. Exercise begins at a slow pace with little resistance for 3 min. The resistance is then increased every 3 min, thus forcing the patient to work harder to maintain the same revolutions per minute. Composite cardiac cycles are acquired at each 3-min stage with each stage processed as a separate study. In this way, regional wall motion and ejection fractions are obtained for each level of work to reveal any myocardial areas that may become ischemic during exercise. Care must be taken to secure the patient during this procedure because motion during the test can cause the patient's heart to shift positions relative to the gamma camera face. This can lead to a blurring of the ventricular blood pool and inaccurate calculation of the ejection fraction. The study is terminated when the patient can no longer continue or until clinical symptoms restrict exercise.

Rest Imaging. Following three-lead ECG placement and radiopharmaceutical administration, the patient is placed supine on an imaging table and the camera is positioned in the 45° LAO or best septal resolution LAO. A 64x64x16 acquisition matrix with either 16, 24, or 32 segments per cardiac cycle is used. Greater pixel depth is required for rest images since a larger number of cardiac cycles and therefore counts will be acquired. The LAO view is acquired for 5 min or a minimum of 300 beats. Additional views (typically, anterior and steep LAO or left lateral) can be obtained with the same time/count parameters. When using the best septal resolution method of positioning, it is preferable to use the angle subtraction technique discussed previously to ensure that image interpretation is consistent from patient to patient.

Data Processing. In both rest and stress studies, the same data will be generated. Global ejection fraction is the percentage of diastolic volume pumped during a cardiac cycle for the entire ventricle. By drawing computerized regions of interest around the ventricle at diastole and systole, global ejection fraction can be calculated using the formula:

$$\%EF = \frac{\text{net diastolic counts} - \text{net systolic counts}}{\text{net diastolic counts}} \times 100.$$

Regional ejection fractions are calculated by dividing the ventricle into areas and applying the same equation to each area. This is very important in stress imaging when ischemia is suspected or in the patient who has suffered a myocardial infarction. In both cases, the area of the myocardium supplied by a blocked blood vessel may demonstrate decreased regional ejection fraction.

Qualitative assessment of the contraction can be visualized by displaying the composite cardiac cycle as a continuous loop running the 16, 24 or 32 segments of the R-R interval in sequence to simulate the beating heart. This display is useful in visualizing regional wall motion abnormalities such as akinesis, dyskinesis and hypokinesis. Left ventricular aneurysms may also be demonstrated with a cine image.

Contraindications. There are no real contraindications to the gated equilibrium imaging technique, but there are some technical pitfalls. Patient motion during a stress procedure can introduce false or misleading information into the images and, consequently, into the calculated ejection fractions. Care should be taken to stabilize the patient's thorax as securely as possible.

A composite cardiac cycle can only be produced if the R-to-R interval is of approximately equal length for each heart beat. Small variations in the length of the R to R interval can be expected in all patients. In patients with severe cardiac arrhythmias, however, it may be impossible to obtain adequate data. The determination of cardiac function for such patients may be better performed using first-pass analysis.

Careful adherence to a standardized RBC labeling protocol will help ensure high labeling efficiency. Excess free pertechnetate in the circulation or concentrated in structures surrounding the heart may obscure cardiac chambers and make it difficult to identify the left ventricular borders. The RBCs of patients on high doses of steroids may be difficult to label with [^{99m}Tc]pertechnetate because steroids interfere with the labeling process; although the mechanism for this interference is not known.

First-Pass Analysis

First-pass radionuclide angiography is a useful tool in the evaluation of patients with left ventricular dysfunction, interventricular shunts or even myocardial infarction or ischemia. This technique is used to record the initial passage of the radiopharmaceutical through the cardiac chambers. An advantage to first-pass analysis is that the tracer activity is limited to one chamber at a time, so it is easier to define ROIs. Also, background interference is minimized since only one structure or chamber is visualized at one time. In addition, this procedure is quick and does not require the patient to lie on an imaging table for prolonged periods of time. It can be used in combination with myocardial perfusion agents or as part of a gated left ventricular study. Although this is a useful study, it is one of the most technically difficult studies that nuclear medicine technologists will be asked to perform.

Patient History and Preparation. As for all studies, the technologist should completely explain the procedure to the patient. One of the most important parts of the patient history is a pretest ECG. Since first-pass studies will be representative of only two or three beats, a good heart beat without ectopic beats or premature ventricular contractions (PVCs) is essential for a successful study. If the radiopharmaceutical bolus enters the right ventricle during a spurious beat, the entire study could be worthless. For patients with frequent PVCs, an equilibrium gated study with bad beat rejection might be a better choice. The patient should be positioned supine on an imaging table that will allow access to the patient's external jugular or antecubital vein with the camera in place over the patient's heart.

Imaging. A large-bore (18-gauge or larger) catheter is placed in an external jugular vein or medial antecubital vein

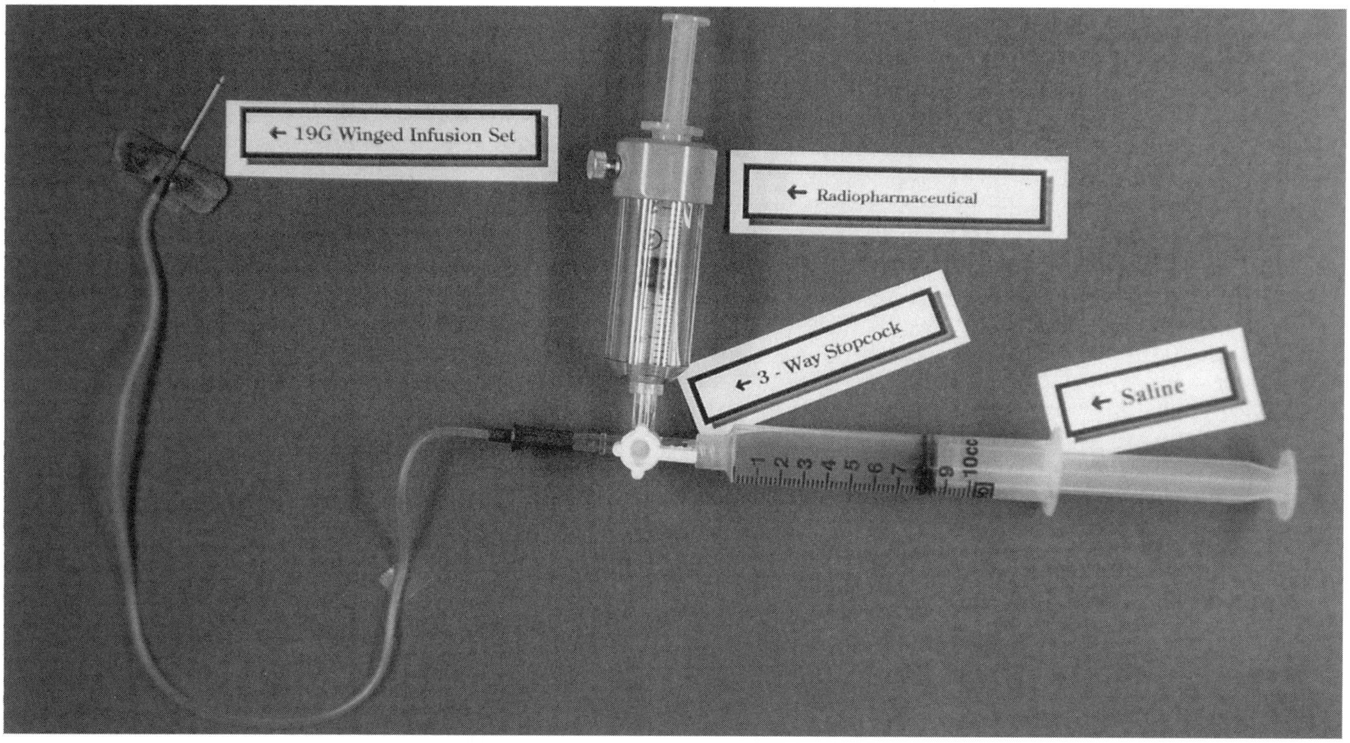

Figure 7.13 Bolus injection set-up.

so that a small bolus of activity is pushed into the system without resistance. The choice of radiopharmaceutical depends on what studies are to follow. If no other studies are planned after the first-pass study, [^{99m}Tc]sodium pertechnetate or ^{99m}Tc-pentetate (DTPA) are preferred tracers. If an equilibrium ventricular function study is planned, the patient's blood should be pre-tinned with stannous pyrophosphate; [^{99m}Tc]pertechnetate will then be administered to perform the first-pass study. Technetium-99m-sestamibi can be used for first-pass angiography if a myocardial perfusion study is planned later. In this way, a single injection can be used to evaluate both ventricular performance and myocardial perfusion. Regardless of the radiopharmaceutical, it must be in as small a volume as possible, preferably less than 1 ml because a small volume will help ensure that the injected bolus will remain intact as long as possible. The volume also should not exceed the volume of the tubing used during the injection. Too large a volume will cause the bolus to be separated during radiopharmaceutical loading into the system. The catheter should be connected to a three-way stopcock with the radiopharmaceutical and 10 ml of normal saline (Fig. 7-13).

The gamma camera should be able to acquire data at a high count rate (200,000 cps or more) and be equipped with a high-sensitivity collimator. Positioning is one of the most difficult aspects of first-pass imaging. Unlike most imaging in nuclear medicine, positioning is performed with no activity in the body. A 1-mCi (37 MBq) spot source can be used to ensure that the sternal notch and the xiphoid process are both in the field of view before injection. By doing this, there will be little doubt as to the position of the heart in the field of view. The camera detector should be placed in the 10° RAO position to separate the ventricles and give the same view as the left ventricular image using contrast angiography. The computer should be set with a 64x64x8 matrix. Dynamic imaging should be set so that about eight frames per cardiac cycle are collected. For a typical patient with a heart rate of 70 bpm, each frame would last for about 0.11 sec. With the patient and camera in position, the radiopharmaceutical is loaded into the tubing and the stopcock turned to allow saline injection. Then the camera is started, the saline is injected as a bolus and data are acquired for 5–7 sec. In this length of time, the bolus will have passed through both ventricles, the lungs and out into the systemic circulation.

Data Processing. First-pass angiography is used many times as a low-cost screening tool for those patients with suspected interventricular shunt. Patients with this shunt, usually neonates, will not be able to oxygenate blood properly because part of each cardiac stroke volume is sent into the systemic circulation instead of the lungs. Following tracer injection, venous blood with the radiotracer will be shunted into the left ventricle and the systemic circulation, an event that is easily detected. If the study is being performed to evaluate a shunt, a region of interest (ROI) is drawn over the right ventricle, lungs and left ventricle or nonpulmonary background region. These regions are applied to the dynamic series. By graphing each region over time, peaks representing the bolus of activity are observed. In shunting, the peak of left ventricular or background activity will occur earlier or be superimposed on the lung peak.

Left ventricular ejection fraction can be calculated by drawing a ROI around the left ventricle. Application of the ROI to the dynamic set should give two to three peaks of bolus act activity representing ventricular contraction. The apex of each of these peaks will represent diastole, while the low points or "valleys" will represent systole. By obtaining the counts of each of these points, ejection fraction can be calculated.

Technical Considerations. A compact tracer bolus and a precise bolus injection technique are the keys to a technically satisfactory first-pass cardiac study. The tracer should be contained in a volume of less than 1 ml. Use of a vein that offers a direct path to the superior vena cava minimizes the possibility of bolus fragmentation as it travels through the circulation. The injection technique itself is as critical as the injection site. The bolus must be delivered rapidly into the circulatory system with a saline flush.

REFERENCES

1. Berman DS, Kiat H, Van Train KF, et al. Comparison of SPECT using technetium-99m agents and thallium-201 and PET for the assessment of myocardial perfusion and viability. *Am J Cardiol* 1990;66:72E–79E.
2. Berman DS. Introduction-Technetium-99m myocardial perfusion agents and their relation to thallium-201. *Am J Cardiol* 1990;66:1E–4E.
3. Berman DS, Kiat H, Friedman JD, et al. Separate acquisition rest thallium-201/stress technetium-99m-sestamibi dual-isotope myocardial perfusion single-photon emission computed tomography: a clinical validation study. *J Am Coll Cardiol* 1993;22:1455–1464.
4. Blust JS, Boyce TM, Moore WH. Pharmacologic cardiac intervention: comparison of adenosine, dipyridamole and dobutamine. *J Nucl Med Technol* 1992;20:53–59.
5. Bonow RO, Dilsizian V. Assessing viable myocardium with thallium-201. *Am J Cardiol* 1992;70:10E–17E.
6. Borges-Neto S, Coleman RE, Jones RH, et al. Perfusion and function at rest and treadmill exercise using technetium-99m-sestamibi: comparison of one- and two-day protocols in normal volunteers. *J Nucl Med* 1990;31:1128–1132.
7. Casale PN, Guiney TE, Strauss HW, et al. Simultaneous low-level treadmill exercise and intravenous dipyridamole stress thallium imaging. *Am J Cardiol* 1988;62:799–802.
8. Christian TF et al. Comparison of reinjection thallium-201 and resting ^{99m}Tc-sestamibi tomographic images for the quantification of infarct size after acute myocardial infarction. *J Nucl Cardiol* 1994;1:17–28.
9. Sodee DB, Port SC, O'Donnell JK, et al. Cardiovascular System. In: Early PJ, Sodee DB, eds. *Principles and practice of nuclear medicine,* 2nd ed. St. Louis: Mosby Year-Book; 1995:420.
10. Guyton AC. *Physiology of the human body,* 5th ed. Philadelphia: WB Saunders; 1979:127.
11. Laarman GJ, Niemyer MG, van der Wall EE, et al. Dipyridamole thallium testing: noncardiac effects, cardiac side effects, electrocardiographic changes and hemodynamic changes after dipyridamole infusion with and without exercise. *Int J Cardiol* 1988;20:231–238.
12. *Introduction to nuclear cardiology,* 3rd ed. N. Billerica, MA: DuPont Pharma; 1993.
13. Patrick ST, Glowniak JV, Turner FE, et al. Comparison of in vitro RBC labeling with the UltraTag RBC kit versus in vivo labeling. *J Nucl Med* 1991;32:242–244.
14. Taillefer R, Gagnon A, Laflamme L, et al. Same-day injections of ^{99m}Tc-methoxy isobutyl isonitrile (hexamibi) for myocardial tomographic imaging: comparison between rest-stress and stress-rest injection sequences. *Eur J Nucl Med* 1989;15:113–117.
15. Verzijlbergen JF, Vermeersch PH, Laarman GJ, et al. Inadequate exercise leads to suboptimal imaging. Thallium-201 myocardial perfusion imaging after dipyridamole combined with low-level exercise unmasks ischemia in symptomatic patients with non-diagnostic thallium-201 scans who exercise submaximally. *J Nucl Med* 1991;32:2071–2078.
16. Zeller FP, Blend MJ. The use of intravenous dipyridamole in thallium-201 myocardial perfusion imaging. *Pharmacotherapy* 1987;7:178–184.

8 Central Nervous System

Robert L. Gladding

Increased advances in SPECT instrumentation and computer technology in conjunction with the development of cerebral imaging agents has resulted in a resurgence of brain imaging in recent years. Regional cerebral blood flow studies have become a powerful tool in the investigation of a wide array of neurological abnormalities.

Although the focus of central nervous system (CNS) imaging today is SPECT brain imaging, this review will also discuss planar brain imaging and cisternography.

PLANAR BRAIN IMAGING

Planar radionuclide brain imaging has become mostly obsolete due to its own limitations and the advancement of other imaging modalities, such as computed axial tomography (CT) and magnetic resonance imaging (MRI). It can, however, still be a useful procedure in certain instances; for example, when the patient's condition requires bedside imaging or when claustrophobia or contrast media sensitivity precludes using MRI or CT. Today, planar brain imaging is most frequently used as an accurate means of determining brain death.

Planar brain imaging is most useful when the following pathologies are suspected: (a) primary or metastatic disease (e.g., glioma, meningioma), (b) Intracranial inflammatory disease (e.g., abscess, encephalitis), (c) cerebrovascular disease (e.g., cerebral hemorrhage, vascular occlusion, hemangioma, arteriovenous malformation) and (d) complications of head trauma (e.g., subdural hematoma).

Radiopharmaceuticals

The radiopharmaceuticals used to perform planar brain imaging do not cross the blood-brain barrier (BBB), a defense mechanism that prevents certain undesirable substances from reaching the brain and cerebral spinal fluid. However, cerebral pathologies such as stroke, abscess or tumor result in disruption of the BBB, which allows a circulating radiopharmaceutical to enter that area of abnormality.

Several ^{99m}Tc-labeled radiopharmaceuticals can be used to perform planar brain imaging. Technetium-99m-pertechnetate is probably the least desirable because it accumulates in the choroid plexus of the brain, making it necessary to administer a blocking agent such as potassium perchlorate. Technetium-99m-pentetate (DTPA) or ^{99m}Tc-gluceptate (GH) are better agents for planar brain imaging because:

1. DTPA and GH are rapidly cleared from the circulation by the kidneys, thus providing lower radiation exposure to the patient and increased target-to-nontarget ratios. Imaging can begin sooner with these agents than with pertechnetate.
2. DTPA and GH do not accumulate in the choroid plexus making pretreatment with potassium perchlorate unnecessary.
3. GH is slightly superior to DTPA due to the slower clearance rate of GH, which yields a better count rate on delayed images.

Clinical Procedure

Patient Preparation. Patient preparation includes those steps common to all imaging procedures: verify the identity of the patient, confirm the written order for the procedure, and obtain medical information relevant to the patient's condition and to the clinical indications for the test. Potassium perchlorate must be administered orally prior to performing brain imaging with [^{99m}Tc]pertechnetate.

Imaging. The scintillation camera is prepared with an appropriate collimator and proper energy settings. Planar brain imaging is typically a three-phase study consisting of a dynamic cerebral blood flow study, followed by static blood-pool images and concluding with static delayed images performed 30–90 min following tracer administration. Additional delayed images up to 3 hr after injection may be necessary for those patients whose initial images suggest an abnormality.

The anterior flow study is routinely performed with the patient sitting in the upright position (if possible). The head is positioned with the forehead and nose touching the collimator. The top of the head should be below the top of the field of view; the anterior neck should also be included to visualize carotid blood flow. It is imperative that the head remain still during imaging. A strip of tape to secure the head to the collimator may be helpful. An intravenous bolus injection of 20–25 mCi (740–925 MBq) of a ^{99m}Tc agent is administered. Imaging begins immediately with images being obtained at 1–2-sec intervals for 30–60 sec.

In patients with suspected cerebellar pathology or in pediatric patients where lesions in the posterior fossa seem to dominate, a posterior blood flow study is indicated. The physician should be consulted prior to positioning the patient.

Sixty-second blood-pool images in the anterior, right and left lateral, and posterior projections should be obtained within 5–10 min after completion of the flow study.

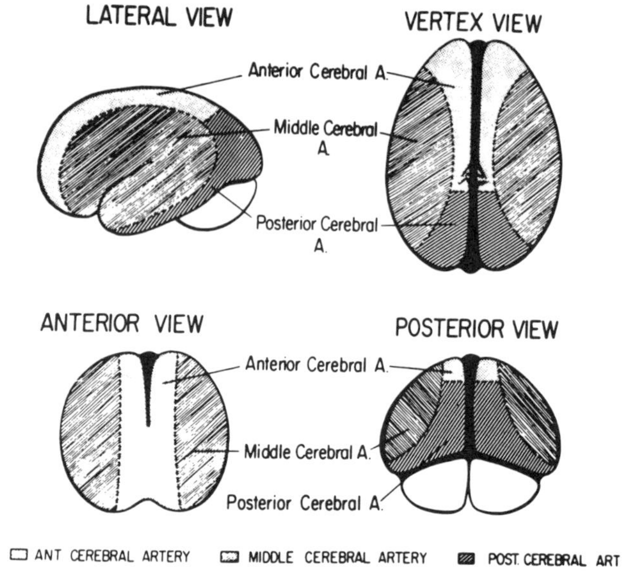

Figure 8.1 Regional cortical distribution of the cerebral arteries. Reprinted with permission from: Freeman LM, Johnson PM, eds. *Clinical scintillation imaging,* 2nd ed. New York: Grune and Stratton; 1972:295.

Delayed views are obtained in the anterior, posterior, right and left lateral, and vertex positions 60–90 min after DTPA or GH administration, or 30–60 min later if pertechnetate is used. If desired, the anterior projection can be acquired for counts and all subsequent images acquired for that same time. The vertex projection should be obtained with a lead cape draped over the patient's shoulders to prevent interference from activity in the rest of the body. On lateral views, a lead shield can be used reduce the counts arising from facial activity. It is important to obtain the immediate and delayed static images in the same projections if there is any suspicion of a lesion or other abnormality on the initial images.

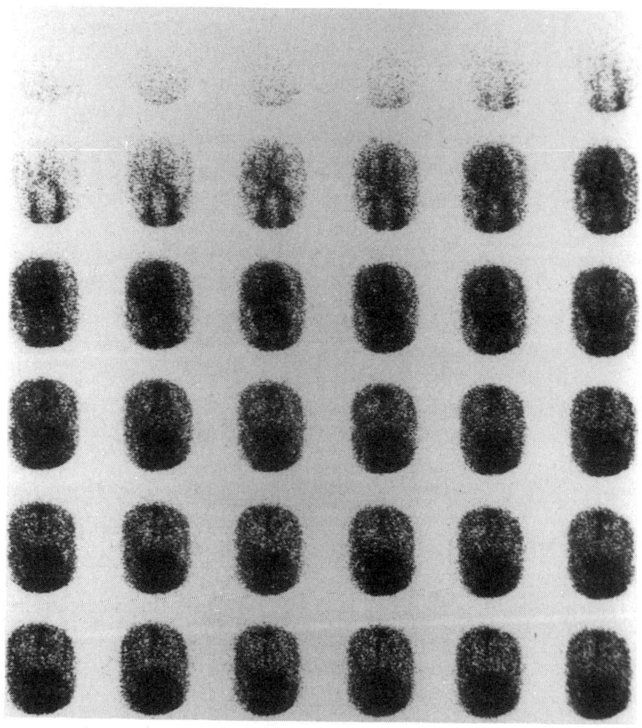

Figure 8.2 Normal anterior cerebral blood flow study. Courtesy of the Hospital of the University of Pennsylvania, Philadelphia, PA.

Image Findings

Knowledge of the gross anatomy of the brain and the cerebral circulatory system is important to understanding tracer distribution patterns (Fig. 8-1).

Normal Tracer Distribution. Approximately 6 sec after tracer administration, there is symmetrical distribution of the radiopharmaceutical in the right and left carotid arteries and visualization of the anterior cerebral artery. Visualization of the superior sagittal sinus after 15 sec indicates that arterial blood has begun to flow into the venous system (Fig. 8-2).

Normal delayed static images usually show symmetrical activity around the entire skull border. Increased activity is observed around the face and base of the skull as well as in the sagittal, transverse and sigmoid sinuses due to blood-pool activity in these areas.

Abnormal Tracer Distribution. Any disruption of the BBB from a lesion in the brain will result in increased localization of the radiopharmaceutical in the area of the pathology (Fig. 8-3). In the case of brain death, the flow study will demonstrate tracer distribution in the carotids, then a complete absence of perfusion in the middle and anterior cerebral arteries (Fig. 8-4).

SPECT BRAIN IMAGING

SPECT brain imaging is proving to be a very useful method to evaluate functional abnormalities in brain tissue. Brain SPECT imaging is clinically indicated when the following abnormalities are suspected:

1. Cerebrovascular disease: acute stroke, transient ischemic attacks.
2. Dementia: Alzheimer's disease, multi-infarct dementia.
3. Psychiatric disorders: affective disorders (e.g., depression), schizophrenia.
4. Seizure disorders: identification and location of sites focal epilepsy.
5. Head trauma.

Radiopharmaceuticals

The three primary radiopharmaceuticals used for regional cerebral blood flow imaging are [^{123}I]iofetamine (IMP), ^{99m}Tc-exametazime (HMPAO) and ^{99m}Tc-bicisate (ECD). Only the two ^{99m}Tc-labeled radiopharmaceuticals are currently approved for use in the U.S.

Both agents are lipid soluble and therefore, can cross the BBB. Although the exact mechanism is not known, the solubility of each agent changes once inside the cell, making it dif-

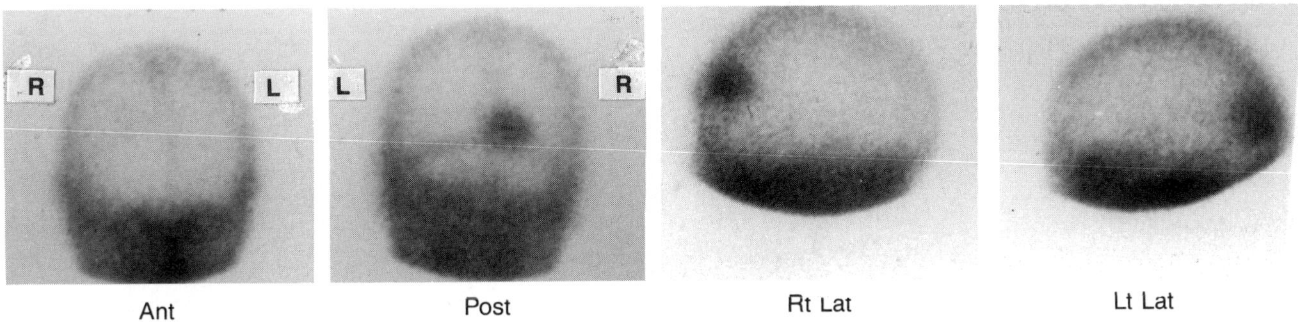

Figure 8.3 Abnormal static brain image depicts a primary brain tumor in the midoccipital region. Courtesy of the Hospital of the University of Pennsylvania, Philadelphia, PA.

ficult for the tracer to diffuse back into the circulation. Thus, the agent becomes "fixed" within the brain cells. Tracer uptake is believed to be proportional to cerebral blood flow. Imaging may take place up to 6 hr after tracer injection.

Clinical Procedure

Patient Preparation. Explain the entire procedure to the patient. If possible, it is best to place the patient supine in a quiet, dimly lit room for radiopharmaceutical administration. A butterfly needle should be placed into an antecubital vein of either arm. After 5–10 min, the tracer may be administered through the butterfly, followed by a saline flush. Following removal of the butterfly, the patient should remain supine for at least 10–15 min to allow the tracer to localize in the brain. Imaging may begin 30–60 min after tracer administration.

Imaging. Optimally, a triple-head tomographic camera system with ultra-high resolution, fan-beam collimators should be used. The patient should be resting as comfortably as possible with the head secured to minimize movement. The detectors should be placed as close as possible to the patient's head which should be positioned far enough into the detector array to image the entire cerebellum.

Image acquisition takes 20–40 min, depending on how well the technologist thinks the patient can tolerate the procedure. A 128 x 128 matrix is used and the technologist should acquire 4–8 continuous images of the brain, which may be added together during data reconstruction. The advantage of continuous dynamic imaging is that valuable information may still be obtained from the previously collected data should the study need to be terminated before the predefined time. In addition, if for some reason the patient moves suddenly during the acquisition, that particular image may be deleted.

If a single detector camera system is used, a parallel- or slant-hole collimator may be used. Since the camera detector must rotate 360° around the patient's head, a slant-hole collimator eliminates the problem of shoulder interference and allows the detector to rotate closer to the organ of interest, thereby improving image resolution.

To begin imaging, position the detector perpendicular to the floor at the side of the head, as if acquiring a lateral view. Adjust the camera to rotate under the patient's head first, before the camera begins to come over the patient's face. This allows 180° of data to be acquired in the event that imaging must be stopped due to patient agitation or panic when the camera rotates over the patient's face. Typical acquisition parameters are 64 views, 40 sec per view for a 360° rotation.

Image Findings

After the data are acquired, computer reconstructed images in the transaxial, sagittal and coronal planes are obtained. Knowledge of cross-sectional anatomy is necessary to process the data and present the necessary information to the physician for interpretation (Fig. 8-5).

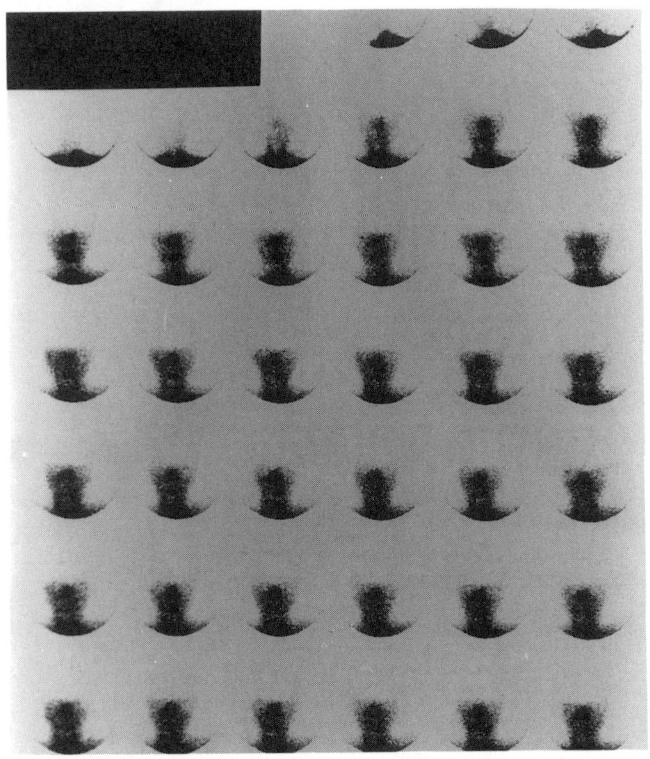

Figure 8.4 Anterior cerebral flow study demonstrates brain death. Note absence of activity over cerebral hemispheres. Courtesy of Children's Hospital, Philadelphia, PA.

TRANSAXIAL VIEWS

1. Falx cerebri
2. Body of corpus callosum
3. Putamen
4. Hippocampus
5. Glomus in trigone of lateral ventricle
6. Superior vermis of cerebellum
7. Thalamus
8. Fornix
9. Insula (Isle of Reil)
10. Septum pellucidum

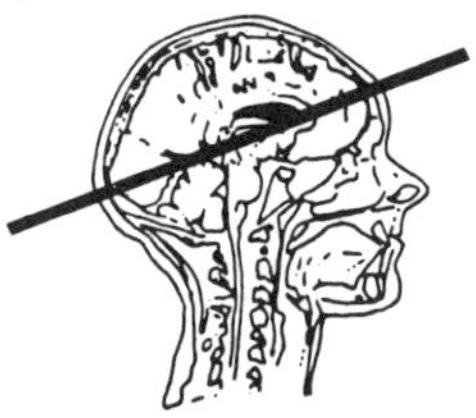

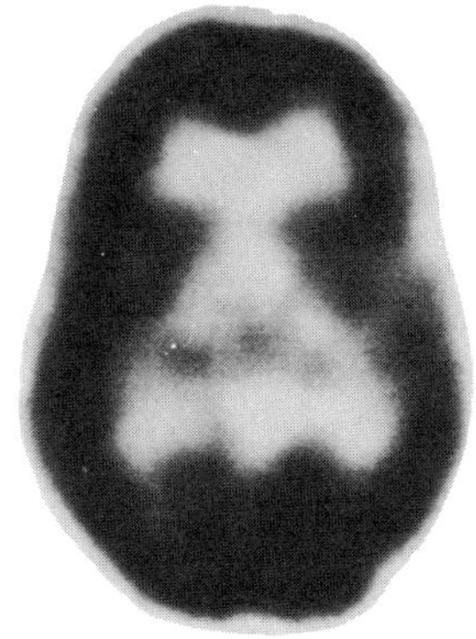

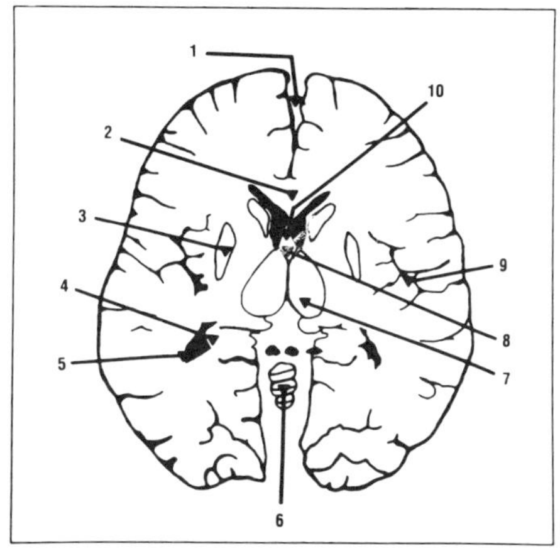

CORONAL VIEWS

1. Caudate nucleus
2. Putamen
3. Temporal lobe of cerebrum
4. Lateral (Sylvian) fissure
5. Genu of corpus callosum

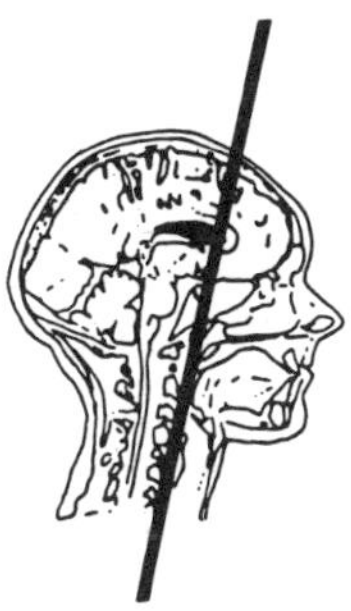

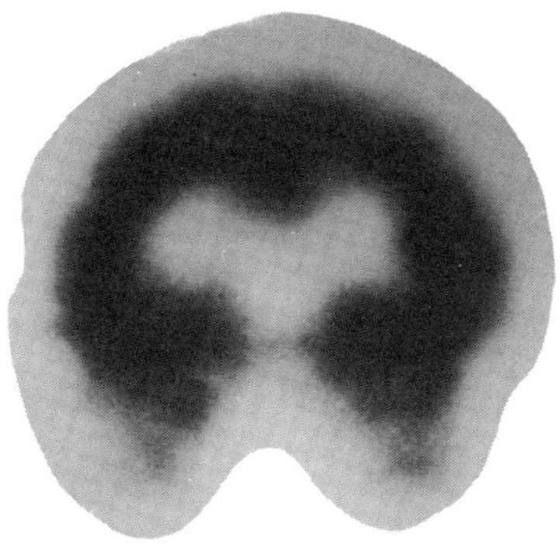

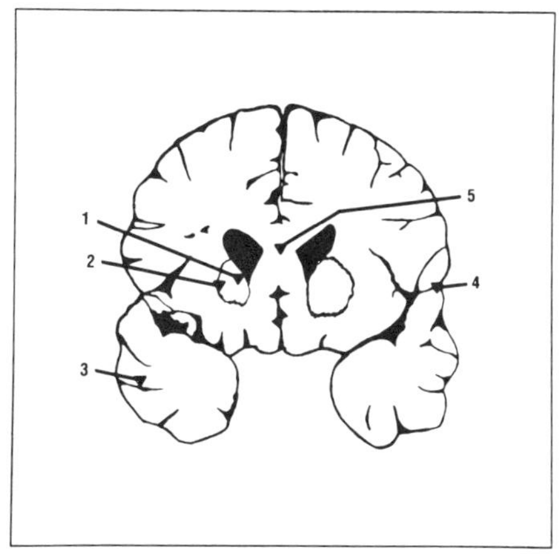

SAGITTAL VIEWS

1. Precentral gyrus
2. Posterior limb of internal capsule
3. Lenticular nucleus
4. Uncinate-fasciculus (frontotemporal)
5. Amygdala
6. Hippocampus
7. Tentorium cerebelli
8. Visual radiations (temporal)
9. Visual radiations (parietal)
10. Central sulcus (of Rolando)

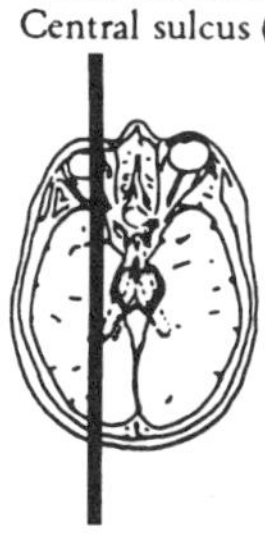

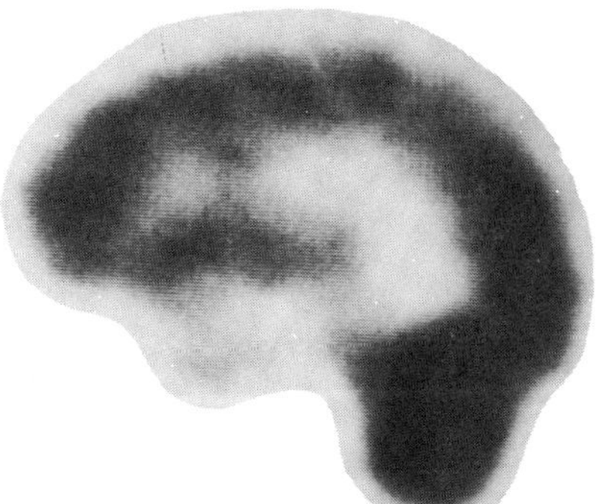

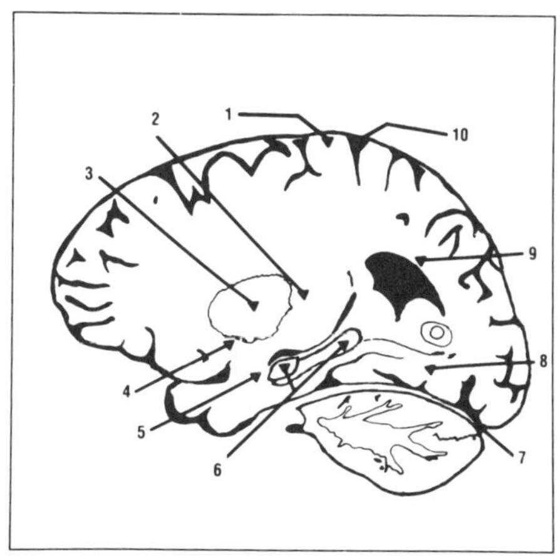

Figure 8.5 Representative anatomical cross-sections of the brain. Reprinted with permission from: *A clinician's guide: SPECT brain*

1. Genu of corpus callosum
2. Lateral fissure (of Sylvius)
3. Lenticular nucleus
4. Cerebral peduncle
5. Parahippocampal gyrus
6. Cerebellar hemisphere
7. Superior cerebellar vermis
8. Red nucleus
9. Subthalamic nucleus
10. Head of caudate nucleus

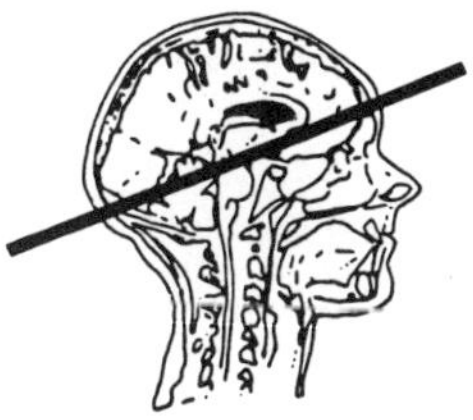

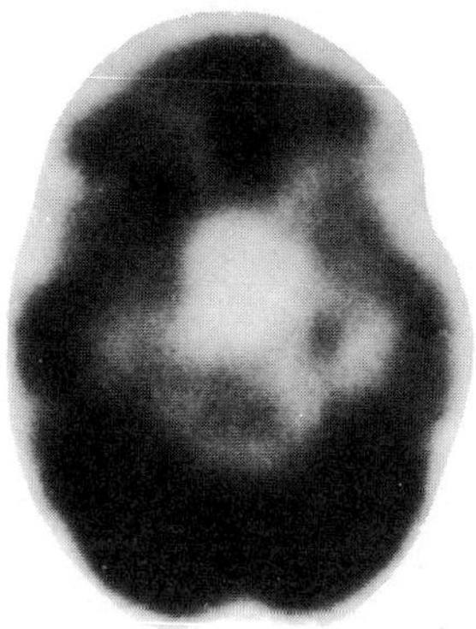

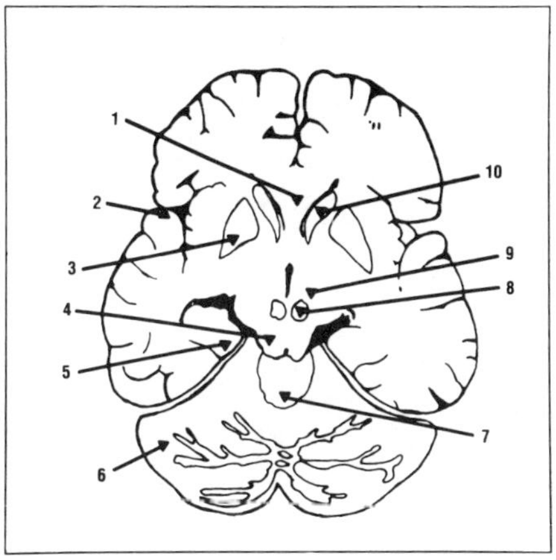

1. Corpus callosum
2. Caudate nucleus
3. Internal capsule
4. Thalamus
5. Lenticular ventricle
6. Hippocampus
7. Substantia nigra
8. Cerebral peduncle
9. Pons
10. Third ventricle
11. Fornix
12. Cingulate gyrus
13. Falx cerebri
14. Superior sagittal sinus

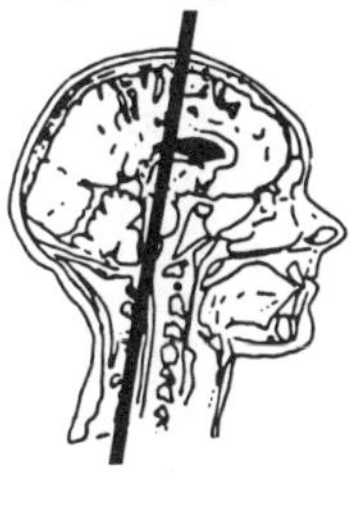

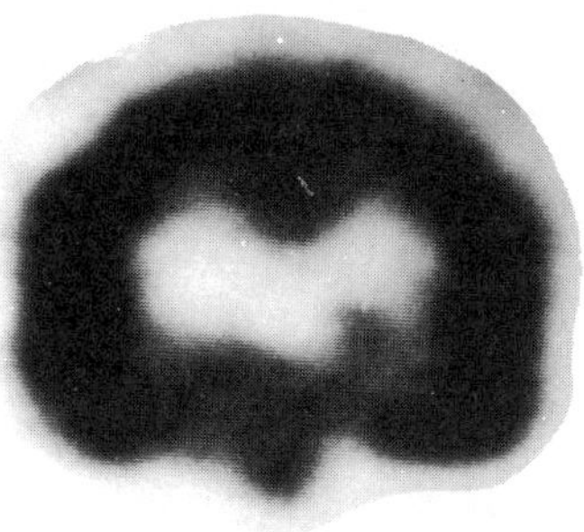

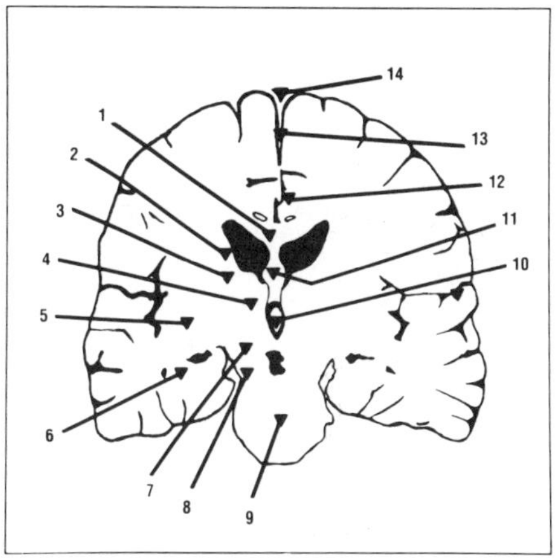

1. Genu of corpus callosum
2. Caudate nucleus
3. Hypothalamus
4. Red nucleus
5. Tectum of mesencephalon
6. Tegmentum of pons
7. Parieto-occipital fissure
8. Paracentral lobule

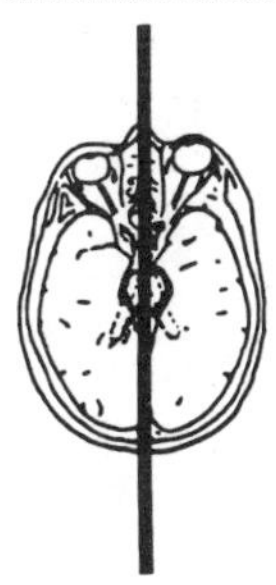

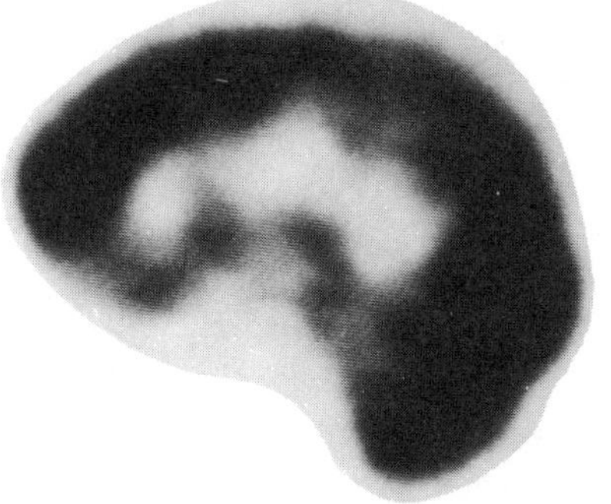

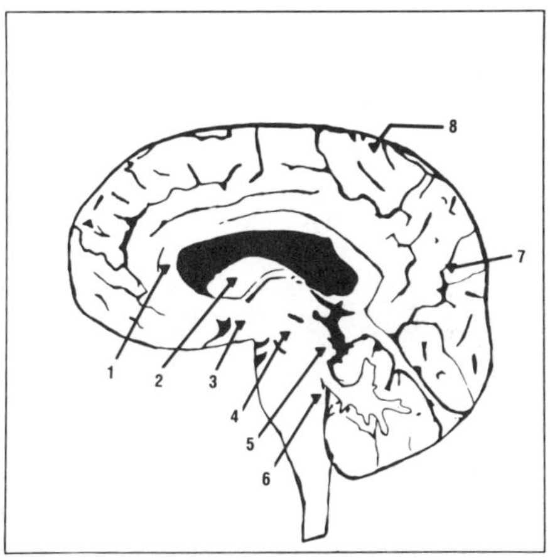

imaging with Ceretec™. Arlington Heights, IL: Amersham Corp.; 1989:3–9. Images courtesy of Nuclear Medicine Services, Harry S. Truman Memorial Veterans Hospital and the University of Missouri Hospitals and Clinics, Columbia, MO.

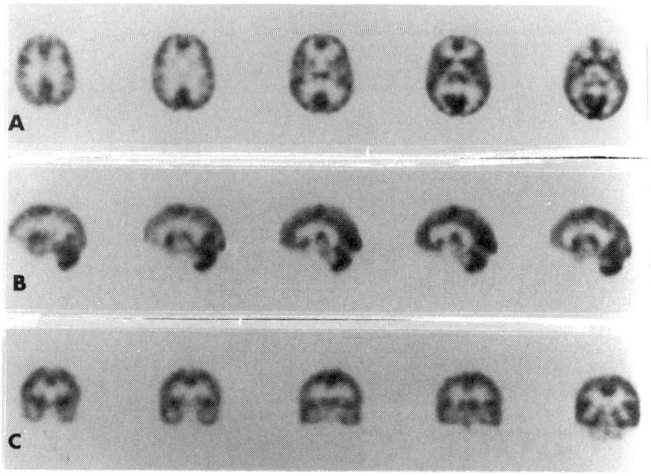

Figure 8.6 Representative transaxial (A), sagittal (B) and coronal (C) slices of a normal brain SPECT study. Courtesy of the Hospital of the University of Pennsylvania, Philadelphia, PA.

Normal Tracer Distribution. Usually there is symmetric distribution of the tracer in both cerebral hemispheres. Since blood flow to gray matter structures is much greater than to white matter, some structures, such as the basal ganglia and the thalamus, will show greater intensity due to increased tracer uptake. White matter typically presents as an area of decreased or no uptake (Fig. 8-6).

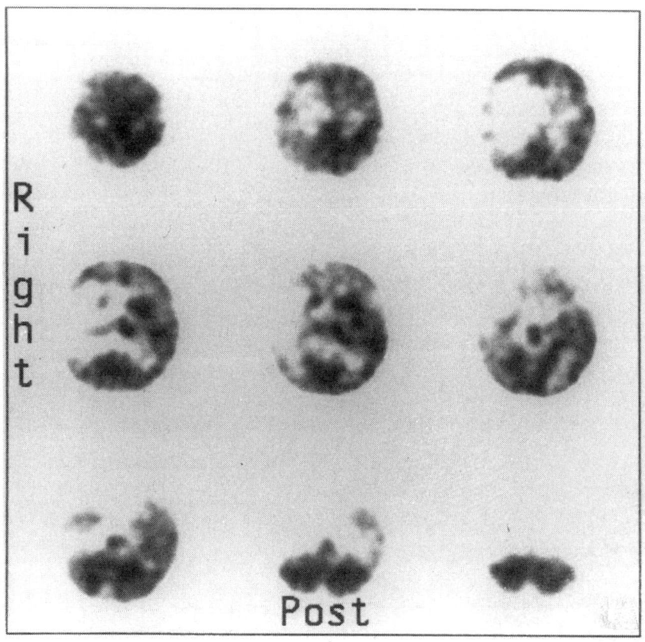

Figure 8.7 HMPAO images of a patient with a history of stroke show significantly reduced blood flow distribution of the middle cerebral artery on the right side. Reprinted with permission from: Alavi A, Hirsch L. Studies of central nervous system disorders with single-photon emission computed tomography and positron emission tomography: evolution over the past two decades. *Semin Nucl Med* 1991;21:67.

Abnormal Tracer Patterns. The site of acute cerebral infarct is usually observed as a large defect (absence of tracer uptake in that area) and is directly related to the cerebral artery affected by the stroke (Fig. 8-7).

Alzheimer's disease findings are usually consistent with decreased perfusion in the parietal and temporal lobes of both hemispheres. This contrasts with multi-infarct dementia, which usually shows random areas of decreased or absent uptake due to multiple areas of infarction.

Patients diagnosed with schizophrenia typically show areas of decreased perfusion in the frontal lobes. Other significant findings include increased activity in the area of the basal ganglia and temporal lobes. In general, clinically depressed patients tend to show decreased tracer uptake over the entire cerebral cortex, while manic patients seem to have greatly increased overall perfusion. During active seizure activity, an area of intense focal uptake of the radiopharmaceutical can be observed.

Acetazolamide (Diamox®)

Acetazolamide stimulation is used in patients with transient ischemic attacks, carotid artery disease and cerebrovascular disease and in other conditions, such as Alzheimer's disease, in which cerebral perfusion is decreased. This test may be used to identify ischemic areas in the brain in much the same way dipyridamole is used to demonstrate this same condition in the heart. Acetazolamide is a drug that induces cerebral vasodilatation. Following oral or intravenous administration of this drug, normal blood vessels dilate but diseased ones do not.

A baseline brain image without acetazolamide is obtained first. The next day, acetazolamide (1 g.) is administered, followed by ^{99m}Tc-exametazime or bicisate 25 min later. Imaging begins 15 min after tracer administration. The baseline and acetazolamide images are compared. Areas of induced ischemia are visualized as areas of decreased tracer uptake on the acetazolamide images.

Side effects of acetazolamide include flushing, tingling sensations in the extremities and around the mouth, lightheadedness, blurred vision, headache, mild confusion, nausea and urinary urgency. These effects are usually mild, subsiding within 10–15 min. Administering the tracer slowly over a period of 2 min can minimize these effects. Contraindications for acetazolamide use include allergy to sulfa drugs, increased cerebral pressures and hepatic cirrhosis.

CISTERNOGRAPHY

Cerebral spinal fluid (CSF) imaging or cisternography is performed to evaluate the flow of CSF through its normal pathways. The CSF circulates around the brain and spinal cord and acts as a shock absorber for the CNS. CSF is produced in the choroid plexus of the ventricles in the brain. The lateral ventricles, located in the cerebrum, connect with the third ventricle, which is located near the thalamus. The third ventricle is connected to the fourth which lies between the brain stem and the cerebellum. The fourth ventricle empties CSF into the subarachnoid space where it flows around the spinal cord and brain. CSF is absorbed from the subarachnoid space into the venous circulation (Fig. 8-8). Total CSF volume is 125–140 ml. Under normal conditions, CSF is formed at the same rate as absorption.

Clinical indications for CSF imaging include: diagnosis of normal pressure hydrocephalus, detection of CSF leaks and evaluation of ventricular shunt patency. Cisternograpy is performed by administering ^{111}In-DTPA intrathecally into the subarachnoid space between the third and fourth lumbar vertebrae. Indium-111 has two major gamma emissions, 173 keV and 247 keV, and a physical half-life of 2.8 days. After introduction of the tracer into the subarachnoid space, the tracer follows the normal pathway of the CSF, until it is reabsorbed into the blood from the CSF and is excreted by the kidneys. The major advantage of using ^{111}In for CSF imaging is that its relatively long half-life permits delayed imaging of up to 72 hr, if necessary.

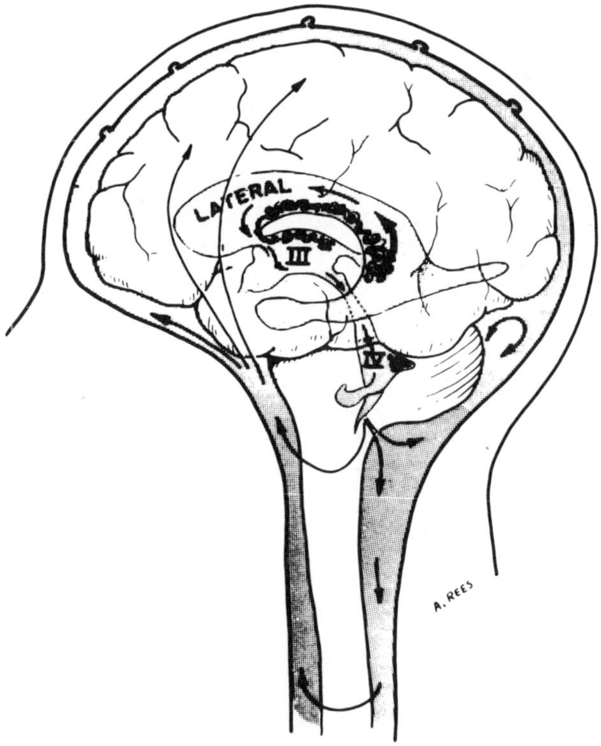

Figure 8.8 Diagrammatic representation of normal CSF flow. Reprinted with permission from: Freeman LM, Johnson PM, eds. *Clinical scintillation imaging,* 2nd ed. New York: Grune and Stratton; 1975:251.

Clinical Protocol

Patient Preparation. The radiopharmaceutical is introduced into the subarachnoid space of the spine by lumbar puncture, an invasive procedure that is always performed by a physician. The patient should remain supine for several hours after the lumbar puncture to prevent headache or other side effects due to temporary CSF imbalance. If a CSF leak is suspected, cotton swabs should be placed in the nose, to rule out rhinorrhea, or in the ears, to rule out otorrhea. Approximately every 2 hr following tracer administration, the swabs should be removed and counted in a well counter to detect any CSF leaks.

Imaging. Adjust the energy settings on the scintillation camera for ^{111}In. Use a medium-energy collimator matched to the higher energy emissions of ^{111}In. Obtain images in the anterior, posterior and lateral projections at 4–6 hr following tracer administration. Activity should be seen in the spinal cord ascending into the basal cisterns of the brain. If no activity is observed in the basal cisterns, it may mean that extravasation of the radiopharmaceutical has occurred at the site of the lumbar puncture. Imaging the injection site first can help rule out tracer extravasation. Activity in the kidneys also confirms extravasation into the surrounding soft tissue, which may be cause for terminating the examination.

If introduction of the tracer is successful, acquire additional images at 24, 48, and if needed, 72 hr postinjection. Be certain to include the entire skull and as much of the spinal tract as possible in the field of view.

Normal Image Findings

At 4–6 hr, the radiopharmaceutical should have completed its ascent. At 24 hr, activity should be seen in the subarachnoid spaces surrounding the cerebral hemispheres as well as in the interhemispheric cisterns. Also, at this time, the tracer should be visualized in the superior sagittal region, the site at which reabsorption of CSF occurs. Failure of the tracer to complete its ascent by 24 hr indicates the need for delayed images at 48 and, possibly, 72 hr. Tracer clearance from the basal cisterns should also be observed at 24 hr (Fig. 8-9).

Abnormal Image Findings

Normal Pressure Hydrocephalus. Visualization of the lateral ventricles at any point in the study, especially if it persists, is a typical finding in cases of normal pressure hydrocephalus. This finding, in conjunction with abnormal delay of the tracer in reaching the superior sagittal region, is cause for concern (Fig. 8-10).

CSF Leaks. Cotton swabs can be used to measure abnormal activity in the nose or the ears, which is indicative of a leak. In addition, imaging the site of the suspected leak while the radiopharmaceutical is passing through the suspected area (1–3 hr postinjection) may be helpful in localizing the CSF leak. CSF leaks may be intermittent, therefore, negative findings by either cotton swab counting or imaging do not necessarily rule out a leak.

Evaluation of Ventricular Shunts. In many cases, ventricular shunting of the CSF into the circulatory system or abdominal cavity is used to treat cases of normal pressure hydrocephalus. Injection of ^{111}In-DTPA or [^{99m}Tc]pertechnetate directly into the shunt reservoir will clearly demonstrate shunt patency. Persistent radiopharmaceutical uptake in the shunt can indicate partial or complete obstruction of the shunt.

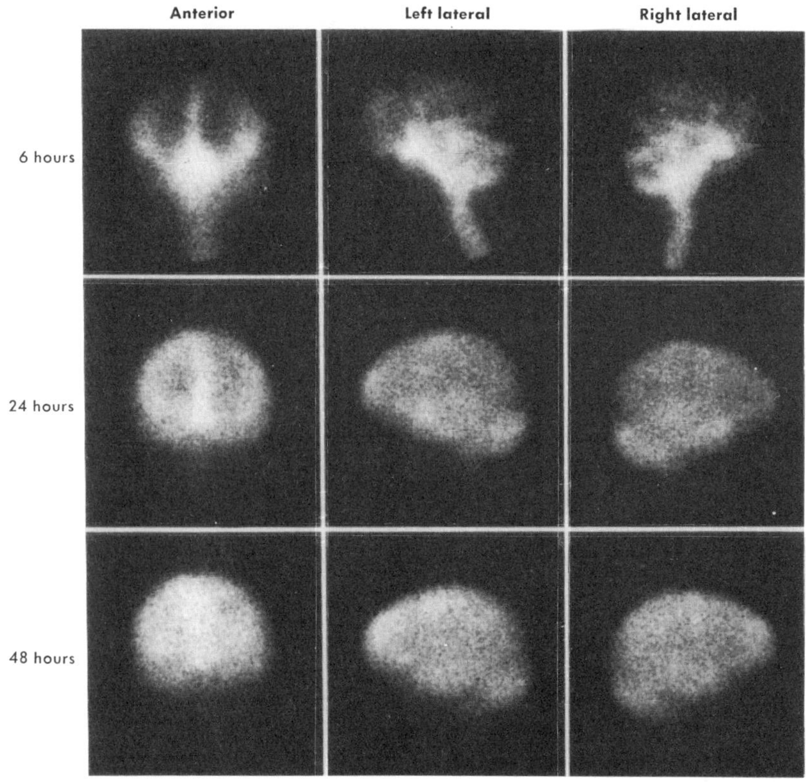

Figure 8.9 Normal cisternogram showing anterior and both lateral views at 6, 24 and 48 hr after intrathecal administration. Reprinted with permission from: Bernier DR, Christian PE, Langan JK, Wells LD, eds. *Nuclear medicine technology and techniques,* 2nd ed. St. Louis: CV Mosby; 1989:293.

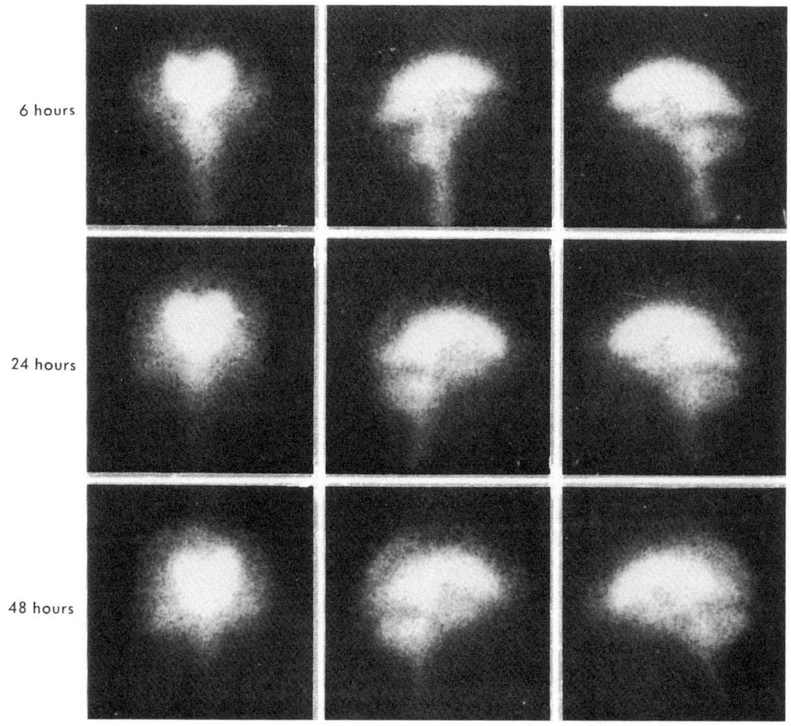

Figure 8.10 Communicating hydrocephalus (normal pressure hydrocephalus) with lateral ventricular reflux on 6-hr images and no significant ventricular clearing on the 24- and 48-hr images. Reprinted with permission from: Bernier DR, Christian PE, Langan JK, Wells LD, eds. *Nuclear medicine technology and techniques,* 2nd ed. St. Louis: CV Mosby; 1989:294.

REFERENCES

1. Carter JC, Burt RW. Acetazolamide intervention for technetium-99m-HMPAO SPECT brain imaging. *J Nucl Med Technol* 1992;20:131–133.

2. Freeman LM, Johnson PM, eds. *Clinical scintillation imaging,* 2nd ed. New York: Grune and Stratton; 1975:295.

3. Harkness B. Computer applications in brain imaging. In: Rowell K, ed. *Clinical computers in nuclear medicine.* Reston, VA: Society of Nuclear Medicine; 1992:51–59.

4. Holman BL, ed. *Radionuclide imaging of the brain.* New York, NY: Churchill Livingstone; 1985.

5. Holmes RA, Hoffman KA. Central nervous system. In: Early PJ, Sodee DB. *Principles and practice of nuclear medicine,* 2nd ed. St. Louis: Mosby Year-Book, Inc.; 1995:549–578.

6. Matin P. *Clinical nuclear medicine imaging.* New York, NY: Elsevier; 1986:1–47.

7. Mettler FA, Guiberteau MJ. *Essentials of nuclear medicine imaging,* 3rd ed. Philadelphia: WB Saunders; 1991:55–74.

8. Park HM, Duncan K. Nonradioactive pharmaceuticals in nuclear medicine. *J Nucl Med Technol* 1994;22:240–249.

9. *SPECT brain imaging with Ceretec: a clinician's guide.* Arlington Heights, IL: Amersham Corp.; 1989.

10. Tikofsky RS, Tremblath L, Voslar AM. Radiopharmaceuticals for brain imaging: the technologist's perspective. *J Nucl Med Technol* 1993;21:57–60.

11. VanHeertum RL, Tikofsky RS, eds. *Advances in cerebral SPECT imaging.* New York: Trivirum; 1989.

12. Velchik MG. SPECT: An update and review of clinical indications. *Del Med J* 1990;62:873–888.

13. Walker JM, Margouleff D, eds. *A clinical manual of nuclear medicine.* Norwak, CT: Appleton-Century-Crofts; 1984:23–52.

9 Endocrine System

Ann M. Steves

Radionuclide imaging of the endocrine system includes imaging of the thyroid, parathyroid and adrenal glands.

THYROID IMAGING

The thyroid gland is located in the anterior neck between the suprasternal notch and the thyroid cartilage (Fig. 9-1). The gland consists of two lobes, each 3–4 cm long from pole to pole. The isthmus, thyroid tissue connecting the right and left lobes of the gland, overlies the trachea. The highly vascular thyroid gland is supplied with blood from the superior and inferior thyroid arteries.

Thyroid imaging, one of the earliest nuclear medicine imaging procedures to be developed, is based on the physiological process of thyroid hormone production. The thyroid hormones, T_3 (triiodothyronine) and T_4 (tetraiodothyronine or thyroxine), are manufactured from iodine absorbed into the blood from the digestive tract. The absorbed blood transports the iodine, in the form of iodide, to the thyroid gland where it is trapped by the thyroid follicular cells. The process of concentrating iodide in the follicles is referred to as the iodide pump. Through the use of a catalyst present in the thyroid follicles, the iodide is then oxidized to form one or two molecules, monoiodotyrosine (MIT) or diiodotyrosine (DIT). T_3 is formed from the coupling of one MIT molecule and one DIT molecule, while T_4 is formed from the combination of two DIT molecules. These hormones are stored in the thyroid gland until they are required by the body for a wide variety of metabolic processes including growth and development, body temperature regulation, and the metabolism of proteins, lipids, carbohydrates, vitamins, and minerals.

Thyroid hormone production and secretion is controlled by a negative feedback mechanism (Fig. 9-2). Thyroid stimulating hormone (TSH), secreted by the anterior pituitary gland, regulates thyroidal iodide uptake and release of the hormones into the circulation. Low levels of circulating hormone cause more TSH to be produced, thereby stimulating the thyroid gland to produce more T_3 and T_4 for release. Increased levels of circulating hormone signal the anterior pituitary to suppress TSH secretion. The levels of these circulating hormones may also affect the hypothalamus, which secretes thyrotropin releasing factor (TRF), a hormone that stimulates the anterior pituitary gland to produce TSH.

Radiopharmaceuticals

All radiopharmaceuticals used for thyroid imaging localize the same way that iodine is trapped in the gland. Table 9-1 compares the commonly used radiopharmaceuticals. Because of its significantly higher radiation dose to the thyroid gland, [^{131}I]sodium iodide has been almost totally replaced by either [^{123}I]sodium iodide or [^{99m}Tc]pertechnetate for routine imaging.

Clinical Indications

Thyroid imaging is performed to evaluate gland size and palpable nodules or masses in the anterior neck. It is also used to identify ectopic thyroid tissue that may be located at the base of the tongue or below the sternum.

Clinical Procedure

Before dose administration, the patient should always be questioned concerning prior thyroid problems or symptoms, neck surgery, medications and recent radiographic procedures. Several medications and radiographic procedures affect radioiodine uptake in the thyroid and can influence both uptake and image results (Table 9-2). Certain thyroid medications may need to be discontinued. Laboratory values for thyroid hormone levels in the blood aid in the interpretation of both the thyroid image and thyroid uptake.

The radiopharmaceutical is administered orally if radioiodine is being used, or intravenously if [^{99m}Tc]pertechnetate is the tracer of choice. Imaging is performed 20–30 min after [^{99m}Tc]pertechnetate administration or 6–24 hr after [^{123}I]sodium iodide administration. The patient is placed in the supine position with the neck hyperextended. Using a scintillation camera with a pinhole collimator, the thyroid is centered in the field of view at a distance from the face of the collimator that will produce an image corresponding to the actual size of the thyroid gland. Images are acquired in the anterior and oblique projections. Images with markers placed on the suprasternal notch or over palpable nodules may also be useful. To enhance structural detail, magnified views may be obtained by moving the collimator closer to the surface of the neck. An anterior view of the mediastinum is indicated if ectopic thyroid tissue is suspected.

When radioiodine is used as the tracer, a thyroid uptake is usually performed immediately before or after imaging. The thyroid uptake procedure and calculations are discussed in Chapter 15.

Image Findings

The normal thyroid gland appears as a "butterfly-shaped" structure with a uniform, symmetrical distribution of activ-

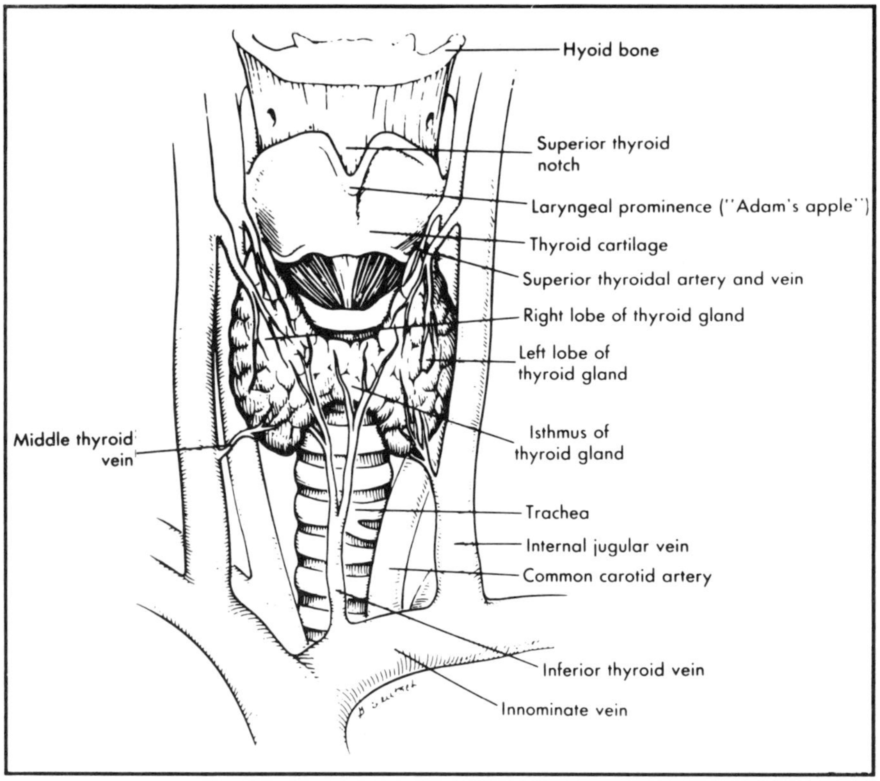

Figure 9.1 Gross anatomy and location of the thyroid gland. Reprinted with permission from: McClintic JR. *Human anatomy.* St. Louis: CV Mosby; 1983:500.

ity (Fig. 9-3). The right lobe is often slightly larger than the left, and the isthmus is usually not visualized.

Abnormal findings include gland enlargement and visualization of functioning or nonfunctioning thyroid nodules. Thyroid imaging is not usually performed to detect nodules, but rather to determine whether a nodule concentrates tracer (Fig. 9-4). Whether a nodule is functioning as well as whether there are single or multiple nodules are important pieces of diagnostic information that have implications for management of the thyroid condition. Nonfunctioning nodules, known as cold nodules, can represent benign adenoma, cyst, hematoma and inflammatory conditions, as well as carcinoma. Generally, hot nodules are benign.

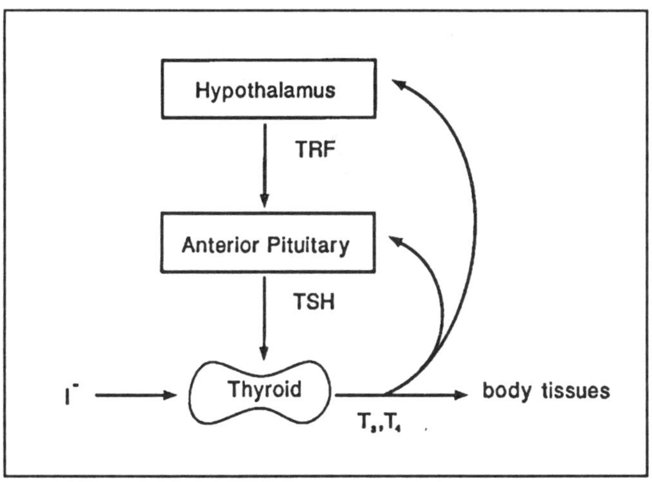

Figure 9.2 Feedback mechanism to control thyroid hormone production.

Technical Considerations

It is important to identify prescribed and over-the-counter medications, food supplements and other diagnostic tests that may interfere with tracer uptake. Determination of such interferences is best accomplished when the patient is scheduled for thyroid imaging.

As with any imaging procedure, patient movement during data acquisition will introduce a motion artifact into the diagnostic image. During thyroid imaging, moving the head, swallowing, coughing or talking should be avoided.

PARATHYROID IMAGING

The four parathyroid glands are located on the posterior aspects of the poles of the thyroid gland (Fig. 9-5). Sometimes a fifth gland is present outside the thyroid. The parathyroid glands produce and secrete parathyroid hormone (PTH), the hormone responsible for regulating the level and distribution of calcium and phosphorus.

Radionuclide imaging of the parathyroid is useful when primary hyperparathyroidism is suspected. This condition results from a tumor in one of the parathyroid glands or from hyperplasia of all four glands, both of which lead to excess secretion of PTH. Excess PTH stimulates removal of large amounts of calcium from the bones, causing weakening and increased fracture risk. The excess calcium level in the blood affects nervous system function and muscle con-

Table 9.1
Thyroid Radiopharmaceuticals

Radiopharmaceutical	$T_{1/2}$	Principal E_γ (keV)	Recommended dose	Thyroid absorbed radiation dose (mrad/μCi)
[^{99m}Tc]pertechnetate	6 hr	140	5-10 mCi	0.20
[^{123}I]sodium iodide	13 hr	159	10-20 μCi (uptake only) 100-400 μCi (imaging)	11
[^{131}I]sodium iodide	8 d	364	6 μCi (uptake only) 30 μCi (imaging)	1100

traction. The excess calcium may also be deposited in various tissues as calcium phosphate. Death may result in extreme cases.

The treatment for primary hyperparathyroidism is surgical removal of the hyperplastic glands or the tumor. Radionuclide imaging is a method of determining the location of the parathyroid tissue prior to surgical intervention. Definitive localization of ectopic tissue or tumor is particularly useful.

Parathyroid imaging is accomplished using a dual-tracer technique. Technetium-99m-pertechnetate is administered to distinguish normal thyroid uptake of ^{201}Tl from abnormal parathyroid uptake. The latter is identified through computer subtraction of the technetium and thallium images.

Table 9.2
Common Drugs and Chemical Substances Influencing Thyroid Uptake of Iodine

Substance	Duration of effect
Iodine-Containing Products	
Lugol's solution, SSKI	2–4 wk
Topical iodine products	2 wk or longer
Kelp	2–4 wk
Certain vitamin/mineral supplements	2–4 wk
Some cough medicines	2–4 wk
Radiographic Contrast Media	
Water-soluble intravascular contrast media	2–4 wk
Other oral and fat-soluble contrast media	4 wk or longer
Thyroid Medications	
Thyroxine	4–6 wk
Triiodothyronine	2–3 wk
Antithyroid Medications	
Propylthiouracil	2–8 d
Methimazole	2–8 d
Other Drugs	
Salicylates	Unknown
ACTH, adrenal steroids	8 d
Competing Anions	
Perchlorate	1 wk
Pertechnetate	1 wk

Clinical Procedure

No special patient preparation is required. The patient is placed in the supine position with the neck hyperextended. Since the patient must remain in the same position throughout the entire imaging procedure, patient comfort should be optimized. The use of sandbags about the head or some type of restraining device to immobilize the head and neck is recommended. An intravenous line is placed into an arm vein to permit easy tracer administration.

After 2.5–3.0 mCi (92.5–111 MBq) [^{201}Tl]thallous chloride are administered intravenously and allowed to clear from the major vessels, an anterior image of the mediastinum is acquired, using a low-energy, all-purpose, parallel-hole collimator, to rule out the presence of a mediastinal tumor. This image should include the area between the mandible and the top of the heart. After the collimator has been changed to a pinhole, an anterior image of the neck that includes the thyroid is acquired.

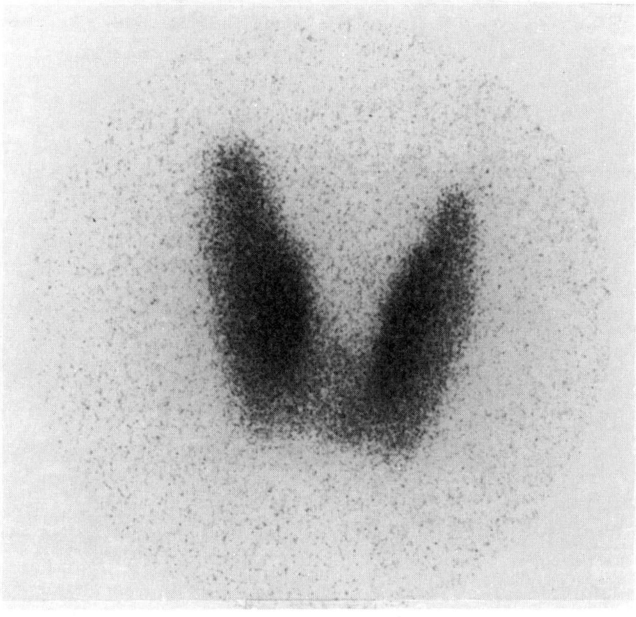

Figure 9.3 Normal thyroid image obtained 24 hr after administration of [^{123}I]sodium iodide. Courtesy of St. Luke's Episcopal Hospital, Houston, TX.

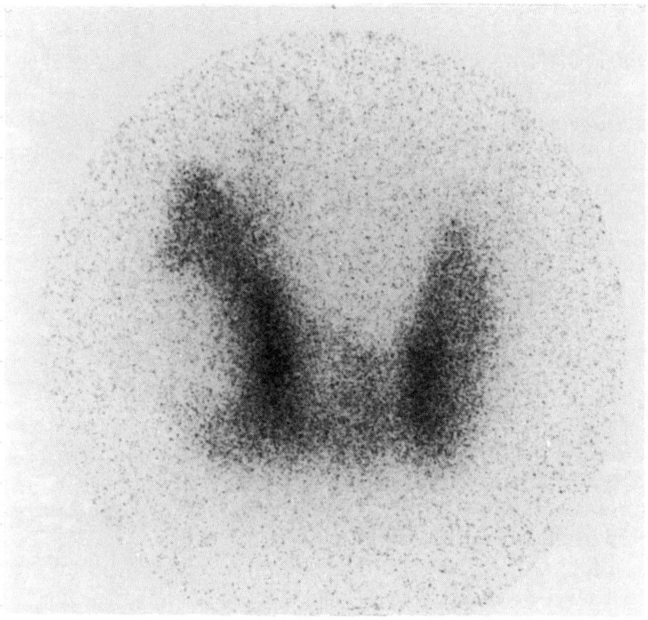

Figure 9.4 Thyroid image demonstrates single cold nodule in right lobe. Courtesy of St. Luke's Episcopal Hospital, Houston, TX.

Following completion of the thallium images, 5–10 mCi (185–370 MBq) [^{99m}Tc]pertechnetate are administered through the intravenous line. After 5–10 min, an anterior image of the neck is acquired for the same number of counts as the thallium image.

All images should be stored in the computer. Computer subtraction of the two pinhole images may assist in image interpretation.

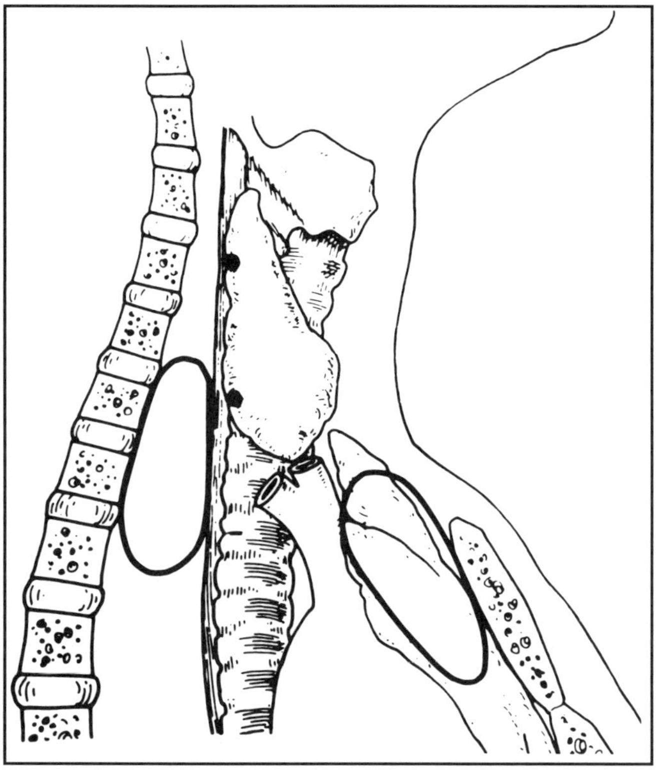

Figure 9.5 Parathyroid glands, represented as solid circles, are located behind the thyroid. Open circles depict common location of ectopic parathyroid glands. Reprinted with permission from: Ratliff B, Soon P, MacFarlane S, Hanelin L. Parathyroid scanning. *J Nucl Med Technol* 1986;14:35.

Image Findings

Both tracers distribute uniformly throughout normal thyroid tissue. Thallium-201 concentrates in parathyroid adenomas to a greater extent than normal thyroid tissue.

Technical Considerations

Thyroid disease is common in patients with hyperparathyroidism. Such disease may cause nonuniform uptake of both tracers in the thyroid gland and lead to false-positive results when the images are processed with computer subtraction.

The diagnostic quality of the images is dependent on patient cooperation. Movement during data acquisition can have adverse effects.

Technetium-99m-pertechnetate may be administered first to minimize the length of time the patient must remain in one position. After ^{99m}Tc administration, the patient does not need to be positioned until the tracer has concentrated in the thyroid and imaging is ready to begin. This method necessitates correction of the ^{201}Tl image for ^{99m}Tc downscatter.

Technetium-99m-Sestamibi

Recently, ^{99m}Tc-sestamibi has been used for parathyroid imaging. Sestamibi is taken up by both thyroid and parathyroid tissue, but it washes out of hyperfunctioning parathyroid tissue more slowly than from thyroid tissue. An early image, 10–15 min after tracer administration, is obtained, which demonstrates tracer uptake in the thyroid gland. A second image obtained 2–3 hr later will show decreased tracer uptake in the thyroid but persistent tracer activity in the parathyroid adenoma (Fig. 9-6).

There are several advantages to this method. Only one tracer and one intravenous injection are required and computer subtraction is not required. Also, the radiation dose to the patient is decreased with the use of a single ^{99m}Tc-labeled agent.

ADRENAL IMAGING

The adrenal glands are located at the superior poles of the kidneys. They are small glands, weighing only 6–7 g and consist of an outer cortex and inner medulla. The cortex produces steroid hormones (aldosterone, cortisol, etc.). Cholesterol, a precursor or building block of these hormones, has been radiolabeled with ^{131}I to image adrenal adenomas and certain other adrenal pathologies. Iodocholesterol is under an IND (investigational new drug) and is not available commercially.

The adrenal medulla manufactures catecholamines (epinephrine and norepinephrine), hormones that control the body's response to stress. Tumors of the adrenal medulla

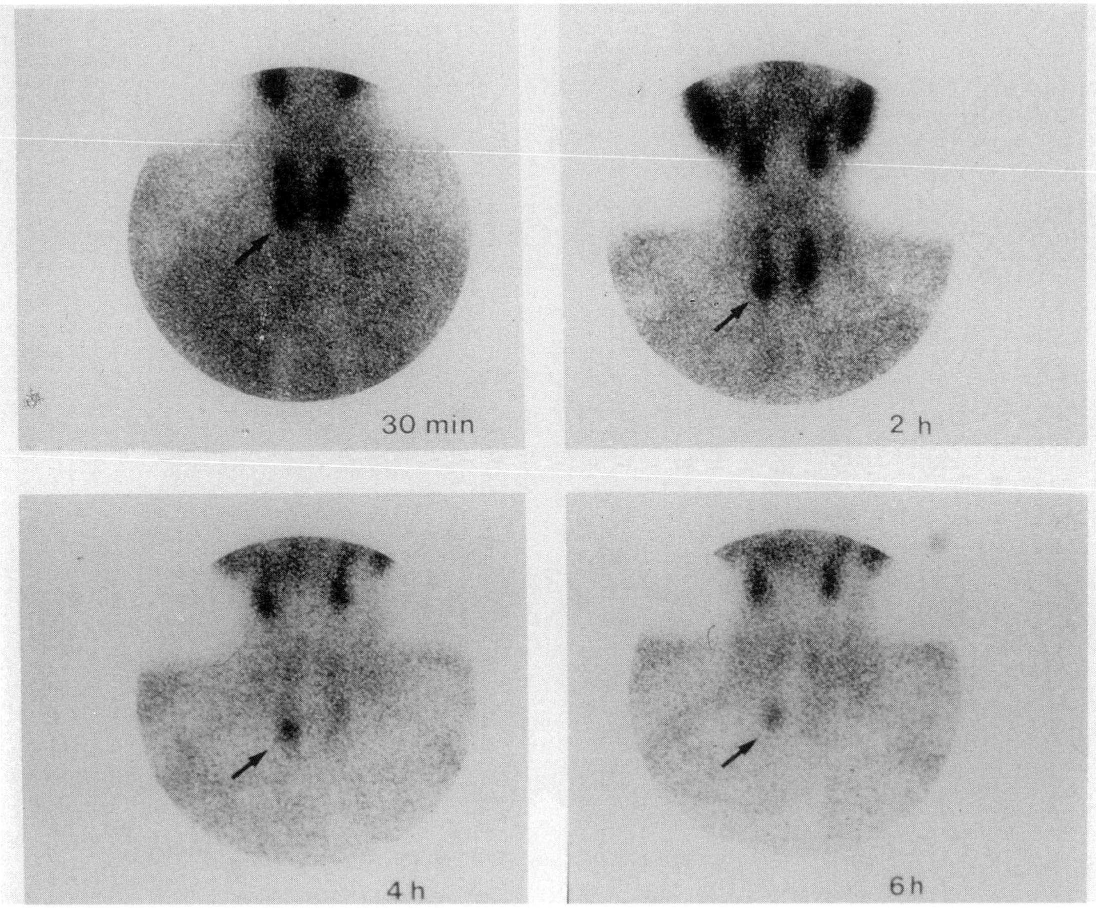

Figure 9.6 Difference in ^{99m}Tc-sestamibi washout from a parathyroid adenoma (arrow) and the surrounding thyroid parenchyma. At 30 min postintravenous injection, slightly increased focal uptake is visualized in the lower right neck (arrow), but the target-to-background ratio is still low. This ratio progressively increases over time and the parathyroid adenoma is well visualized on the 2-, 4- and 6-hr images. Reprinted with permission from: Taillefer R, Strashun AM. Double-phase ^{99m}Tc-sestamibi parathyroid scintigraphy. *Pocket Lecture Series.* Reston VA; Society of Nuclear Medicine; 1994.

are called pheochromocytomas. These tumors secrete excessive amounts of catecholamines and may be benign or malignant. Symptoms of pheochromocytoma include increased catecholamine levels in the blood and urine and hypertension. Nuclear medicine imaging can be used to identify sites of excessive catecholamine secretion within the adrenal bed or in metastatic sites outside of this area. The radiopharmaceutical used to image the adrenal medulla is [^{131}I]MIBG (methyliodobenzylguanidine). This compound is structurally similar to norepinephrine but does not exert any pharmacologic effect.

Clinical Procedure

In preparation for imaging, the patient should receive Lugol's solution at least 1 day before tracer administration and for 6–7 days thereafter. Lugol's solution is a concentrated solution of potassium iodide. The solution saturates the thyroid gland with cold iodine, preventing the uptake of any "free" radioiodine (radioiodine not attached to MIBG) that may be present in the tracer and minimizing unnecessary radiation exposure to the thyroid gland.

Approximately 0.5 mCi (18.5 MBq) [^{131}I]MIBG is administered intravenously. Anterior and posterior imaging from the top of the skull to the pelvis is performed at 1, 3 and 7 days after tracer administration. The patient should be asked to void immediately before imaging because free iodine is excreted through the urine.

Image Findings

Normally, [^{131}I]MIBG uptake is visualized in the liver, spleen and heart. The salivary glands and bladder may also be visualized due to uptake of free iodine in the tracer. Areas of abnormal uptake persist over time. Pheochromocytomas may occur in the adrenal bed or in other places in the thorax and abdomen (Fig. 9-7). Metastases from a malignant pheochromocytoma may be visualized in the liver, bone, lymph nodes, heart, lungs or other sites.

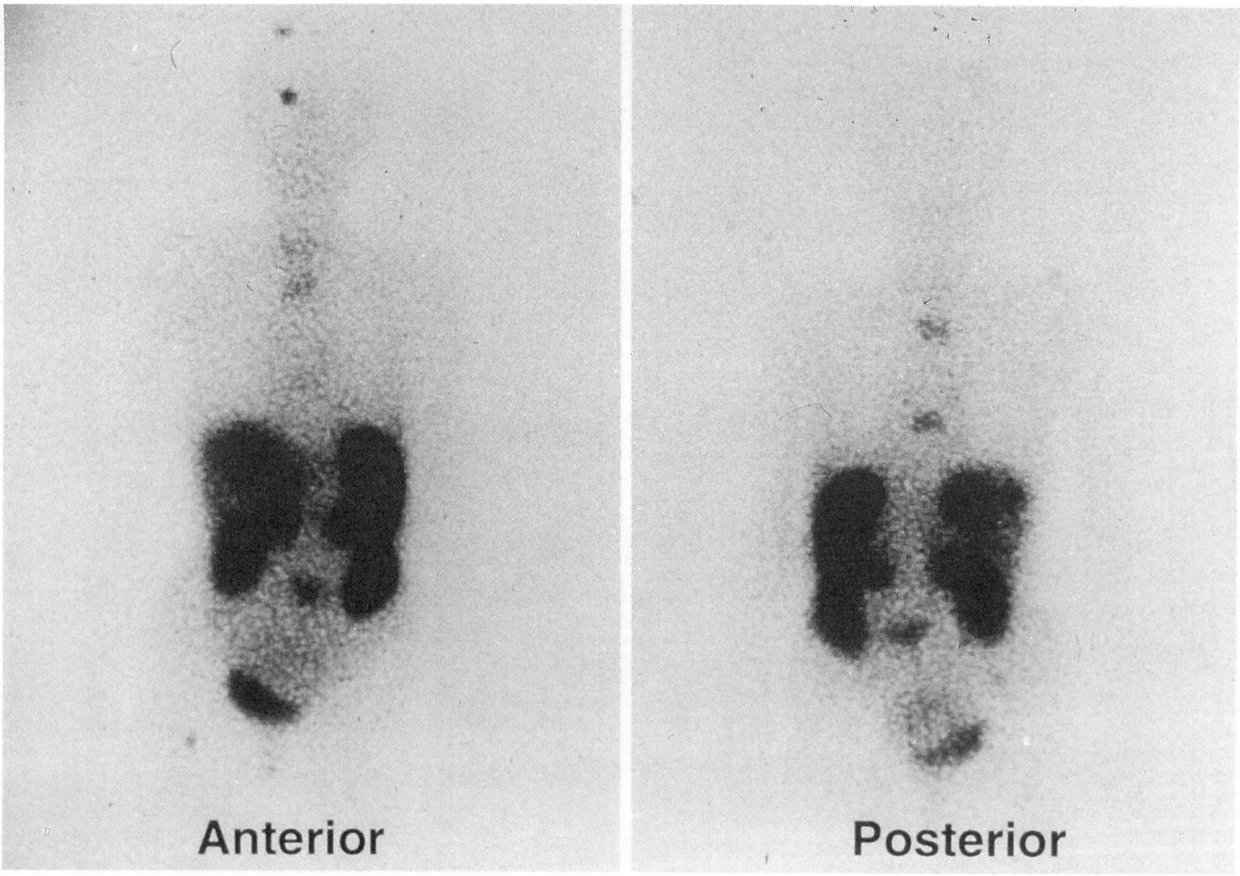

Figure 9.7 OctreoScan® whole-body images 24 hr postinjection. Multiple carcinoid metastases are visible in the liver, pelvis, thoracic and lumbar vertebra and abdomen. Two previously unknown brain metastases are visible on the anterior image. Reprinted with permission from: *Somatostatin receptor imaging for neuroendocrine tumors.* St. Louis: Mallinckrodt Medical Inc.; 1994.

REFERENCES

1. Beierwaltes WH. Endocrine imaging: parathyroid, adrenal cortex and medulla and other endocrine tumors. part II. *J Nucl Med* 1991;32:1627–1639.
2. Christian PE. General imaging applications. In: Rowell K, ed. *Clinical computers in nuclear medicine.* Reston, VA: Society of Nuclear Medicine; 1992:16–19.
3. Drew HH, LaFrance ND, Chen JJS. Thyroid imaging studies. *J Nucl Med Technol* 1987;15:79–87.
4. Early PJ, Sodee DB. *Principles and practice of nuclear medicine,* 2nd ed. St. Louis: Mosby Year-Book.; 1995:617–677.
5. Ferlin G, Borsato N, Camerani M, et al. New perspectives in localizing large parathyroids by technetium-thallium subtraction scan. *J Nucl Med* 1983;24:438–441.
6. Goldsmith S. Endocrine system. In: Bernier DR, Christian PE, Langan JK, eds. *Nuclear medicine technology and techniques,* 3rd ed. St. Louis: Mosby Year-Book; 1994:222–251.
7. O'Doherty MJ, Kettle AG, Wells P, et al. Parathyroid imaging with technetium-99m-sestamibi: preoperative localization and tissue uptake studies. *J Nucl Med* 1992;33:313–318.
8. Ratliff B, Soon P, MacFarlane S, Hanelin L. Parathyroid scanning. *J Nucl Med Technol* 1986;14:34–39.
9. Taillefer R. Double-phase ^{99m}Tc-sestamibi parathyroid scintigraphy. *Pocket lecture series,* vol. 2. Reston, VA: Society of Nuclear Medicine; 1994.

10 Gastrointestinal System

Ann M. Steves

LIVER/SPLEEN IMAGING

The liver is the largest solid organ in the body, weighing 1.5–2 kg in an adult. It is located on the right side, underneath the ribs directly below the diaphragm. While the shape of the liver may vary widely, the right lobe is generally larger than the left.

The liver is composed of two cell types, the reticuloendothelial (RE) cells (Kupffer cells) and hepatocytes. The RE cells account for about 15% of the liver's mass. They are responsible for phagocytosis of particulate matter. Approximately 80% of the body's RE cells are in the liver; the remainder are found in the spleen, bone marrow and lymph system. The hepatocytes, the cells that comprise most of the liver's mass, perform a variety of functions including bile formation.

The liver is a highly vascular organ with a dual blood supply (Fig. 10-1). The hepatic artery, a branch of the abdominal aorta, supplies the liver with oxygenated blood. The hepatic portal vein carries blood containing nutrients absorbed from the intestines into the liver for processing.

The spleen is retroperitoneally located in the left upper quadrant of the abdomen. Although it does contain RE cells, it is not considered part of the gastrointestinal (GI) system.

Clinical Indications

Liver/spleen imaging is performed to determine the size, configuration and position of either organ. It is also useful for the detection of tumor, hematoma, cyst, abscess and trauma. Functional liver diseases such as cirrhosis and hepatitis also can be evaluated with liver/spleen imaging.

Radiopharmaceutical

Liver/spleen imaging is performed with ^{99m}Tc-sulfur colloid. Labeled colloidal particles, averaging 1 micron in size, are engulfed by the RE cells in the liver, spleen and bone marrow.

Clinical Procedure

There is no special patient preparation required for liver/spleen imaging. A medical history should be obtained and include the following information:

1. Patient diagnosis.
2. Pertinent laboratory values: serum bilirubin level, liver enzyme levels (SGOT, SGPT), serum alkaline phosphatase, total serum protein levels (including globulin and albumin), prothrombin time and urine bilirubin level.
3. Previous abdominal surgery.

In addition, liver/spleen imaging should be performed before barium or other contrast agents are used for radiographic studies of the GI tract. These agents may cause photon-deficient artifacts to appear on the nuclear medicine images.

Imaging

Five to 10 mCi (185–370 MBq) ^{99m}Tc-sulfur colloid are administered intravenously. If a flow study is indicated, the patient should be positioned under the scintillation camera prior to tracer administration. The flow images are useful in demonstrating the vascularity of any defects that may be visualized on the static images.

After allowing sufficient time for tracer localization within the liver and spleen (usually 10–15 min), static imaging can begin. Standard views include anterior, posterior, right lateral, RAO and LAO projections. An anterior image with a reference marker placed along the right costal margin is also obtained. Additional views may be required depending on the clinical problem.

Image Findings

Approximately 85% of the ^{99m}Tc-sulfur colloid administered is localized in the liver, 10% in the spleen and the remainder in the bone marrow. The small amount of tracer concentrated in the bone marrow is not normally visualized. The normal size liver is usually located above the right costal margin and can have a variety of shapes (Fig. 10-2). One normal variant is a Riedel's lobe, a greatly elongated right lobe, which may extend down into the pelvis. The left lobe of the liver is relatively thin and anteriorly situated; therefore, it is best visualized on the anterior projection. The normal size spleen is located in the left upper quadrant above the left costal margin. Since the spleen lies more posteriorly, splenic size is best determined from the posterior view.

Other surrounding anatomic structures may cause artifacts that are commonly seen on liver/spleen images. The heart, right kidney, porta hepatis and gallbladder may distort the shape of the liver. Additional views can help distinguish these artifacts from true defects. Certain conditions such as expansion of the lungs, as in emphysema, subphrenic abscess or an enlarged left hepatic lobe, cause the liver to be displaced below the level of the costal margin.

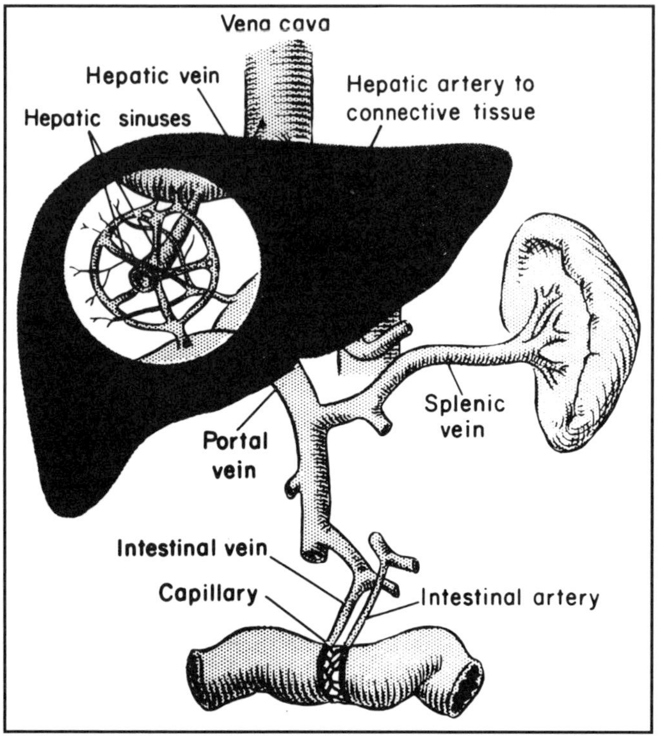

Figure 10.1 Portal and hepatic circulations. Reprinted with permission from: Guyton AC. *Textbook of medical physiology,* 5th ed. Philadelphia: WB Saunders; 1976:375.

Tumors, cysts and abscesses appear as single or multiple areas of decreased or absent tracer uptake. Diffuse liver disease such as cirrhosis and hepatitis is demonstrated by decreased tracer concentration or uneven tracer distribution throughout the liver (Fig. 10-3). In severe cases, the bone marrow is visualized and the tracer concentration in the spleen is greatly increased.

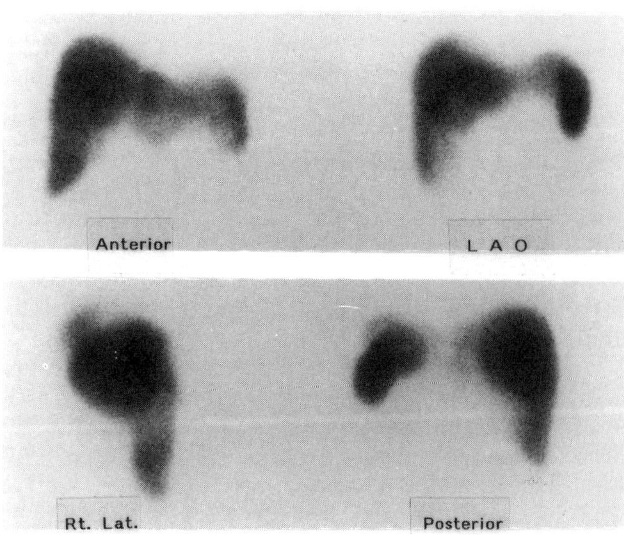

Figure 10.2 Normal liver/spleen images obtained with ^{99m}Tc-sulfur colloid. Courtesy of St. Luke's Episcopal Hospital, Houston, TX.

Technical Considerations

Imaging too soon after injection of ^{99m}Tc-sulfur colloid may demonstrate cardiac blood-pool activity on the images. Allow sufficient time for the tracer to be extracted from the blood by the Kupffer cells.

Attenuation artifacts may appear as a result of residual barium in the GI tract, particularly in the hepatic and splenic flexures, or from female breast tissue overlaying the superior portion of the liver's right lobe. Liver/spleen imaging should be performed before radiographic procedures using contrast agents. Breast shadow artifacts can be eliminated by taping the breast out of the way.

HEPATOBILIARY IMAGING

The biliary tract begins with the microscopic canaliculi that surround each hepatocyte and carry bile from the hepatocytes to the larger branches of the biliary tree. The bile is eventually discharged into the duodenum or stored in the gallbladder until it is needed in the digestive process (Fig. 10-4).

Bile is a product of erythrocyte breakdown and hepatocyte metabolism. It is used to emulsify fats (facilitating their digestion), stimulate peristalsis and enhance absorption of fatty acids. Cholecystokinin, a hormone produced by the duodenum, stimulates the gallbladder to secrete bile when fatty foods enter the duodenum.

Clinical Indications

One of the more important uses of hepatobiliary imaging is the evaluation of patients experiencing upper abdominal pain to rule out cystic duct obstruction (acute chole-

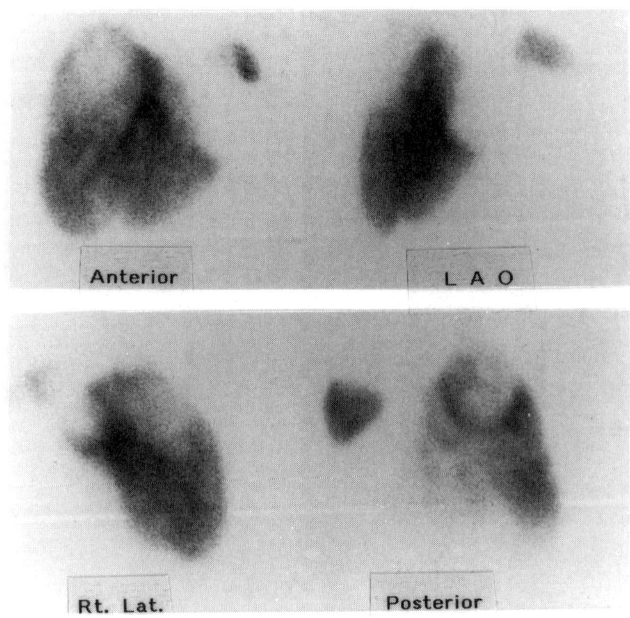

Figure 10.3 Abnormal ^{99m}Tc-sulfur colloid liver/spleen images demonstrate hepatomegaly and multiple areas of space-occupying disease. Courtesy of St. Luke's Episcopal Hospital Houston, TX.

cystitis). Failure to visualize the gallbladder increases the probability of acute cholecystitis. In the case of jaundice, hepatobiliary imaging can help differentiate the cause by ruling out obstruction of the biliary tract. Similarly, such imaging can delineate bile drainage and reflux following surgery. When cold defects are visualized on ^{99m}Tc-sulfur colloid liver/spleen images, subsequent hepatobiliary imaging may identify such defects as normal or abnormal variations of the biliary system.

Pediatric applications include the detection of choledochal cysts, biliary atresia or other congenital abnormalities of the biliary tree.

Radiopharmaceuticals

Mebrofenin, disofenin and lidofenin, which are ^{99m}Tc-labeled derivatives of iminodiacetic acids (IDA), are the commercially available agents used for hepatobiliary imaging. Following intravenous administration, these compounds are carried to the liver where they are extracted from the blood by the hepatocytes. From the hepatocytes, the IDA compounds are transported into the canaliculi along with the bile and follow the path of bile flow.

The amount of hepatic tracer uptake is dependent on several factors, including the chemical structure of the IDA compound, hepatic blood flow, the viability of the hepatocytes and the bilirubin level. Bilirubin, the byproduct of hemoglobin breakdown, competes with the uptake of ^{99m}Tc-IDA compounds. For this reason, patients with elevated bilirubin levels require higher doses of the tracer than do patients with normal or only slightly elevated bilirubin levels.

Clinical Procedures

Pertinent information from the patient's medical history includes the following.

1. Patient diagnosis and/or clinical indication for the imaging procedure.
2. Serum bilirubin level.
3. Previous gallbladder or other GI surgery.
4. Medications which may affect the transit of the tracer through the biliary tract.

Certain steps are required in the preparation of the patient to promote bile flow into the gallbladder. If bile does flow into the gallbladder, cystic duct obstruction can be ruled out. First, narcotics, sedatives or other drugs that relax the sphincter of Oddi, the muscle between the common bile duct and the duodenum, should be discontinued for 6–12 hr prior to hepatobiliary imaging. When the sphincter is relaxed, bile flows preferentially into the small intestine rather than the gallbladder. Morphine or other opiates that increase the muscle tone of the sphincter and promote gallbladder filling may be prescribed in certain instances. Second, the patient should fast 2–4 hr before tracer administration. Again, gallbladder filling is more likely to occur if the duodenum is not stimulated to release cholecystokinin.

The adult dose of ^{99m}Tc-IDA, ranging from 2 to 8 mCi (74–296 MBq), is determined from the serum bilirubin level.

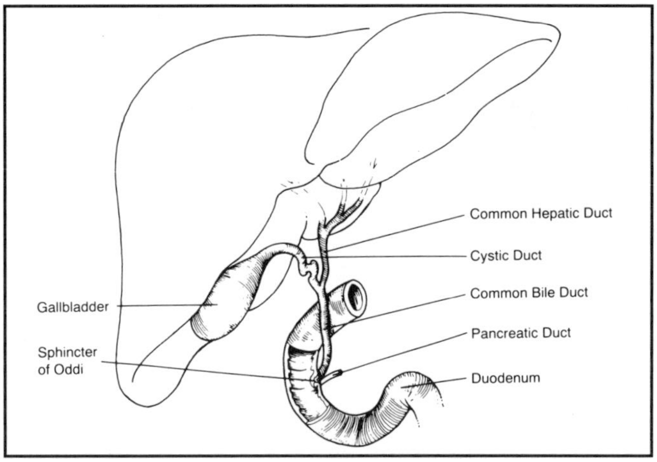

Figure 10.4 Anatomy of the hepatobiliary system.

Imaging

Imaging begins immediately after the tracer is administered intravenously. Images are obtained with a scintillation camera equipped using a low-energy, all-purpose, parallel-hole collimator. The patient is placed in a supine position beneath the detector so that the liver appears in the upper left corner of the field of view. Positioning the patient in this manner permits visualization of the entire biliary tract and the small intestine in a single anterior image. Sequential 5-min images are acquired for 1 hr.

After the first hour, anterior oblique or right lateral projections may be useful to delineate bowel activity or other structures such as the kidneys. If the gallbladder or biliary ducts are not visualized by 1 hr after tracer administration, delayed images should be obtained at intervals up to 24 hr, as necessary. Likewise, if the gallbladder and common bile duct are visualized, but there is no evidence of tracer in the small intestine, delayed views of the abdomen are indicated.

Cholecystokinin

Sincalide, a synthetic form of cholecystokinin (CCK), is used in conjunction with hepatobiliary imaging for two purposes. In patients who have fasted for prolonged periods (greater than 24 hr) or who are on hyperalimentation, the gallbladder is full at the beginning of hepatobiliary imaging. Therefore, the radioactive bile produced during imaging will not be able to enter the gallbladder and cystic duct patency will not be confirmed. Administering sincalide before the tracer will cause the gallbladder to contract, leaving it empty in preparation for hepatobiliary imaging. Sincalide may also be administered near the end of the imaging study when the gallbladder is filled with tracer to determine the gallbladder ejection fraction.

Morphine Sulfate

If the gallbladder is not visualized within 60 min after tracer administration, morphine sulfate may be administered intravenously as an alternative to delayed imaging. Since acute cholecystitis is usually associated with cystic duct obstruction, visualizing the gallbladder effectively rules out this condition. Morphine causes contraction of

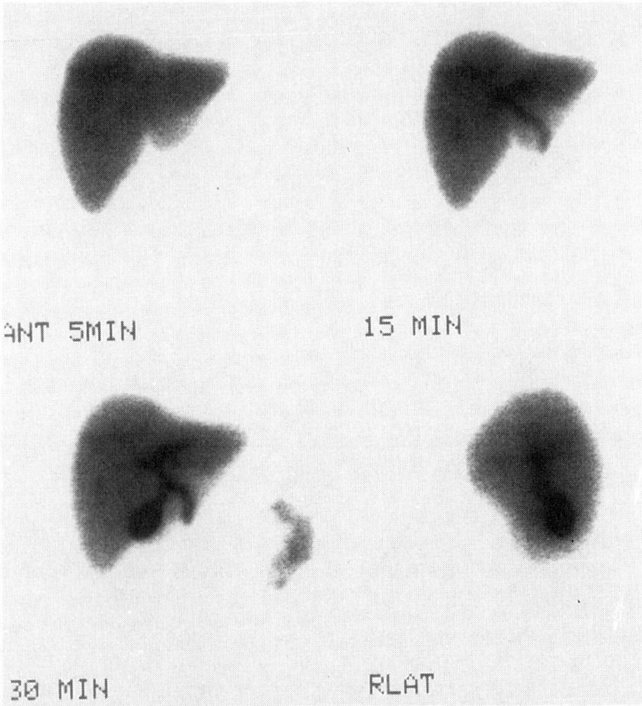

Figure 10.5 Normal hepatobiliary study. Anterior images taken following administration of ^{99m}Tc-mebrofenin demonstrate visualization of common bile duct at 15 min. Gallbladder and small bowel activity are visualized 30 min following tracer administration. Courtesy of Department of Veterans Affairs Medical Center, Nashville, TN.

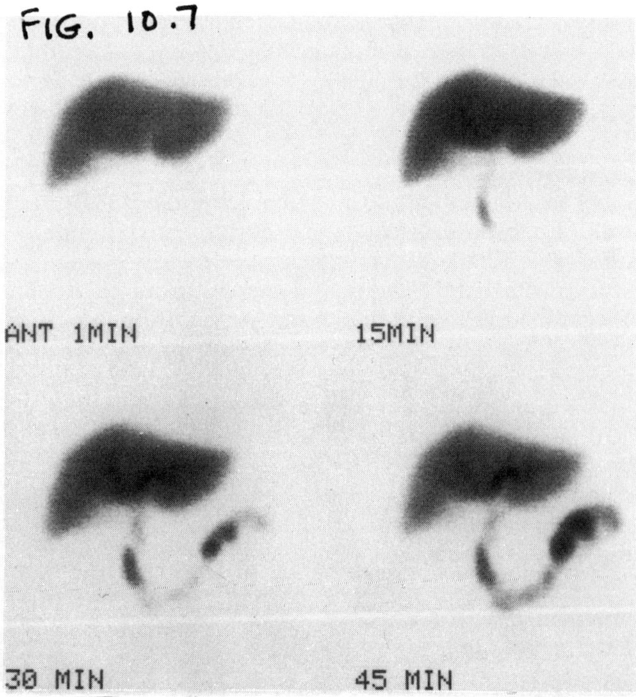

Figure 10.6 Positive Meckel's diverticulum study performed on a young child. Note small area of increasing tracer concentration medially located between stomach and bladder. Courtesy of The Children's Hospital of Alabama, Birmingham, AL.

the sphincter of Oddi which in turn increases the pressure in the bile ducts. The increased pressure forces tracer through the cystic duct, if it is patent, into the gallbladder. Nonvisualization of the gallbladder following administration of morphine increases the likelihood that the patient has acute cholecystitis. By using morphine, the length of the study is shortened and the specificity of the findings is increased.

Image Findings

Normally, there is rapid tracer uptake by the hepatocytes within several minutes after tracer administration. Visualization of the tracer within the hepatic ducts and gallbladder occurs by 15–30 min. The gallbladder is well visualized by 45–60 min and tracer activity appears in the small intestine by 30 min after injection (Fig. 10-5).

Abnormal findings include nonvisualization or markedly delayed visualization of the gallbladder and absence of radioactivity in the GI tract (Fig. 10-6).

Technical Considerations

Prolonged fasting (longer than 24 hr) or hyperalimentation may cause nonvisualization of the gallbladder. In patients with extremely elevated bilirubin levels, clearance of ^{99m}Tc-IDA by the hepatocytes is delayed and the tracer is excreted through the kidneys.

DETECTION OF MECKEL'S DIVERTICULUM

A Meckel's diverticulum is an outpouching of the intestine, usually located in the distal ileum. It is a remnant of an embryonic duct at the point where the yolk sac is attached to the intestine of the fetus. It is formed when the duct fails to close completely during fetal development. Meckel's diverticulum is found in 2% of the population, and only 25% of these individuals ever display symptoms. Imaging for this abnormality is most commonly performed in children.

The diverticulum may contain gastric mucosa. Just as the gastric mucosa lining of the stomach secretes hydrochloric acid and pepsin so does the ectopic gastric mucosa in the diverticulum. Gastrointestinal bleeding can result when the secretions of the gastric mucosa cause ulceration of the adjacent normal intestine. Patients may experience lower abdominal pain as well as GI bleeding.

Technetium-99m-pertechnetate concentrates in gastric mucosa and has been useful in localizing the Meckel's diverticulum in patients with unexplained GI bleeding.

Clinical Procedure

The patient should be fasting and should not have received any laxatives or diagnostic tests that might irritate the intestinal tract for at least 3 days prior to imaging. Potassium perchlorate is often administered to children to prevent thyroid uptake of [^{99m}Tc]pertechnetate. It should not be used in this instance because it also blocks gastric mucosa secretions and may cause false-negative results.

Administration of certain drugs may enhance visualization of the Meckel's diverticulum. Pentagastrin stimulates gastric secretion, thereby increasing pertechnetate secretion in the stomach and diverticulum. It is administered subcutaneously 15 min before the tracer. Alternatively, cimetidine may be administered as it helps retain pertechnetate in the gastric mucosa. The patient receives cimetidine orally every 6 hr for 24 hr before imaging.

Imaging

The patient is placed supine beneath the scintillation camera so that the area between the xiphoid and symphysis pubis is centered in the field of view. After intravenous administration of [^{99m}Tc]pertechnetate, static images are acquired at 5–10-min intervals for 1 hr. Precise localization of a site of increased activity can be accomplished with additional views.

Image Findings

A Meckel's diverticulum containing functioning gastric mucosa should be visualized by 10–15 min after injection, at the same time tracer activity appears in the stomach (Fig. 10-7). It is usually seen in the right lower quadrant but can appear anywhere in the abdomen.

Technical Considerations

Failure to image the entire abdominal area can result in a false-negative examination. False-negative results can also be caused by an absence of gastric mucosa in the diverticulum, insufficient gastric mucosa to permit detection or the removal of pertechnetate by bowel secretions. False-positive results are also possible and are most often caused by other pathologies.

LOCALIZATION OF GASTROINTESTINAL BLEEDING

Detection and localization of the site of GI bleeding can be accomplished with ^{99m}Tc-sulfur colloid or ^{99m}Tc-labeled red blood cells. Sulfur colloid is best used in cases of active bleeding, since it leaves the blood pool rapidly and may be cleared before the next bleeding episode. However, bleeding in the right upper quadrant may be obscured by sulfur colloid uptake in the liver. Labeled red blood cells are the better choice when the bleeding is intermittent, since the tracer remains in the blood pool for a long period and allows delayed imaging.

Clinical Procedure

No special patient preparation is required. The patient is placed under the scintillation camera in the supine position with the abdomen centered in the field of view.

Rapid sequential images are acquired as the tracer is administered. Following the dynamic study, short static images are obtained at intervals, up to 1 hr following injection. If no areas of tracer accumulation are visualized and ^{99m}Tc-labeled red blood cells have been used, delayed images may be obtained at intervals.

Image Findings

In ^{99m}Tc-labeled red blood cell imaging, the liver, spleen, abdominal vessels, kidneys, bladder, genital organs, and stomach are normally visualized. Progressive tracer accumulation in other areas indicates a bleeding site (Fig. 10-8).

If ^{99m}Tc-sulfur colloid is the tracer, an area of active bleeding is demonstrated within the first 5 min of imaging and may become more intense as background activity decreases.

GASTROESOPHAGEAL REFLUX

In adults, recurring or continual reflux of gastric or duodenal contents into the esophagus can lead to esophagitis and dysphagia. In infants, chronic reflux may cause failure to thrive and aspiration pneumonia. Gastroesophageal scintigraphy is a sensitive method for detecting reflux.

Clinical Procedure

The patient should fast for several hours before imaging. For adults, ^{99m}Tc-sulfur colloid is mixed with 150 ml orange juice and 150 ml dilute hydrochloric acid and administered orally. For infants, the tracer is mixed with the infant formula and administered through a nasogastric tube or orally through a baby bottle. It is important that the entire volume be consumed.

Following tracer administration, the patient is placed in a supine position under the scintillation camera. The stomach is positioned low in the field of view to ensure that the esophagus and lung fields are included. Serial images are obtained as varying amounts of pressure are applied to the abdomen using an abdominal binder. Delayed images of the

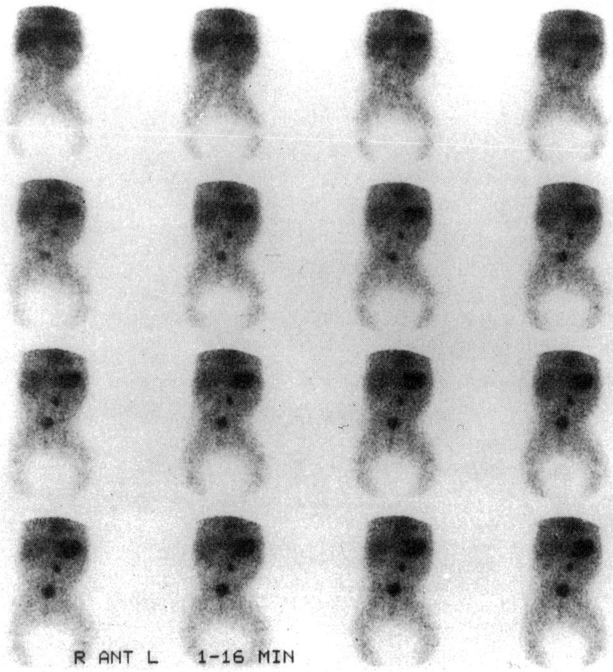

Figure 10.7 Abnormal hepatobiliary study obtained with ^{99m}Tc-mebrofenin. There is prompt excretion of tracer into the biliary tree and small bowel with no evidence of obstruction. The gallbladder, however, is not visualized on the initial images or on the 2-hr delayed images (not shown). Courtesy of Department of Veterans Affairs Medical Center, Nashville, TN.

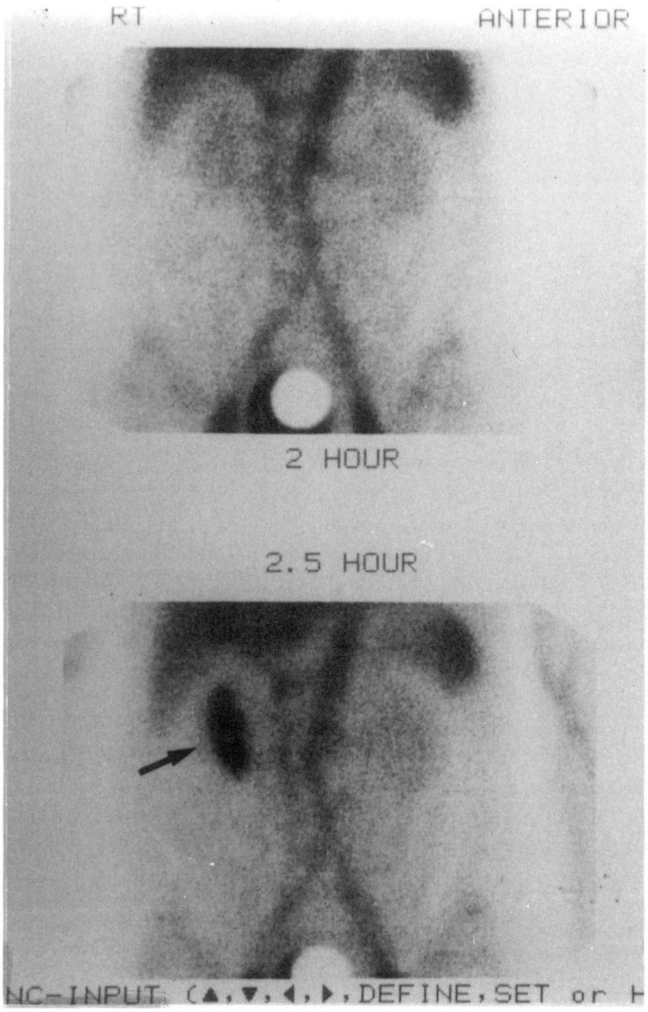

Figure 10.8 Positive GI bleeding study obtained with ^{99m}Tc-RBCs. Arrow indicates area of active bleeding in the upper right quadrant first visualized 2.5 hr following tracer administration. Courtesy of Baptist Memorial Hospital East, Memphis, TN.

lung fields up to 24 hr after tracer administration are useful for detecting intermittent reflux, which leads to aspiration of the tracer into the lungs.

Image Findings

A normal study demonstrates no esophageal reflux. The stomach is visualized, but no radioactivity is observed in the esophagus. Esophageal reflux is confirmed by the presence of activity in the esophagus or in the lungs (Fig. 10-9).

Technical Considerations

The patient may experience emesis. The technologist should take steps to minimize possible radioactive contamination before the procedure begins.

GASTRIC EMPTYING

Abnormal gastric emptying rates can be caused by diseases or surgical procedures. Patients experience nausea, vomiting, weight loss or abdominal fullness and distention.

Clinical Procedure

The patient should fast for at least 8 hr before the procedure. A meal consisting of both liquids and solids, to which ^{99m}Tc-sulfur colloid or ^{111}In-DTPA has been added, is consumed by the patient. One of a variety of meals may be used. It is important that the patient consume the meal within 5 min, alternating liquids and solids.

Immediately after eating, the patient is positioned supine under the scintillation camera with the stomach in the middle of the field of view. An immediate image is obtained, followed by images acquired at 15-min intervals for 2 hr. Data are stored in a computer.

Quantitative analysis yields an emptying half-time for both solid and liquid phases. Normal half-time values depend on the type of meal consumed. The images by themselves are not diagnostic.

LEVEEN SHUNT PATENCY

The LeVeen shunt is used to control ascites by draining the fluid in the peritoneal cavity through a tube implanted through the internal jugular vein into the superior vena cava. A patency study is performed to ensure that the tube is functioning and that it is not blocked.

Clinical Procedure

No special patient preparation is required. The patient is placed in a supine position under the scintillation camera with the shunt tube in the field of view. The tube is palpable in the thoracic wall and lateral neck. One to 2 mCi ^{99m}Tc-sul-

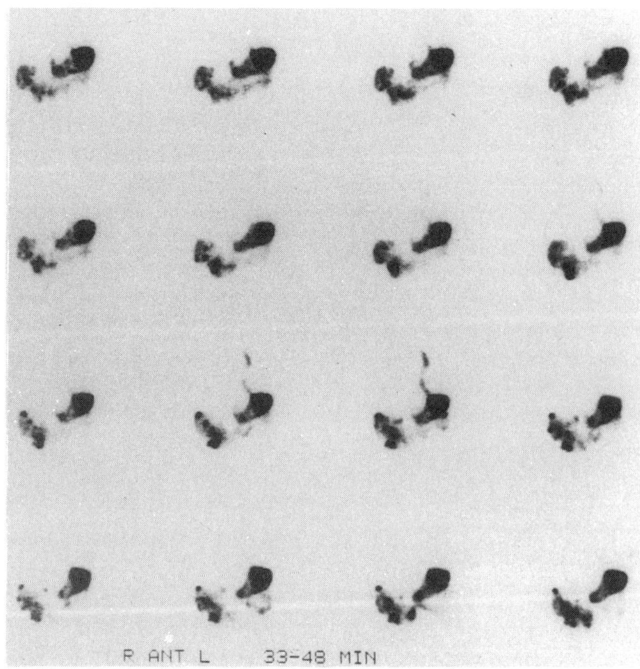

Figure 10.9 Serial images of gastroesophageal reflux study in an infant demonstrate intermittent reflux (second and third images in third row) into the esophagus approximately 42 min post-tracer injection into the stomach. Courtesy of The Children's Hospital of Alabama, Birmingham, AL.

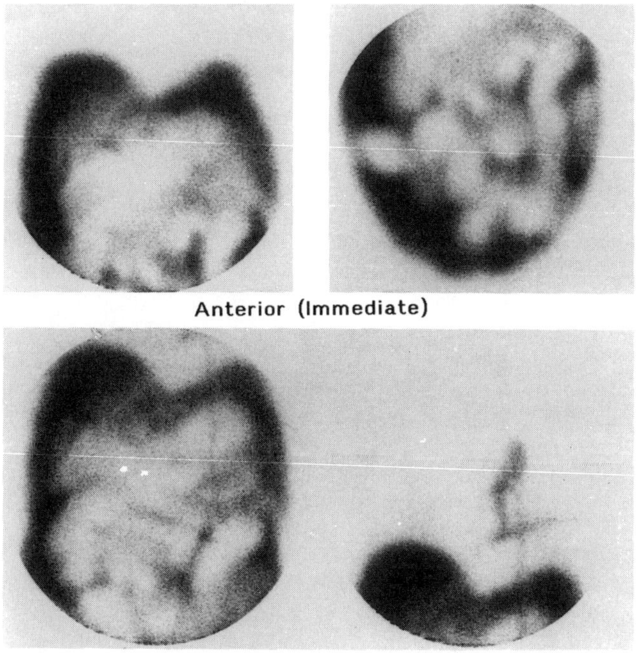

Figure 10.10 LeVeen shunt study performed by intrapertioneal administration of ^{99m}Tc-sulfur colloid. Delayed abdominal images demonstrate visualization of the shunt tubing along the left midclavicular line. Courtesy of St. Luke's Episcopal Hospital, Houston, TX.

fur colloid is introduced into the peritoneal space with a needle. Serial imaging begins when the radioactivity appears in the lower portion of the tube. Liver/spleen imaging is performed 1 hr following tracer administration. If the tube is not visualized, delayed views are performed as necessary.

Image Findings

A patent shunt is demonstrated by early visualization of the tube. Liver/spleen visualization occurs within 20 min of tracer administration (Fig. 10-10). Lack of tube visualization and delayed tracer concentration in the liver and spleen indicate shunt malfunction.

REFERENCES

1. Chester M, Glowniak J. Hepatobiliary imaging update. *J Nucl Med Technol* 1992;20:3–7.
2. Christian PE, Datz FL, Moore JG. Technical considerations in radionuclide gastric emptying studies. *J Nucl Med Technol* 1987;15:200–207.
3. Gilbert SA, Brown PH, Krishnamurthy GT. Quantitative nuclear hepatology. *J Nucl Med Technol* 1987;15:38–43.
4. Park HM, Duncan K. Nonradioactive pharmaceuticals in nuclear medicine. *J Nucl Med Technol* 1994;22:240–249.
5. Sodee DB, Velchik, MG, Noto RB, et al. Gastrointestinal system. In: Early PJ, Sodee DB. *Principles and practice of nuclear medicine,* 2nd ed. St. Louis: Mosby Year-Book; 1995:476–534.
6. Spencer RP. The spleen. In: Early PJ, Sodee DB. *Principles and practice of nuclear medicine,* 2nd ed. St. Louis: Mosby Year-Book: 1995:535–548.
7. Thrall JH, Ziessman HA. *Nuclear medicine—the requisites.* St. Louis: Mosby Year-Book; 1995:191–204.
8. Vitti RA, Malmud LS. Gastrointestinal system. In: Bernier DR, Christian PE, Langan JK, eds.: *Nuclear medicine technology and techniques,* 3rd ed. St. Louis: Mosby Year-Book; 1994:302–334.
9. Weiss SC, Conway JJ. Pediatrics. In: Bernier DR, Christian PE, Langan JK, eds. *Nuclear medicine technology and techniques,* 3rd ed. St. Louis: Mosby Year-Book; 1994:432–435.

11 Genitourinary System

Melanie A. Stepherson and Ann M. Steves

RENAL IMAGING

Renal imaging is a reliable method of evaluating the structure, location and function of the kidneys. This can be easily accomplished without danger of allergic reaction and with little or no patient discomfort.

Anatomy and Physiology

The kidneys regulate the volume and composition of the body's extracellular fluid through their excretory function. The kidneys are retroperitoneal organs located between the twelfth thoracic and fourth lumbar vertebrae (Fig. 11-1). The right kidney is positioned slightly lower than the left due to the presence of the liver superiorly. The ureters and the blood vessels attach at the hilus, an indention on the medial border of the kidneys. The kidneys receive blood from the right and left renal arteries, which branch directly off the descending aorta.

Each kidney consists of an outer renal cortex and an inner renal medulla (Fig. 11-2). The cortex contains the majority of the nephrons which are the microscopic functional units of the kidney. Each kidney contains more than one million nephrons. The nephron consists of a renal corpuscle and its attached tubule. The corpuscle is composed of a glomerulus surrounded by Bowman's capsule. The glomerulus receives blood from the afferent arteriole, which also helps regulate blood pressure through the juxtaglomerular apparatus. The tubules consist of the proximal convoluted tubule, the loop of Henle and a distal convoluted tubule. The renal medulla contains the renal pyramids, which empty urine into the minor and major calyces of the renal pelvis.

There are three processes involved in urine formation: glomerular filtration, tubular reabsorption and tubular excretion. Glomerular filtration involves the filtration of water and solutes out of the glomeruli and into Bowman's capsule. Tubular reabsorption occurs in the walls of the renal tubules and collecting systems, where most of the water and other physiologically important substances are reabsorbed into the blood. Tubular secretion also occurs in the tubular cells and involves the secretion of certain substances out of the blood and into the filtrate.

The urine passes into the renal calyces, the renal pelvis and into the ureters. Peristalsis forces urine down the ureters and into the bladder. The urine exits the body through the urethra.

Clinical Indications

Renal imaging is most often used to determine renal function rather than morphology. Functional imaging is indicated in the evaluation of the following conditions:

1. Relative blood flow and renal function.
2. Obstructive uropathy.
3. Renal transplant function.
4. Renal function of potential kidney donors.
5. Renovascular hypertension.

Renal morphology usually is better demonstrated with other imaging modalities such as ultrasound or radiography; however, static renal imaging may be useful in the following instances:

1. Evaluation of renal trauma.
2. Demonstration of congenital abnormalities, tumors and cysts.
3. Patients allergic to radiographic contrast media.

Radiopharmaceuticals

Radiopharmaceutical choice depends upon the reason for renal imaging. Renal radiopharmaceuticals are localized in the kidneys by glomerular filtration, tubular secretion, tubular binding or a combination of one or more of these processes.

Technetium-99m-Pentetate (DTPA). DTPA is cleared by glomerular filtration with minimal binding to the renal parenchyma. Due to its rapid clearance rate, it is useful to demonstrate glomerular filtration capabilities as well as relative blood flow to each kidney.

Orthoiodohippurate (OIH). Hippurate may be labeled with ^{131}I or ^{123}I. Approximately 80% of the tracer is secreted by the tubules, while the remainder is filtered by the glomeruli. This tracer is commonly used to assess relative blood flow, differential tubular function and urinary tract patency.

Technetium-99m-Mertiatide (MAG$_3$). MAG_3 is handled solely by tubular secretion and has an overall clearance that is less than that of OIH. It has the better physical characteristics of ^{99m}Tc. Millicurie amounts of MAG_3 can be administered to patients, thus resulting in higher counting statistics and better image resolution.

Technetium-99m-Succimer (DMSA). DMSA binds to the tubules in the renal cortex. Approximately 50% is bound within 2 hr of administration. Since this tracer remains fixed in the renal parenchyma for a relatively long period of time, it is most useful for imaging space-occupying lesions or gross renal anatomy.

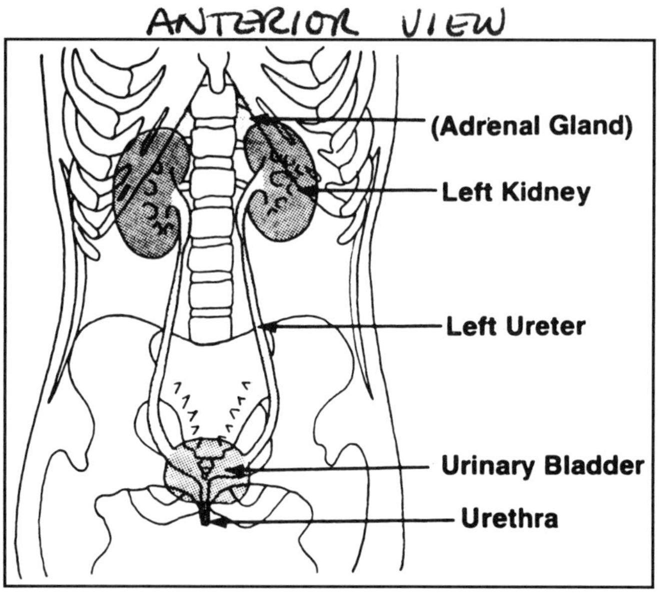

Figure 11.1 Urinary system. Reprinted with permission from: Bontrager A. *Textbook of radiographic positioning and related anatomy,* 2nd ed. St. Louis: CV Mosby; 1987:442.

Technetium-99m-Gluceptate (GH). GH is excreted primarily by glomerular filtration with some tubular secretion. It is retained in the tubules for several hours after administration. Since the tracer is cleared rapidly by the kidneys, it can be used for dynamic renal imaging as well as delayed static imaging.

Clinical Procedure

Prior to the start of the study, fully explain the procedure to the patient to elicit full cooperation. A medical history should be obtained that includes the following:

1. Patient's diagnosis.
2. Pertinent laboratory values: Laboratory analysis of blood chemistry is useful in determining renal function. Creatinine, urea and nitrogen are metabolic waste products that the kidneys normally remove from the circulation. Elevated BUN (blood urea nitrogen) and creatinine levels may indicate poor renal function.
3. Previous abdominal surgery, particularly to the kidneys.
4. Patient's blood pressure to determine if renovascular hypertension is a consideration.

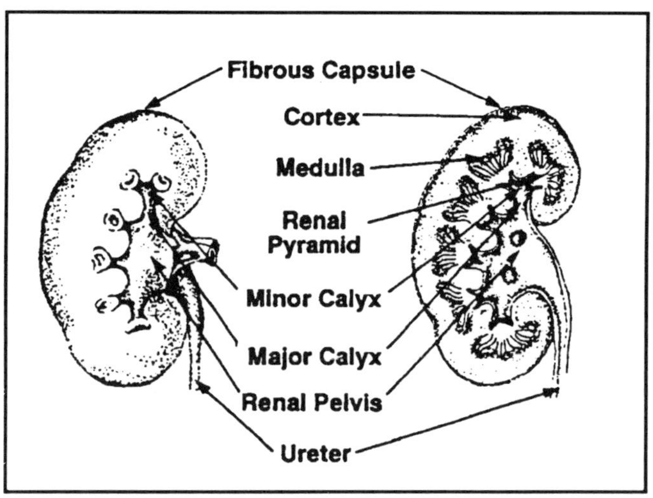

Figure 11.2 Renal structure. Reprinted with permission from: Bontrager A. *Textbook of radiographic positioning and related anatomy,* 2nd ed. St. Louis: CV Mosby; 1987:444.

Perfusion Imaging

Renal blood flow imaging can be performed with a number of ^{99m}Tc-labeled agents. The procedure is conducted as follows:

1. Position the patient supine with the kidneys centered over the detector to obtain a posterior projection.
2. Administer 10–15 mCi (370–555 MBq) of the technetium imaging agent intravenously using a bolus injection technique.
3. Obtain sequential images every 2 sec for 30–60 sec.
4. Obtain a blood-pool image immediately following the flow study acquisition, as necessary.

Normal Findings. Soon after its arrival in the aorta, the radiopharmaceutical bolus perfuses each kidney in a vascular blush. The activity should arrive in each renal area at approximately the same time with equal intensity (Fig. 11-3). Subsequent concentration levels and disappearance of the tracer depend on the ^{99m}Tc agent used. Pertechnetate will promptly visualize the renal bed and then fade to background body activity over the first few minutes. DTPA will demonstrate a gradual increase in concentration of the agent due to glomerular filtration. Activity will then be seen in the renal collecting system, ureters and bladder. If DMSA is used, there will be gradual accumulation of the activity outlining the tubular cells. Little of the agent is excreted in the urine and therefore the collecting systems will not concentrate the radiopharmaceutical.

Abnormal Findings. Areas of increased activity during the flow sequence are demonstrated by vascular tumors and arteriovenous malformations (AVMs). Areas of relative decreased activity due to cysts or avascular tumors may also be seen in the flow sequence.

Technical Considerations. Positioning errors are a common pitfall. They may be minimized by:

1. Placing the iliac crests in the lower one-third of the field of view to ensure that both kidneys are included.
2. Positioning the detector over the patient's right or left iliac fossa when performing a flow study on a renal transplant patient. The aortic bifurcation, iliac artery and urinary bladder should be included in the field of view. For an accurate flow study, it is also important that the tracer be given as a compact bolus and that it not be infiltrated.

Static Imaging

Delayed static imaging to demonstrate the renal cortical outline, size, shape and contour is performed 2–3 hr after the flow study. The patient is positioned for a posterior projection. Left and right posterior oblique images are obtained as required.

Normal Findings. Normal static images obtained 1 hr or more after injection of gluceptate or DMSA demonstrate a smooth renal contour. Tracer distribution within each kidney should be uniform and both kidneys should have equal tracer concentration.

Abnormal Findings. Congenital malformations such as fetal lobulations and horseshoe kidneys are easily identified on the images as areas of activity outside the normal renal outline. Areas of increased or decreased radioactivity may represent cysts, neoplasms, infarcts or renal trauma.

Technical Considerations. If the patient is in severe renal failure, images obtained with DMSA may need to be delayed up to 24 hr to improve visualization of the kidneys. Horseshoe kidneys and pelvic kidneys are located more anteriorly than the normal renal position. If these anomalies are a consideration, an anterior projection may be helpful.

Renal Function Imaging (Renogram)

Renal function imaging is performed with [^{131}I]OIH, [^{123}I]OIH or ^{99m}Tc-mertiatide. Along with a set of sequential images, a time-activity curve called a renogram is generated to demonstrate renal function. It is important that the patient be well hydrated before the study begins. Also, the patient should void immediately prior to the study. Data are acquired as follows.

1. Position the patient prone or supine to obtain a posterior projection over the kidneys. In the case of a renal transplant, the patient should be placed supine with the detector over the iliac fossa where the kidney is located.
2. Administer the tracer intravenously.
3. Acquire sequential 30–60 sec images for 20–30 min in a computer for later processing.
4. Administration of furosemide (Lasix®) may be indicated to rule out ureteral obstruction if tracer activity does not clear from the renal pelvis or ureteropelvic junction after the initial acquisition is completed. (See Diuresis Renography.)

Normal Findings. Normal kidneys demonstrate prompt tracer uptake with peak uptake at 3–5 min. The kidney activity then gradually decreases as the tracer is excreted. Renal pelvis and bladder activity is usually seen by 3–6 min.

The computer-generated curves represent three phases: vascular, secretory and excretory (Fig. 11-4). The vascular phase reflects the arrival of the bolus of activity at the renal area. In the secretory phase, the tracer is extracted from the renal tubules and to a smaller extent filtered by the glomerulus. The peak transit time, usually 3–5 min following injection, is the time at which the tracer reaches its maximum concentration in the kidneys. The excretory phase follows with a fairly rapid drop in the activity curve as the tracer is excreted from the kidney into the bladder.

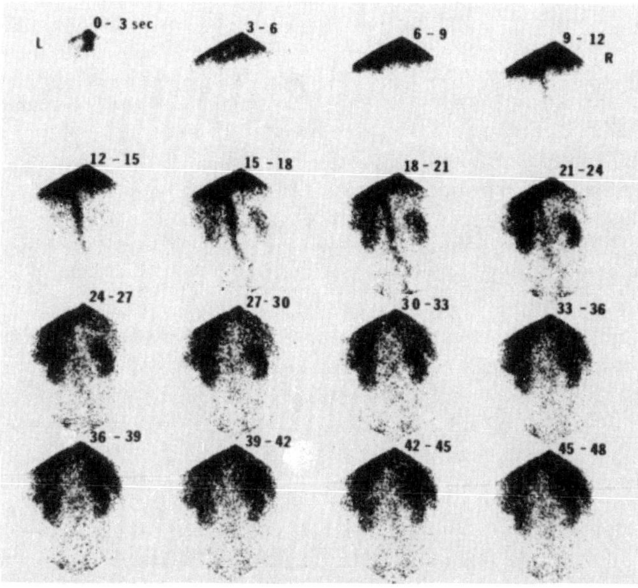

Figure 11.3 Normal perfusion study with 15 mCi ^{99m}Tc-DTPA obtained as a posterior view. Note the significant amount of activity in the liver and spleen. Reprinted with permission from: Bernier DR, Christian PE, Langan JK, Wells LD, eds. *Nuclear medicine technology and techniques,* 2nd ed. St. Louis: CV Mosby; 1989:428.

Abnormal Findings. Abnormalities of the renogram curve are usually reflected in the second and third phase of the renogram curve. An activity curve that exhibits an adequate upslope but no subsequent fall in activity is usually due to obstruction and indicates that the renal tubules take up the material but cannot excrete the activity. A curve that displays a below normal level of activity throughout the curve denotes poor renal function. Serial images corresponding to the curve provide additional visual demonstration of the abnormalities.

Technical Considerations. Be sure to ascertain the patient's state of hydration, since a dehydrated patient may exhibit delayed transit time.

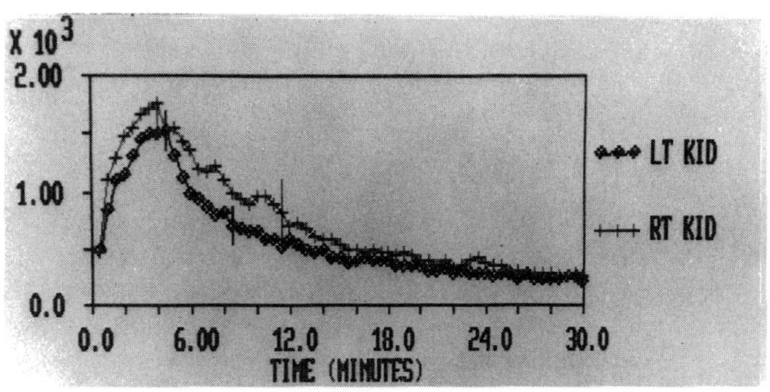

Figure 11.4 Normal renogram curves for left and right kidneys. Courtesy of Department of Veterans Affairs Medical Center, Buffalo, NY.

Diuresis Renography

If, at the conclusion of renal function imaging, tracer is retained in the renal pelvis or calyces, the administration of a diuretic to rule out a urinary tract obstruction may be indicated. Furosemide is administered intravenously to increase urine production. Increased urine flow will promptly washout the residual tracer activity if there is no obstruction (Fig. 11-5).

The patient should be well hydrated as required for functional imaging and empty the bladder before furosemide is administered. Patients who are unable to void voluntarily should be catheterized. Increased bladder pressure may diminish the effect of the diuretic. Data acquisition is the same as for a renal function study. The diuretic is injected slowly over 60 sec while images are acquired and should have an effect within 30–60 sec. Imaging is continued for about 20 min.

QUANTITATIVE RENAL STUDIES

Quantitative techniques provide numerical values that indicate the level of tubular and glomerular function. In addition to the renogram curve and nuclear medicine images, such values are useful in monitoring the course of patients with many different types of renal pathology. Quantitative studies are based on either a blood sampling technique to estimate tracer clearance from the blood or a camera method to determine the amount of tracer accumulated in the kidneys. The advantage of radionuclide techniques over chemical measurements, such as creatinine clearance, is that the function of each kidney (differential function) can be determined.

Effective Renal Plasma Flow

Effective renal plasma flow (ERPF) is a measurement of renal tubular function and is performed with OIH or ^{99m}Tc-mertiatide. Renal plasma flow was first measured using a nonradioactive substance, *p*-aminohippuric acid (PAH). The term "effective" is used to describe the measurement of renal plasma flow with OIH and mertiatide because their urinary clearance is slightly different than that of PAH. This is a small difference that does not grossly affect the calculation.

Several methods have been developed to estimate ERPF. Some require imaging and computer data processing, while others also require the collection of blood and urine samples.

Glomerular Filtration Rate

The glomerular filtration rate (GFR) is defined as the volume of plasma filtrate produced in 1 min by the renal glomeruli of both kidneys. The normal value is 125 ml/min. Usually, ^{99m}Tc-DTPA is used to determine GFR. Several methods, utilizing either a single blood sample or imaging with computer data processing, have been developed to determine GFR.

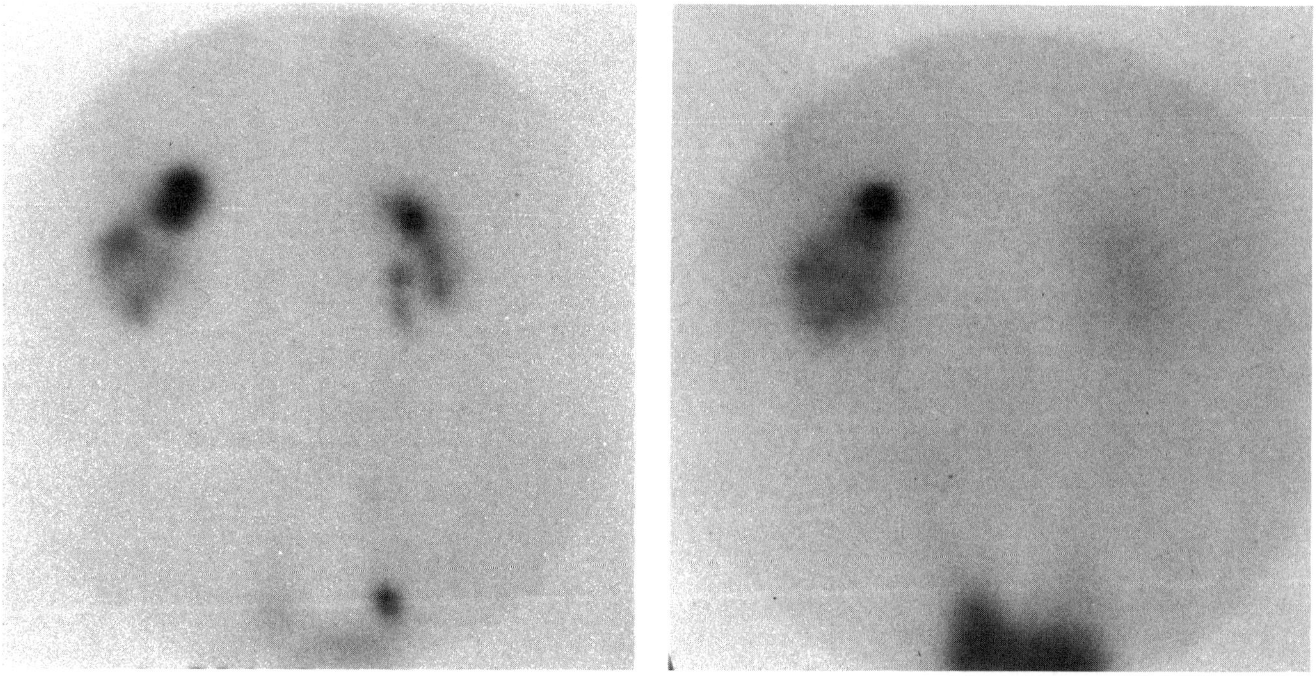

Figure 11.5 Approximately 12 min after administration of ^{99m}Tc-DTPA, tracer activity remains in the pelvis and calyces of the right kidney and in the calyces of the upper pole of the left kidney. Following intravenous administration of furosemide, activity drains from the right kidney but remains in the upper pole of the left kidney. Courtesy of Department of Veterans Affairs Medical Center, Buffalo, NY.

RADIONUCLIDE CYSTOGRAPHY

Radionuclide cystography is performed for the evaluation of vesicoureteral reflux, which is common in children. This condition is often responsible for recurrent urinary tract infections, which may damage the kidneys.

Two methods are available to perform radionuclide cystography. The indirect method involves intravenous administration of a renal agent. After the agent is cleared from the kidneys into the bladder, the patient is asked to void while being imaged. Reflux that occurs during voiding can then be observed. The more commonly used direct method is described in the following section.

Clinical Procedure

1. Have patient void before the study begins.
2. Catheterize the patient.
3. Connect the catheter to a bottle of normal saline to which 1 mCi (37 MBq) [^{99m}Tc]pertechnetate has been added.
4. Position the patient supine on the imaging table with the upper portion of the bladder in the lower part of the field of view.
5. Obtain multiple sequential images as the bladder is being filled with the radioactive saline solution.
6. Discontinue saline infusion when bladder capacity is reached. Obtain a posterior prevoid image that includes the entire bladder and upper urinary tracts.
7. Obtain voiding images with the patient in the seated position and the camera against the patient's back. Remove the catheter and encourage the patient to void into a bed pan or urinal.
8. Obtain a postvoid image that includes the entire bladder and upper urinary tracts.

Image Findings

The normal exam will demonstrate increasing activity in the bladder without reflux into the ureters. The abnormal exam will demonstrate ureteral reflux, especially during micturition. Reflux usually increases as the study progresses, although transient reflux may occur (Fig. 11-6).

Certain quantitative information, such as the reflux bladder volume and volume of reflux into the kidney, can also be calculated.

Technical Considerations

1. Equipment and the surrounding area should be covered with absorbent paper to prevent contamination with radioactive urine.
2. It is important to establish adequate bladder filling before the voiding portion of the exam. An increase in patient discomfort, leakage of urine around the catheter or cessation of flow from the saline infusion bottle may all indicate sufficient bladder filling. Bladder capacities vary according to age and condition of the bladder.
3. If quantitative results are desired, note that any loss of urine will cause inaccuracies in the calculations.
4. Children may not cooperate when asked to void, depending on their age.
5. Catheterization should be performed by someone who is well trained in the technique to ensure correct placement and to avoid physical or psychological trauma to the child.

SCROTAL IMAGING

Scrotal imaging is most often performed to differentiate acute torsion (twisting) of the spermatic cord and epididymitis. Torsion of the spermatic cord is often spontaneous and occurs most commonly in young men, with an acute onset of pain. The distinction is important since torsion requires immediate surgical intervention while epididymitis requires antibiotic therapy.

Clinical Procedure

With the patient in the supine position, the penis is taped to the pubic symphysis out of the field of view. The scrotal sac is supported on towels or a sling to permit close placement to the anteriorly placed camera. The testes should be positioned as symmetrically as possible. With the scrotum positioned in the lower center of the field of view, dynamic images are obtained at 2–3-sec intervals after the intravenous injection of 5–15 mCi (185–555 MBq) [^{99m}Tc]pertechnetate. Following dynamic imaging, several immediate static images are acquired.

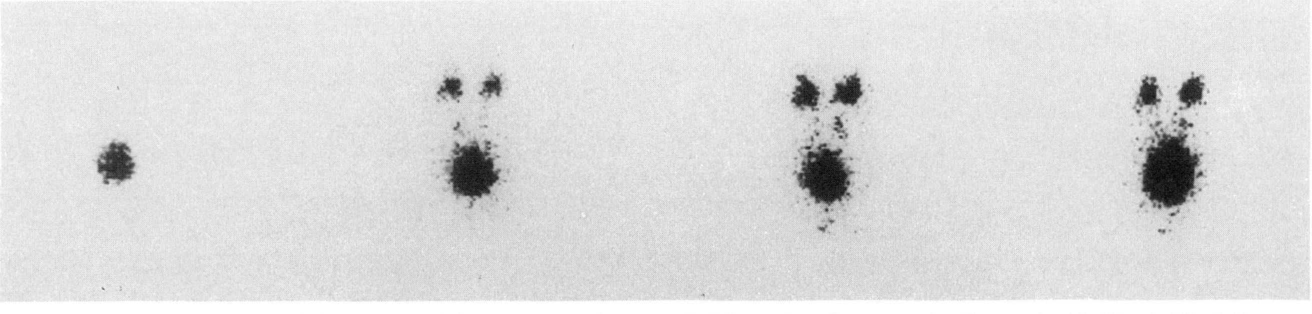

Figure 11.6 Positive radionuclide cystogram demonstrates increase in bilateral vesicoureteral reflux as the bladder is filled. Courtesy of The Children's Hospital of Alabama, Birmingham, AL.

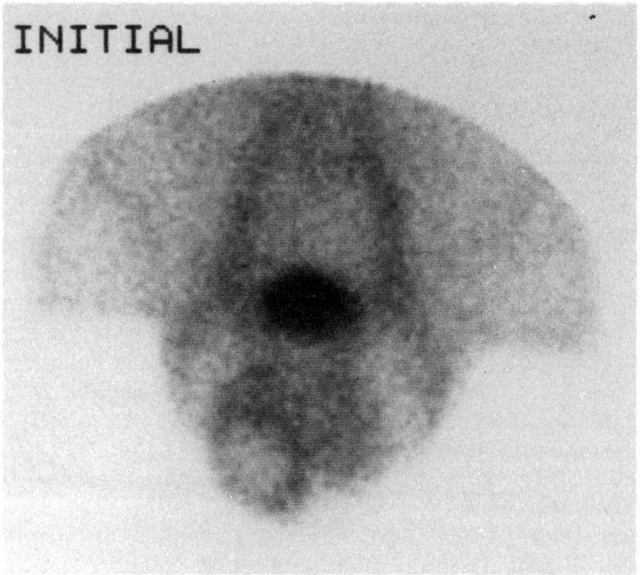

Figure 11.7 Testicular torsion. Scrotal image obtained with [^{99m}Tc]pertechnetate shows decreased activity in the right testicle surrounded with an intense halo of activity. Courtesy of The Children's Hospital of Alabama, Birmingham, AL.

Image Findings

Normal. The normal flow study demonstrates symmetrical activity distribution. Scrotal perfusion, if seen at all, is of minimal intensity. The static images will demonstrate the scrotum and contents to have homogenous areas of activity of similar intensity to the thigh.

Abnormal. Acute torsion will present on the dynamic images as normal or absent perfusion of the affected side. The static images will demonstrate an area of absent or decreased activity when compared to that of the opposite testicle or the thigh (Fig. 11-7). Epididymitis is demonstrated by increased blood flow to the affected side. The static images will also demonstrate increased activity.

REFERENCES

1. Alazraki NP, Mishkin FS. *Fundamentals of nuclear medicine.* 2nd ed. Reston: Society of Nuclear Medicine; 1988:102–111.
2. Beschi RJ, Dubovsky E, Kontzen FN. Genitourinary system. In: Bernier DR, Christian PE, Langan JK, eds. *Nuclear medicine technology and techniques,* 3rd ed. St. Louis: Mosby-Year Book; 1994:335–360.
3. Datz FL. *Handbooks in radiology: nuclear medicine.* Chicago: Yearbook Medical Publishers; 1988:185–219.
4. Rowell KL, ed. *Clinical computers in nuclear medicine.* Reston, VA: Society of Nuclear Medicine; 1992:39–50.
5. Rowell KL, Stutzman ME, Scott JW. Quantitation of renal function. *J Nucl Med Technol* 1987;15:146–152.
6. Sfakianakis GN, Georgiou M, Cavagnaro F, et al. Fast protocols for obstruction (diuretic renography) and for renovascular hypertension (ACE inhibition). *J Nucl Med Technol* 1992; 20:193–206.
7. Solomon EP, Phillips GA. *Understanding human anatomy and physiology.* Philadelphia: Saunders; 1987.
8. Taylor A, Ziffer J. Urinary tract. In: Early PJ, Sodee DB. *Principles and practice of nuclear medicine,* 2nd ed. St. Louis: Mosby Year-Book; 1995:579–616.
9. Thrall JH, Ziessman HA. *Nuclear medicine-the requisites.* St. Louis: Mosby Year-Book; 1995:283–320.
10. Vogel JM, Matin P. Genitourinary tract scintigraphy. In: Matin P, ed. *Clinical nuclear medicine imaging.* New York: Medical Examination Publishing Co.; 1986:117–140.
11. Weiss SC, Conway JJ. Radionuclide cystography. *J Nucl Med Technol* 1987;15:66–74.

12 Respiratory System

Ann M. Steves

Radionuclide lung imaging can be used to evaluate pulmonary physiology. The most common clinical indications for lung imaging include:

1. Evaluation of pulmonary emboli (PE): initial screening to rule out PE, follow-up to evaluate response to therapy. Diagnosing a pulmonary embolism is the primary use of radionuclide lung imaging.
2. Evaluation of chronic obstructive pulmonary disease (COPD), such as emphysema.

Figure 12-1 shows the anatomic relationship of the lungs to other structures in the thoracic cavity. The major airways, the bronchi, divide into successively smaller branches called bronchioles and terminate with the alveoli (Fig. 12-2). In the alveoli, carbon dioxide and oxygen are exchanged. Each alveolus is surrounded by approximately 1000 capillaries of the pulmonary circulation.

Respiration is the transport of oxygen and carbon dioxide to and from the cells of the body. Four processes are involved in respiration: (a) ventilation, the flow of air into and out of the lungs; (b) gas exchange, the diffusion of oxygen and carbon dioxide between the alveoli and the blood; (c) gas transport, the movement of oxygen and carbon dioxide to and from the cells through the circulation; and (d) regulation of ventilation. In the healthy lung, ventilation and perfusion (blood flow) are matched for efficient and complete exchange of oxygen and carbon dioxide. Pulmonary disease upsets this balance.

PERFUSION IMAGING

Perfusion imaging demonstrates blood flow to the lungs. Technetium-99m-MAA particles are injected intravenously and are trapped in the vasculature of the lungs. The majority of these particles are 10–90 microns in diameter and thus will block arterioles of this size within the lung. Areas of the lung where perfusion is decreased or absent will receive little or no tracer. The number of arterioles that are blocked with tracer depends on the number of particles injected. An adult patient should receive 100,000–500,000 tracer particles, which will occlude less than 1% of the lung arterioles while providing a uniform tracer distribution.

Clinical Procedure

Relevant medical history includes the following:

1. Factors predisposing the patient to PE: recent surgery, cancer, COPD, immobility, obesity or prior history of PE.
2. Symptoms of PE: shortness of breath, chest pain, fever, cough, syncope, tachycardia, jugular venous distension or hemoptysis. These signs and symptoms are not specific to PE and can occur in a variety of conditions.
3. Recent chest radiograph findings.

Chest radiograph findings are needed for interpretation of the lung images. Since the symptoms of PE are common to many other conditions, it is necessary to rule out other pathology which may mimic PE or obscure its diagnosis.

The patient should be placed in the supine position for injection of the radiopharmaceutical. When the patient is supine, the effect of gravity, which hinders blood flow to the lung apices, is minimized, allowing uniform tracer distribution throughout the lung. Two to 4 mCi (74–148 MBq) ^{99m}Tc-MAA are administered intravenously.

Imaging

Imaging can begin immediately following tracer administration. Acquire static images for the following anatomic views: anterior, posterior, laterals and posterior or anterior obliques.

Image Findings

The radiopharmaceutical is normally distributed evenly throughout the lungs (Fig. 12-3). Because the lung apices are thinner than the lower portions of the lungs, tracer distribution may appear to be somewhat decreased at the apices. The cardiac impression may be seen on the anterior and left lateral views. Decreased areas of tracer uptake indicate a disruption of blood flow, which can be due to a variety of conditions.

Technical Considerations

Common technical errors associated with perfusion imaging include the following.

1. Extravasation of the tracer at the injection site, which may cause an insufficient number of particles to be delivered to the lungs, resulting in nonuniformities not related to pathology in the lungs.
2. Small blood clots in the syringe, formed when blood is withdrawn into the syringe and allowed to stand for a period of time. When these clots are injected into the patient, they may result in hot spots on the images, again, not related to pathology.
3. Failure to remove attenuating objects such as jewelry and ECG leads results in cold spot artifacts on images.
4. Tracer administration with the patient in an upright position, which causes decreased tracer concentration in the lung apices.

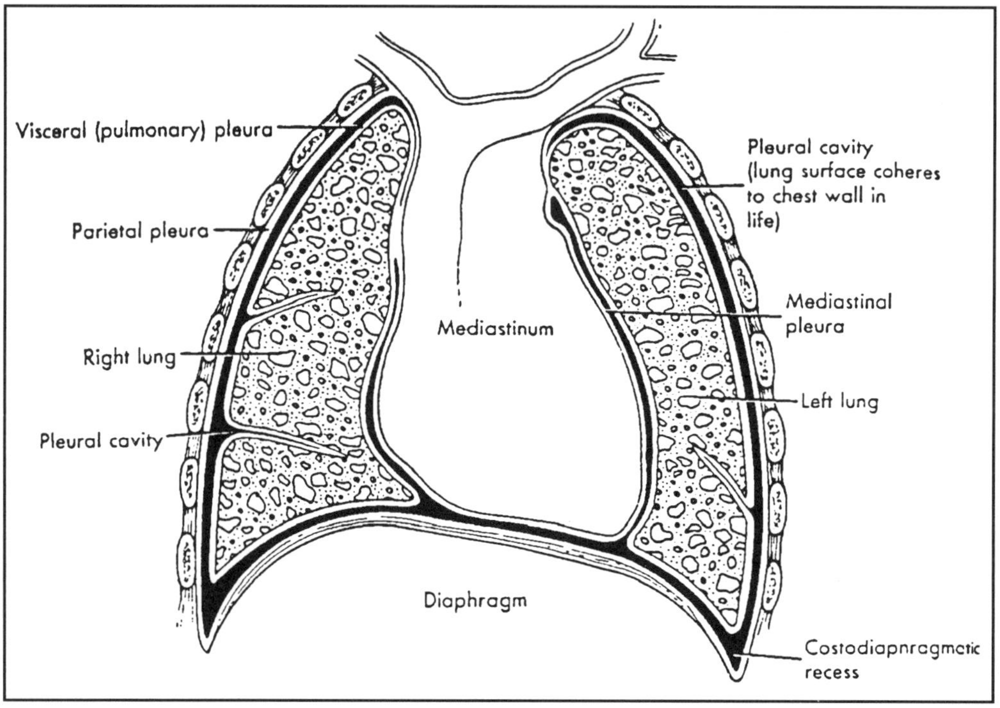

Figure 12.1 Mediastinum (heart, its great vessels, trachea and bronchi have been removed). Reprinted with permission from: McClintic JR. *Human anatomy.* St. Louis: CV Mosby; 1983:412.

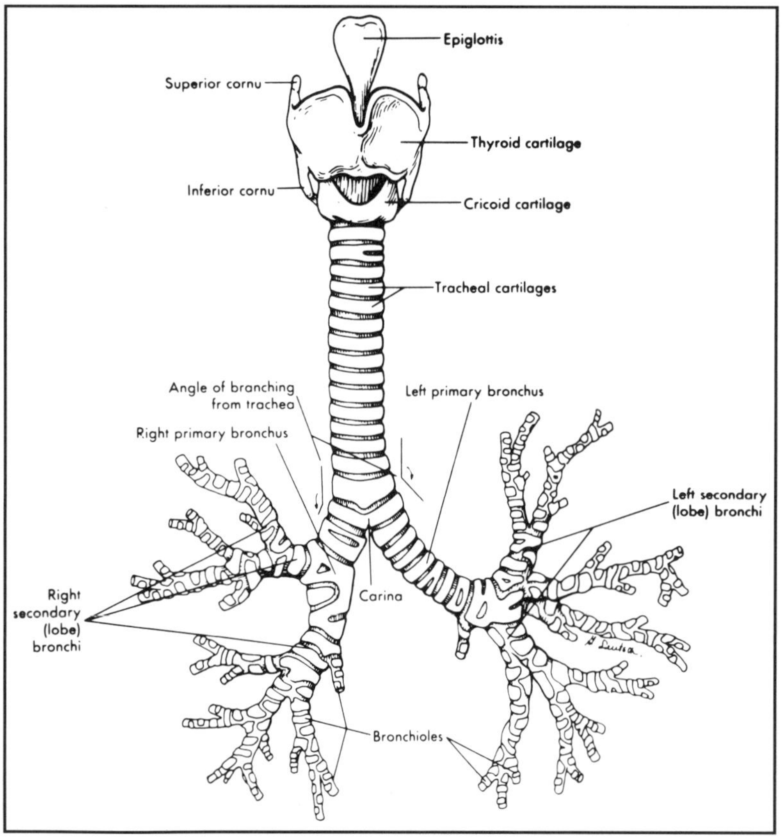

Figure 12.2 Larynx, trachea and bronchi. Reprinted with permission from: McClintic JR. *Human anatomy.* St. Louis: CV Mosby; 1983:411.

VENTILATION IMAGING

Ventilation imaging demonstrates the flow of air into and out of the lungs. Whereas perfusion imaging is very sensitive for detecting changes in blood flow, it is unable to specify the cause of the change. Ventilation imaging, performed in conjunction with perfusion imaging, can increase the specificity of the perfusion study by differentiating perfusion defects that are due to PE from those that are due to obstructive lung disease.

Ventilation imaging may be performed with radioactive inert gases such as ^{133}Xe, ^{127}Xe or ^{81m}Kr or radiolabeled aerosol particles such as ^{99m}Tc-DTPA. All are administered via inhalation: the patient breathes through a facemask or mouthpiece attached to a spirometry system or nebulizer.

Clinical Procedure

Relevant medical history includes the same items obtained for perfusion imaging.

Patient Preparation

The procedure should be reviewed thoroughly with the patient to elicit full cooperation. The administration apparatus should be placed on the patient for a practice run before the tracer is inhaled. If radioactive gas is used as the tracer, the patient should be positioned prior to administration. The patient may be placed in a supine or upright position, whichever is more comfortable for the patient.

Imaging

Xenon. The standard view is the posterior because more lung area is exposed in this projection. Other views, however, may be appropriate if a particular segment of the lung is of interest and would be better visualized with a different projection. The following images are obtained: single-breath, acquired during initial inhalation of the gas; washin or equilibrium, collected while the xenon distributes throughout the aerated portions of the lungs; and washout, taken while the radioactivity is cleared from the lungs. The length of time for which equilibrium and washout images are obtained varies from department to department.

Krypton-81m. Krypton-81m ($T_{1/2}$ = 13 sec) is breathed continuously by the patient as it is eluted with oxygen from its parent nuclide ^{81}Rb. Multiple projections are possible, but single-breath and washout images are not because of the tracer's short half-life.

Technetium-99m-DTPA Aerosol. The tracer is injected into a nebulizer to generate the aerosol particles. Twenty to 30 mCi (740 MBq–1.11 GBq) placed in the nebulizer will deliver 1–2 mCi of activity to the patient. Following a single 5-min inhalation of the aerosolized tracer, multiple projections matching those of the perfusion study can be obtained. Single-breath or washout images are not possible.

Image Findings

Radioxenon is normally distributed uniformly throughout both lungs, with no retention of tracer during the washout phase (Fig. 12-4). Retention of the xenon after 2–3 min of the washout phase indicates obstructive lung disease.

Normal krypton and aerosol images demonstrate symmetric deposition of the tracer from the apex to the base of both lungs. Segments of the lungs that are not ventilated will show decreased or absent tracer activity.

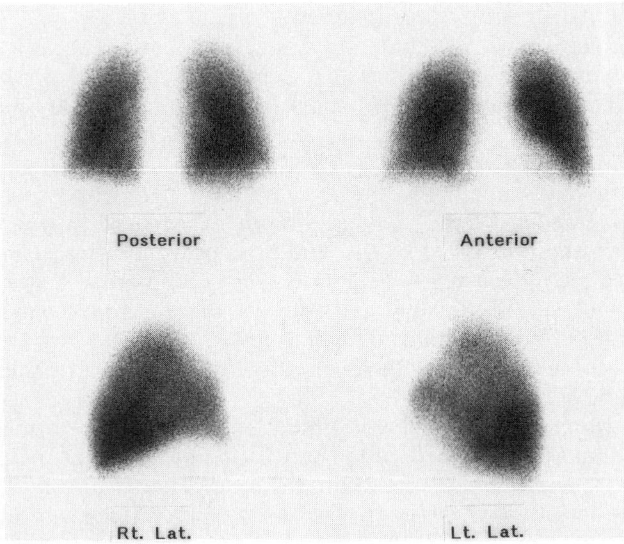

Figure 12.3 Normal lung perfusion images obtained after intraveous administration of ^{99m}Tc-MAA. Courtesy of St. Luke's Episcopal Hospital, Houston, TX.

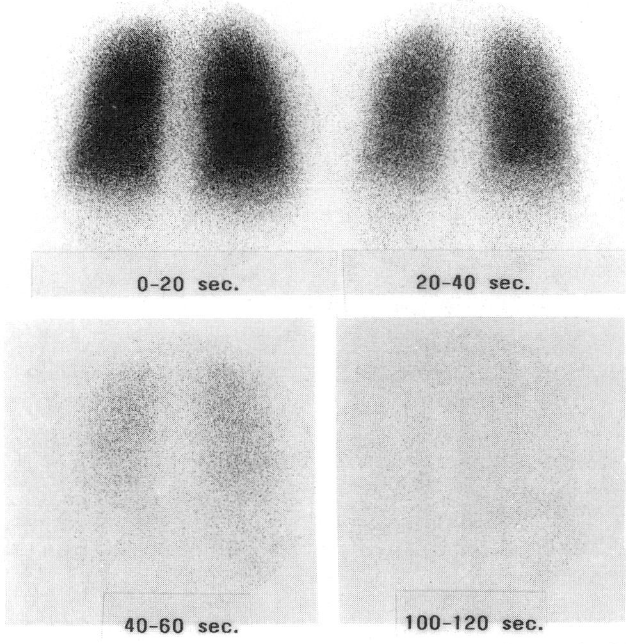

Figure 12.4 Normal lung ventilation images obtained with ^{133}Xe gas in the posterior view demonstrate complete washout of tracer. Courtesy of St. Luke's Episcopal Hospital, Houston, TX.

Technical Considerations

In performing ventilation imaging, the following technical points need to be considered. Certain patients may not be able to tolerate an oxygen mask, mouthpiece or nose clips. They may attempt to remove the apparatus during the procedure, allowing xenon to escape into the room. Patients who have difficulty holding a mouthpiece tightly may cause the same problem. Trapping equipment is necessary to contain xenon exhaled by the patient to prevent unnecessary radiation exposure to personnel. The equipment should be checked periodically to ensure that there are no leaks in the closed system and that the charcoal filter has not become saturated with xenon, thereby decreasing its trapping effectiveness.

Rooms in which xenon ventilation imaging is performed should be equipped with a ventilation system that maintains negative pressure within the room. The system should be activated when xenon is in use to contain the gas inside the room should a leak occur.

When performing aerosol imaging, it is important to maintain the correct oxygen flow rate (9 liters/min) through the nebulizer. Improper flow rate may affect particle size; too large particles will lodge in the central airways rather than being carried throughout the lungs. Also, significant contamination may occur during the performance of aerosol studies. The source of the contamination is the exhaust vent of the aerosol administration device.

VENOGRAPHY

Deep vein thrombosis (DVT) of the lower extremities may cause PE. A radionuclide venogram to visualize the deep veins in the legs and pelvis may be performed in conjunction with perfusion imaging. Technetium-99m-MAA is administered through the pedal veins in the feet to demonstrate blood flow and sites of tracer accumulation. An alternate method is to use ^{99m}Tc-red blood cells to obtain images of the venous system in the pelvis and lower extremities.

Immobility, surgery, certain medications, cancer, congestive heart failure and recent myocardial infarction predispose patients to developing thrombophlebitis and DVT. Symptoms of thrombophlebitis include swelling, redness and pain in one or both legs.

Clinical Procedure

Relevant medical history includes the following:

1. Recent injuries and/or surgeries.
2. History of previous DVT or PE.
3. Other predisposing factors.
4. Results of contrast venogram radiograph, if one was performed.

Patient Preparation

1. Place patient in supine position and tie tourniquets below each knee and at each ankle.
2. Place the legs close together and immobilize them with tape or sandbags. Radioactive markers at the knees and ankles may be positioned at this time.
3. Insert a scalp vein infusion (butterfly) needle into the pedal vein on the top of each foot and attach a three-way stopcock with a saline flush to the infusion line.
4. Position the camera detector anteriorly to include the area from the ankle to the knee.

Imaging

1. Acquire images while bilateral injections of 1–1.5 mCi (37–55 MBq) ^{99m}Tc-MAA are made into each foot, followed by a saline flush.
2. Reposition the detector to include the area from the knees to the lower pelvis and administer another set of injections followed by a saline flush while acquiring an image.
3. Repeat Step 2 after the detector is repositioned over the pelvis. A total of 6–9 mCi (222–333 MBq) will have been administered to the patient.
4. Remove tourniquets and needles and instruct the patient to exercise by walking about or moving the legs.
5. Repeat the series of three images for a preselected time, placing the patient in the same position as for the dynamic imaging.
6. Lung perfusion images may now be obtained.

Image Findings

Normal findings are demonstrated by a smooth, symmetric, uninterrupted flow of the tracer from the ankles to the pelvis through the deep veins. There should be no evidence of dilation or obstruction of the deep veins or of collateral circulation.

Abnormal findings include areas of increased tracer concentration, visualization of collateral circulation or obstruction of flow (Fig. 12-5).

Technical Considerations

1. Extravasation in one or both feet hinders tracer flow, which could be interpreted as decreased flow unilaterally or bilaterally. Also, comparison of contralateral sides is not possible if tracer is infiltrated at one of the injection sites.
2. Wrapping the legs in elastic bandages helps confine flow to the deep veins and may make veins more prominent for ease in placing the needles.
3. Warm towels placed over the injection site may also cause veins to become more prominent.
4. Since hot spots may be caused by blood clots formed in the syringe, avoid drawing blood into the syringe containing the tracer.

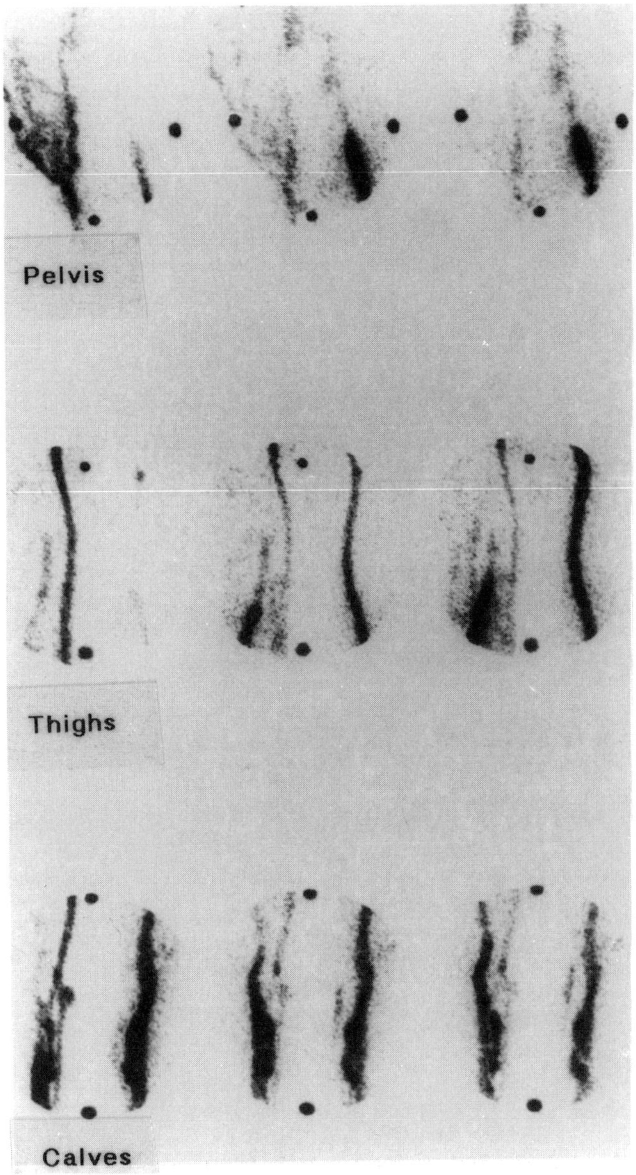

Figure 12.5 Abnormal radionuclide venogram obtained with ^{99m}Tc-MAA. Anterior views of pelvis and thighs demonstrate obstruction in right iliac and right femoral veins. Courtesy of St. Luke's Episcopal Hospital, Houston, TX.

REFERENCES

1. Alazraki NP, Mishkin FS. *Fundamentals of nuclear medicine,* 2nd ed. Reston, VA: Society of Nuclear Medicine; 1988:68–72.
2. Gilworth DL, Donovan BC, Morrison R, et al. Patient management of pulmonary embolism. *J Nucl Med Technol* 1988; 16:33–36.
3. Gottschalk A, Hoffer PB. *Diagnostic nuclear medicine,* 2nd ed. Baltimore: Williams & Wilkins; 1988:458–465, 475–481, 502–537.
4. Hanson PC. Ventilation scintigraphy. *J Nucl Med Technol* 1987; 15:193–197.
5. McGraw RS, Culver CM, Juni JE, et al. Lung ventilation studies: surface contamination associated with technetium-99m-DTPA aerosol. *J Nucl Med Technol* 1992:20:228–230.
6. Mettler FA, Guiberteau MJ. *Essentials of nuclear medicine imaging,* 3rd ed. Philadelphia: WB Saunders; 1991:141–176.
7. Palla A, Tumeh SS, Giuntini C. Lung. In: Early PJ, Sodee DB, eds. *Principles and practice of nuclear medicine,* 2nd ed. St. Louis: Mosby-Year Book, Inc.; 1995:443–475.
8. Phegley DJ, Secker-Walker RH. Respiratory system. In: Bernier DR, Christian PE, Langan JK, eds. *Nuclear medicine technology and techniques,* 3rd ed. St. Louis: Mosby-Year Book, Inc.; 1994:252–270.

13 Skeletal System

Ann M. Steves

Bone imaging is one of the most commonly ordered procedures in nuclear medicine. The clinical indications for performing bone imaging include:

1. Staging of malignant disease: screening of patients with primary tumors (e.g., breast, lung, prostate carcinoma) known to metastasize readily to bone; evaluation of response to therapy; localization of biopsy sites.
2. Evaluation of primary bone neoplasms (e.g., Ewing's sarcoma, osteogenic sarcoma): detection of sites in other bones; detection of soft-tissue metastases.
3. Diagnosis of skeletal inflammatory disease (e.g., osteomyelitis).
4. Evaluation of skeletal pain of unknown cause.
5. Evaluation of elevated serum alkaline phosphatase level of unknown origin.
6. Determination of bone viability when blood supply to the area is in question.
7. Evaluation of painful joint prostheses.
8. Detection of occult fractures (e.g., sports injury) not demonstrated radiographically.

All of the indications listed are important reasons for performing bone imaging, but staging of a malignant disease is the most frequent.

Technetium-99m-medronate (MDP) and ^{99m}Tc-oxidronate (HDP) are currently the two radiopharmaceuticals of choice. Medronate has been shown to have a faster blood clearance compared to other labeled phosphate compounds and oxidronate has greater bone uptake. Approximately 50% of the administered tracer is concentrated in bony tissue. The other 50% is excreted from the body through the kidneys.

Localization of these tracers in the bone is dependent on blood flow and the rate of bone production or remodeling. Blood flow is required to carry the radiopharmaceutical to the bone where an exchange between ions in the bone crystal and the tracer takes place. The crystal structure of the bone is hydroxyapatite. The ratio of elements making up the crystal is represented by the formula $Ca_{10}(PO_4)(OH)_2$. While the mechanism is not completely understood, it is believed that the phosphorus groups of the tracer exchange onto the calcium of the hydroxyapatite crystal.

Throughout life, bone is constantly being destroyed and replaced with new bone; this process is called bone remodeling. Hence, bone tracers will be concentrated in even normal skeletal tissue to some extent. Any process that increases osteoblastic (bone formation) activity will cause increased tracer uptake. Conversely, areas of osteolytic (bone destruction) activity will be visualized as areas of decreased tracer activity.

A thorough knowledge of the gross anatomy of the skeletal system is essential for the technologist. Figures 13-1 and 13-2 illustrate the more important skeletal structures visualized during bone imaging, but the reader is encouraged to review other more comprehensive anatomy texts.

CLINICAL PROCEDURE

Patient History

Relevant medical history should include: patient's diagnosis, if known; recent injuries and/or surgeries; previous injuries to bones; medications (certain medications may alter tracer distribution); location, duration and frequency of pain, if patient is experiencing pain; serum alkaline phosphatase level (alkaline phosphatase is an enzyme involved in the calcification of bone; the serum level may be elevated in certain diseases of bone).

Patient Preparation

1. Explain the reason for the delay between tracer administration and imaging.
2. Administer 15–20 mCi (555–740 MBq) ^{99m}Tc-labeled phosphate compound intravenously. If a flow study is requested, position patient under the scintillation camera prior to tracer administration.
3. Unless contraindicated, encourage the patient to drink four to six 8-oz glasses of liquid and to void frequently during the delay before imaging. Hydration of the patient helps clear the tracer from the body. Frequent voiding decreases the bladder's exposure to radiation.
4. Patient should void immediately before imaging. A large amount of radioactive urine in the bladder can obscure bony structures of the pelvis.

Imaging

1. Technetium-99m imaging can begin 3 hr after tracer administration.
2. Ascertain that patient has voided before proceeding with imaging.
3. Set camera controls (photopeak energy, % window, etc.).
4. Place the patient in a supine or prone position, which ever is better tolerated by the patient. The patient/detector distance should be minimized for each view.

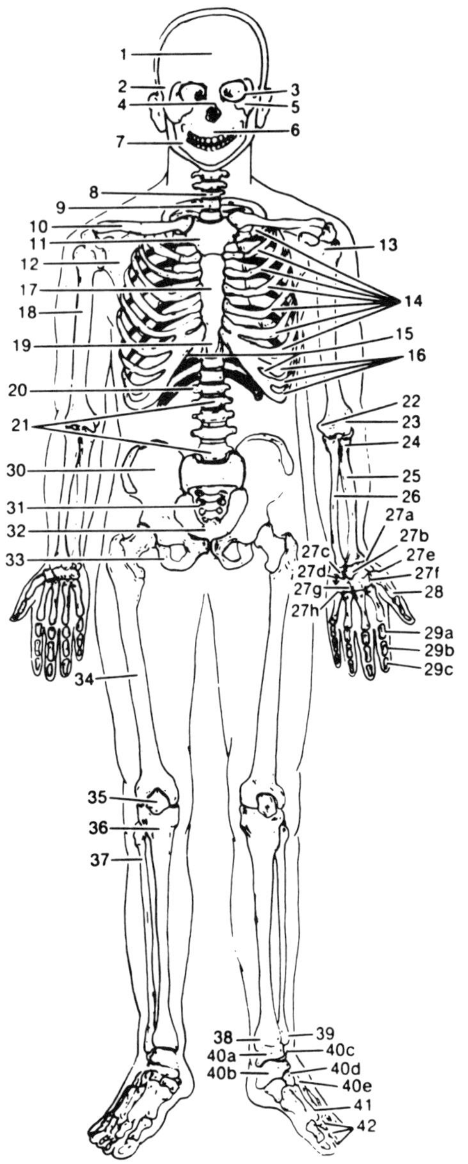

1. Frontal bone
2. Temporal bone
3. Orbit
4. Nasal bone
5. Zygomatic bone
6. Maxilla
7. Mandible
8. Seventh cervical vertebra
9. Thoracic vertebra I
10. Clavicle
11. Manubrium of sternum
12. Scapula
13. Head of humerus
14. True ribs
15. Kidneys
16. False ribs
17. Body of sternum
18. Humerus
19. Xiphoid process
20. Transverse process
21. Lumbar vertebrae
22. Medial condyle of humerus
23. Lateral epicondyle of humerus
24. Capitulum of radius
25. Radius
26. Ulna
27. Carpal bones
    a. Scaphoid bone of hand
    b. Lunate bone
    c. Triangular bone
    d. Pisiform bone
    e. Trapezium
    f. Trapezoid
    g. Capitate bone
    h. Hamate bone
28. Metacarpal bones
29. Phalanges
    a. Proximal phalanx
    b. Middle phalanx
    c. Distal phalanx
30. Iliac bone
31. Sacrum
32. Bladder
33. Ischium
34. Femur
35. Patella
36. Tibia
37. Fibula
38. Medial malleolus
39. Lateral malleolus
40. Tarsal bones
    a. Talus
    b. Navicular bone
    c. Calcaneus
    d. Cuneiform bones
41. Metatarsal bones
42. Phalanges of toes

Figure 13.1 Anterior skeleton. Reprinted with permission from: Early PJ, Sodee DB. *Principles and practice of nuclear medicine.* St. Louis: CV Mosby; 1985:571.

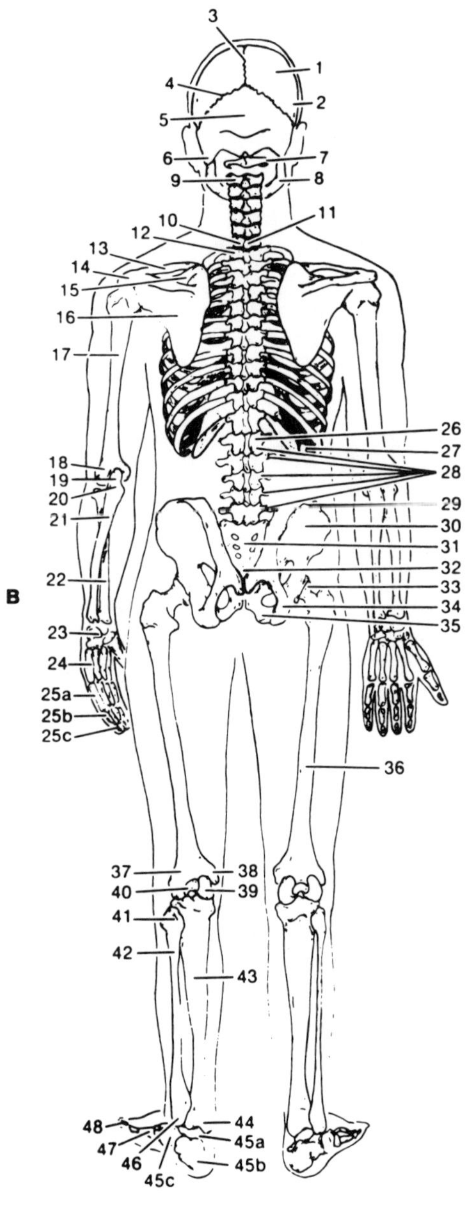

1. Parietal bone
2. Temporal bone
3. Sagittal suture
4. Lambdoidal suture
5. Occipital bone
6. Mastoid process
7. Atlas
8. Mandible
9. Axis or second cervical vertebra
10. Seventh cervical vertebra
11. Spinous process
12. Thoracic vertebra I
13. Clavicle
14. Acromion
15. Spine of scapula
16. Scapula
17. Humerus
18. Lateral epicondyle of humerus
19. Olecranon
20. Head of radius
21. Ulna
22. Radius
23. Carpal bones
24. Metacarpal bones
25. Phalanges
    a. Proximal phalanx
    b. Middle phalanx
    c. Distal phalanx
26. Transverse process
27. Kidneys
28. Lumbar vertebrae
29. Iliac crest
30. Upper part of ilium
31. Sacrum
32. Bladder
33. Head of femur
34. Ischium
35. Pubic bone
36. Femur
37. Lateral epicondyle of femur
38. Medial epicondyle of femur
39. Medial condyle of femur
40. Lateral condyle of femur
41. Head of fibula
42. Fibula
43. Tibia
44. Medial malleolus
45. Tarsal bones
    a. Talus
    b. Calcaneus
    c. Cuboid bone
46. Lateral malleolus
47. Metatarsal bones
48. Phalanges of toes

Figure 13.2 Posterior skeleton. Reprinted with permission from: Early PJ, Sodee DB. *Principles and practice of nuclear medicine.* St. Louis: CV Mosby; 1985:572.

5. Use the spot image technique, whole-body table technique or SPECT imaging to acquire data.

Spot Image Technique

Depending on the size of the field of view, 10–30 separate images may be required to image the entire skeleton. A medium/high-resolution, parallel-hole or diverging-hole collimator can be used. An anterior or posterior view of the chest is imaged for a preset number of counts.

Adequate counting statistics must be achieved. For a standard size field of view camera, 400,000–600,000 counts are collected; for a large field of view camera, 500,000–1,000,000 counts are recommended. All subsequent images are collected for the same time interval. Since all images are collected for the same length of time, the film density in one image can be compared to that of another. For each image, the distance between the patient and the surface of the detector should be minimized to obtain the best possible spatial resolution.

Whole-Body Table Technique

A miniaturized image of the total skeleton is attained with a device that moves either the camera detector or the patient through the scintillation camera's field of view. Depending on the size of the field of view and the type of collimator used, one to three passes are required to cover the width of the patient's body. A medium/high-resolution, parallel-hole or a special type of diverging collimator specifically designed for this application can be used. The speed that the detector travels over the patient depends on the count rate obtained from the anterior or posterior chest. The same scanning speed is used for both anterior and posterior images and is determined from a chart supplied by the camera manufacturer. Total body images should contain greater than 1 million counts. Again, the detector should be as close to the patient as possible for optimum spatial resolution.

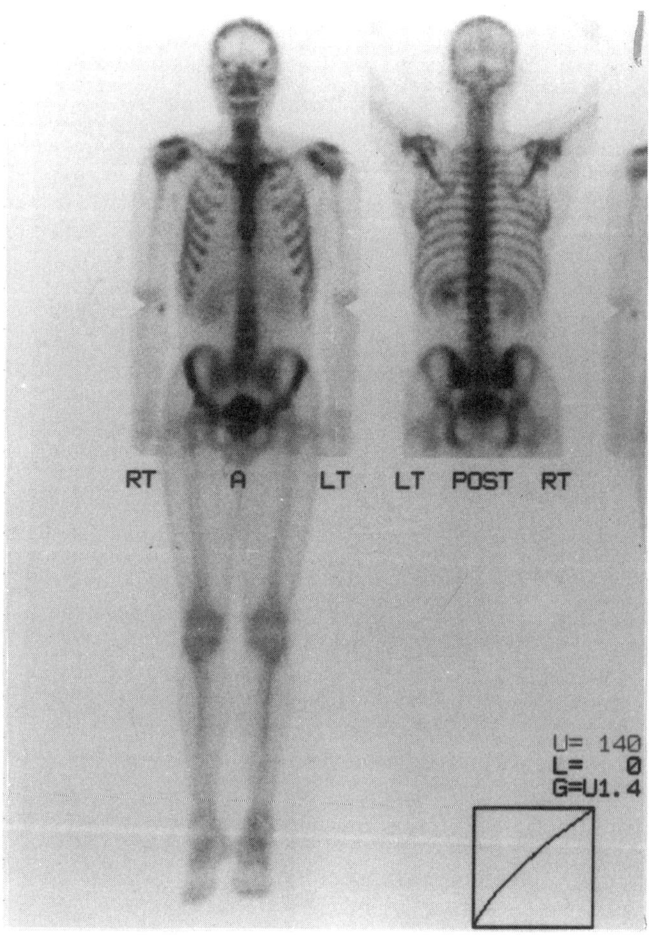

Figure 13.3 Normal adult bone image obtained with ^{99m}Tc-medronate. Courtesy of Baptist Memorial Hospital East, Memphis, TN.

SPECT Imaging

The use of SPECT for bone imaging is a specialized type of spot imaging. SPECT is not appropriate for total-body imaging but can be very useful for imaging limited areas of the skeleton, where bony structures are superimposed on one another. These areas include the knees, hips, lumbar spine and facial bones. Abnormalities not seen on planar imaging are frequently demonstrated with SPECT imaging. A low-energy, all-purpose, parallel-hole collimator is recommended. The detector/patient distance should be minimized. This distance will vary, depending on the area of the body being imaged, since the detector must be able to travel around the patient, unimpeded, for 360° (see Chapter 5).

IMAGE FINDINGS

Normal Tracer Distribution

The radiopharmaceutical is normally taken up symmetrically throughout the skeleton (Fig. 13-3). Areas of normally increased activity include the sacroiliac joints, anterior iliac crests, sternum, nasopharyngeal area, shoulder joints and spine. In children, increased tracer concentration at epiphyseal plates of the long bones and costochondral junctions is due to increased bone production (Fig. 13-4). Conversely, overall skeletal uptake in the elderly is lower than in younger people. Activity in the kidneys is usually less than bone activity but can vary and may even indicate certain types of renal disease. Tracer accumulation can also occur in normal female breast tissue, as well as in certain diseases of the breast.

Abnormal Tracer Distribution

Abnormal tracer distribution can include areas of increased tracer accumulation within the skeleton itself or outside in soft tissue. Increased blood flow and/or bone production are responsible for increased tracer concentration and can occur in the following instances: neoplastic disease, both primary and metastatic; bone trauma; inflammatory processes (e.g., osteomyelitis); metabolic bone disease (e.g., Paget's disease); arthritic changes.

Extraosseous activity is sometimes seen in the following sites: renal abnormalities; soft-tissue inflammation (e.g., surgical sites); neoplastic masses; female breasts; acute myocardial infarction.

Photopenic areas (areas of decreased tracer accumulation) are usually related to diminished blood flow to the area or to complete destruction or replacement of normal bone tissue. The following conditions may result in photopenic areas on images: radiation injury as a result of therapy; bone cyst; disuse atrophy of an extremity; avascular necrosis; artifacts (e.g., pacemaker, prosthesis).

THREE-PHASE/FOUR-PHASE BONE IMAGING

When an inflammatory process, such as osteomyelitis, is suspected, dynamic or multiple-phase bone imaging may be helpful to the physician in making a differential diagnosis. In this technique, the patient is first positioned under the gamma camera with the affected area in the field of view. The standard tracer dose is administered as a bolus injection while dynamic images are acquired beginning at the time of injection and continuing for about 1 min. Immediate static images are then acquired, followed by delayed images at 2–4 hr. The fourth phase consists of 24-hr delay images.

Both cellulitis and osteomyelitis demonstrate increased activity on the early images. With osteomyelitis, however, the tracer concentration persists throughout the delayed images.

TECHNICAL CONSIDERATIONS

Although bone imaging is one of the simplest and most frequently performed nuclear medicine imaging procedures, technical errors sometimes occur. These errors, discussed below, result in a variety of image artifacts.

Extravasation of the tracer at the injection site may be construed as pathology or obscure bony pathology underlying the area of infiltration. Additional images of the affected area may be helpful in confirming the cause of the increased accumulation and in ruling out skeletal disease. Furthermore, there may appear to be overall decreased activity concentration in the bones if a significant amount of the tracer is not administered intravenously. Imaging times may need to be extended in this instance to achieve adequate counting statistics.

Since the tracer is excreted from the body through the urinary tract, radioactive urine contamination is possible with young children or older incontinent patients. Equipment should be protected and the patient should be checked for contaminated garments or linens before imaging begins.

It is important that patients void immediately prior to imaging the pelvis. Excess activity in the bladder can obscure pelvic structures. Images of the pelvis should be obtained first, if the spot view technique is being used. Separate spot images of the pelvis may be necessary when whole-body imaging is performed.

Any attenuating materials such as jewelry, belt buckles, removable prostheses, pocket contents or ECG leads, could cause a photopenic area on the image. Such materials should be removed from the patient prior to imaging.

Close attention to precise patient positioning is essential. Contralateral sides of bony structures (e.g., iliac crests, shoulder joints) must be positioned at the same angle and at the same distance from the detector. Failure to do so may cause one side to appear to have a greater tracer concentration than the other. Asymmetry of contralateral sides may be falsely interpreted as an abnormality. It is equally important to include all areas of interest on the bone images. A problem sometimes arises when certain parts of the skeleton, usually the arms, cannot be positioned within the field of view during whole-body imaging. Greater care should be taken to include the entire skeleton in the field of view or additional spot images of the excluded parts of the skeleton should be obtained to avoid missing any abnormalities.

An unexpected pattern of tracer distribution may indicate improper preparation of the radiopharmaceutical and can degrade the quality of bone images. Excess free

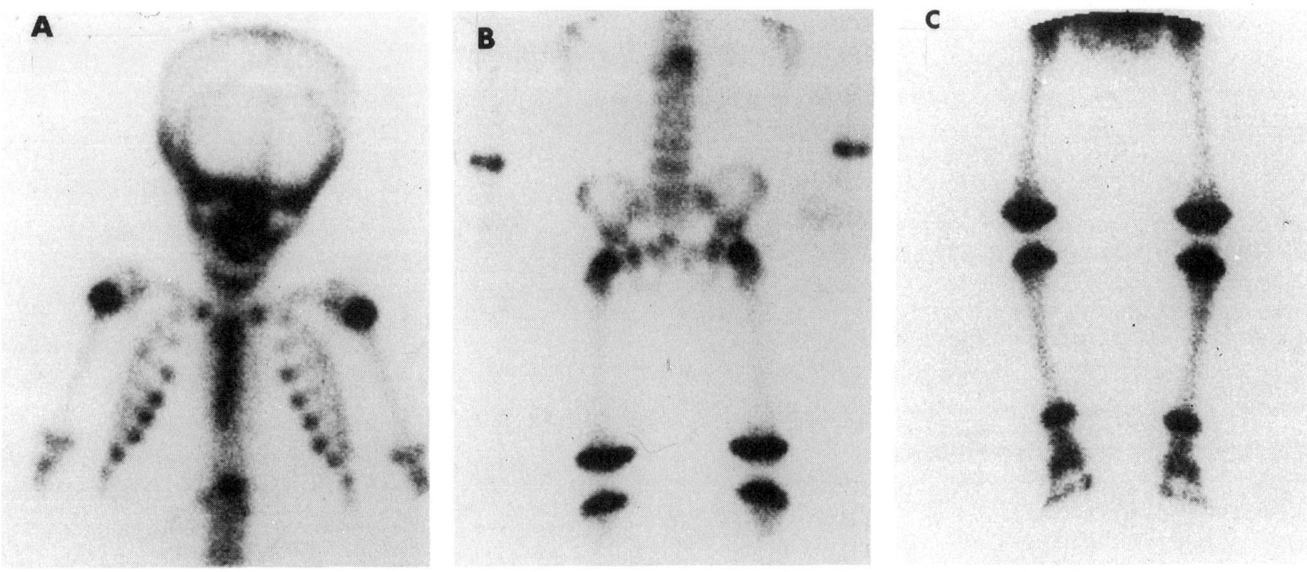

Figure 13.4 Total-body bone images of a young child. Note areas of normally increased tracer accumulation in children in the epiphyseal plates and costochondral junctions. Courtesy of The Children's Hospital of Alabama, Birmingham, AL.

pertechnetate appears as tracer concentration in the thyroid, salivary glands and stomach. Liver uptake or increased soft-tissue and kidney uptake can also be indicators of radiopharmaceutical problems. Adequate and timely radiopharmaceutical quality control is necessary to identify formulation problems before the preparation is administered to patients (see Chapter 3).

REFERENCES

1. Christian PE, Coleman RE. The skeletal system. In: Bernier DR, Christian PE, Langan JK, eds. *Nuclear medicine technology and techniques,* 3rd ed. St. Louis: Mosby Year-Book; 1994:361–385.
2. Collier BD, Sodee DB, Robinson RG. Bone. In: Early PJ, Sodee DB. *Principles and practice of nuclear medicine,* 2nd ed. St. Louis: Mosby Year-Book; 1995:339–369.
3. English RJ, Brown SE. *SPECT: a primer,* 2nd ed. Reston, VA: Society of Nuclear Medicine; 1990:63, 99–100, 103–106.
4. Hladik WB III, Saha GB, Study KT, eds. *Essentials of nuclear medicine science.* Baltimore: Williams and Wilkins; 1987.
5. Nagle CE, Morayati SJ, Carichner S, et al. The whole-body bone scan? Case report. *J Nucl Med Technol* 1988;16:15–16.
6. Thrall JH, Ziessman HA. *Nuclear medicine—the requisites.* St. Louis: Mosby Year-Book; 1995:93–128.

14 Inflammatory Processes and Tumor Imaging

Ann M. Steves

GALLIUM IMAGING

Gallium-67-citrate has been used to image both neoplastic and inflammatory diseases. Although a variety of processes have been suggested, the exact mechanism by which gallium concentrates in tumor or infection sites is not known.

Gallium is useful for assessing the extent of malignancies such as bronchogenic carcinoma, Hodgkin's disease, lymphoma and melanoma and for determining the effectiveness of therapy for these types of cancers. This agent can be used to demonstrate sites of inflammation in conditions such as sarcoidosis, osteomyelitis and pneumocystis pneumonia. Gallium imaging also serves as a screening procedure when occult intra-abdominal abscess is suspected.

Clinical Procedure

There is no special preparation prior to administration of the radiopharmaceutical. Knowledge of the clinical indication for a particular study will assist the technologist in determining the areas of interest to be imaged. The amount of ^{67}Ga-citrate administered ranges from 2 to 10 mCi (74–370 MBq), depending on the pathology being imaged.

Imaging is performed 6–72 hr after intravenous injection of the tracer. Earlier imaging times are favored for abscess detection, while later imaging is preferred for neoplastic disease. Planar or tomographic techniques may be performed.

Gallium-67 has a range of photon energies (93, 184, 296 and 388 keV gamma emissions), so an appropriate choice of collimator is critical to minimize scatter and septal penetration and to obtain optimal resolution. Depending on the individual collimator rating, a medium- or high-energy, parallel-hole collimator typically is used. If the scintillation camera can be set to accept multiple photopeaks, acquiring photons of two or three energies (93 and 184 keV or 93, 184 and 296 keV) decreases imaging time.

Image Findings

The normal distribution of ^{67}Ga-citrate includes tracer uptake in the following areas: nasopharynx, lacrimal glands, salivary glands, bony thorax (ribs, sternum, clavicle, scapulae), external genitalia, liver, kidney (up to 48 hr postinjection), colon contents, pelvis (lumbar spine, sacrum, ileum, ischium) and in children, active epiphyses of long bones.

Liver uptake is intense so the liver is the most prominent structure seen in a normal gallium image (Fig. 14-1). Since the kidneys excrete 20%–30% of the administered dose during the first 24 hr, renal activity is normally visualized up to 48 hr after tracer administration. After 48 hr, persistent renal activity is indicative of disease.

Changes in biodistribution may result from blood transfusions, chemotherapy or iron therapy. These changes cause increased gallium concentration throughout the skeleton. Recent trauma may result in areas of increased uptake.

Technical Considerations

Since gallium is excreted initially through the kidneys, patients who are being imaged earlier than 48 hr should be asked to void before the pelvis is imaged. Gallium is also excreted through the gastrointestinal tract. Images of patients taken after 48 hr postinjection will usually show a concentration of ^{67}Ga within the intestinal contents, particularly within the large bowel. Areas of increased tracer concentration within the bowel may be mistaken for disease. Laxatives or enemas may be prescribed to help bowel clearance. Bowel preparations are contraindicated in patients with diarrhea.

Radiographic examinations of the gastrointestinal tract performed with barium should be scheduled after gallium imaging.

INDIUM-111-LEUKOCYTE IMAGING

Leukocytes, which are white blood cells, accumulate in areas of infection. Labeling these cells with a radiotracer permits detection of infection sites using nuclear medicine imaging techniques.

Indium-111-leukocytes do not normally accumulate in the abdomen, as does ^{67}Ga-citrate. For this reason, ^{111}In-labeled leukocytes are the preferred tracer for the detection of intra-abdominal infection.

Leukocyte Labeling

White cells are isolated from a sample of the patient's blood. Indium-111-oxine is added to the leukocytes; it diffuses into the cells and binds to components within them. The labeling procedure takes 2 hr (Fig. 14-2). Strict aseptic technique must be maintained, since the labeled cells will be reinjected into the patient. Depending on the method used to tag the cells, a white cell labeling efficiency of 70%–90% can usually be achieved. Patients who are taking steroids,

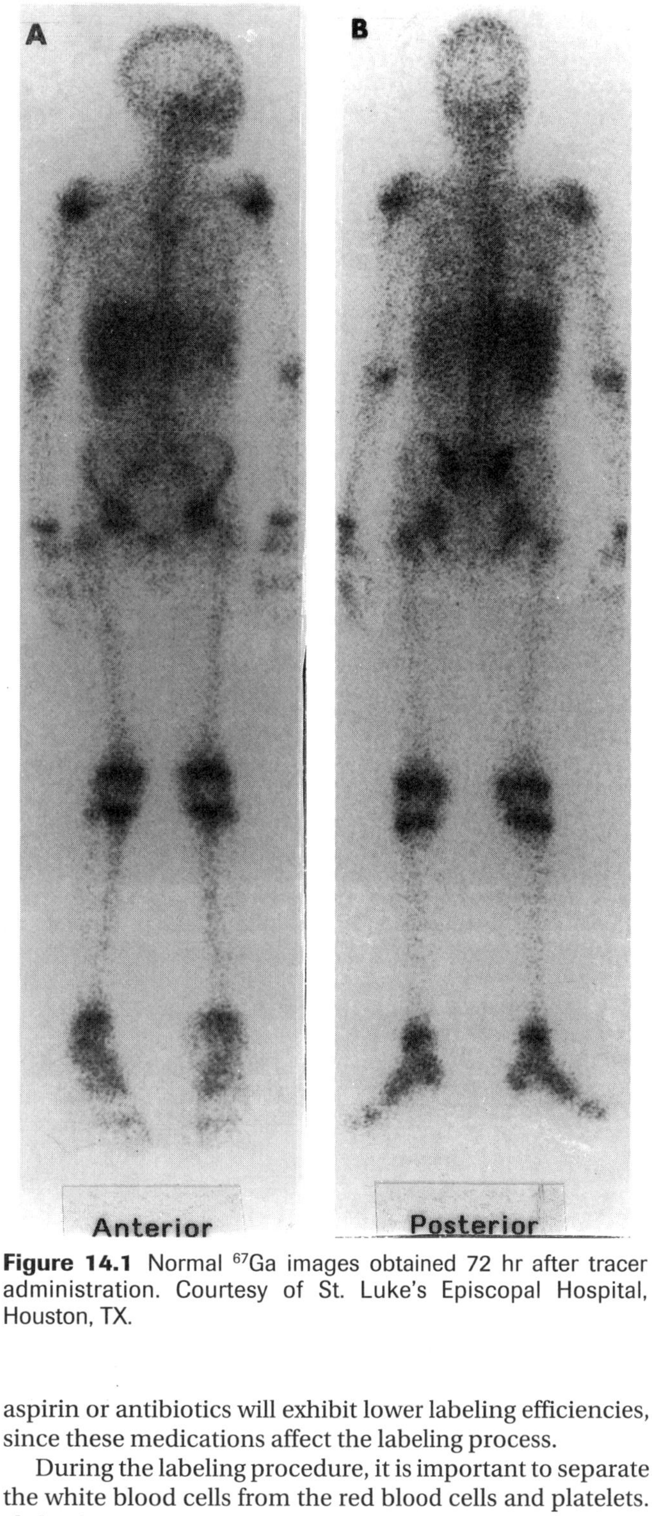

Figure 14.1 Normal ^{67}Ga images obtained 72 hr after tracer administration. Courtesy of St. Luke's Episcopal Hospital, Houston, TX.

aspirin or antibiotics will exhibit lower labeling efficiencies, since these medications affect the labeling process.

During the labeling procedure, it is important to separate the white blood cells from the red blood cells and platelets. If platelets are tagged along with the leukocytes, a false-positive image may result because platelets concentrate in sites of thrombosis, rather than in areas of infection. Use of the proper centrifuge speed when separating the various types of cells minimizes platelet labeling.

Patients with extremely low white cell counts may not be able to provide sufficient white cells for labeling. In such cases, donor cells may be tagged.

Imaging

Imaging is performed at 4 and 24 hr after the labeled leukocytes are administered to the patient. If the infection site is unknown, anterior and posterior views of the head, abdomen, pelvis and chest, as well as views of the extremities should be obtained.

Indium-111 emits two gamma photons with energies of 173 and 247 keV, respectively. Therefore, a medium- or high-energy, parallel-hole collimator should be used. Acquisition of photons from both photopeaks decreases imaging time.

Image Findings

A normal image demonstrates tracer activity in the spleen, liver and bone marrow. The most intense activity occurs in the spleen; there is less activity in the liver and an even smaller amount of activity in the bone marrow. Any other areas of tracer uptake represent infection (Fig. 14-3).

Technical Considerations

Damage to the labeled leukocytes can be avoided by injecting them into the patient slowly through a large-gauge needle. Extravasation of the labeled cells will compromise image quality and may result in a false-negative image if insufficient leukocytes are administered intravenously.

TECHNETIUM-99m-LEUKOCYTE IMAGING

There are many advantages to using ^{99m}Tc as the radioactive tag. Today's gamma cameras are designed to work best with ^{99m}Tc's photon energy. More radioactivity may be administered which results in shorter acquisition times, better quality images and lower absorbed radiation dose to the patient. For these reasons, a method to label white blood cells with ^{99m}Tc had long been pursued.

Leukocytes may be labeled with ^{99m}Tc using ^{99m}Tc-labeled exametazime (HMPAO). Exametazime is available as a radiopharmaceutical kit that is reconstituted with [^{99m}Tc]pertechnetate. The radiolabeled exametazime is then added to white cells isolated from a sample of the patient's whole blood. The procedure is very similar to the ^{111}In labeling process shown in Figure 14-2, but in Step 3, ^{99m}Tc-exametazime is added to the white cell button in place of ^{111}In-oxine. When ^{99m}Tc-exametazime is prepared for white cell labeling, the stabilizer, methylene blue, supplied in the radiopharmaceutical kit is not added to the preparation.

The imaging protocol is similar to that for ^{111}In-WBC imaging. With ^{99m}Tc-leukocytes, however, a low-energy, all-purpose or high-resolution, parallel-hole collimator or pinhole collimator should be used. SPECT imaging is also possible with ^{99m}Tc-leukocytes.

It has been suggested that 4-hr imaging be performed if abdominal or retroperitoneal inflammation is suspected. Early imaging will avoid visualization of renal, biliary and intestinal excretion of the tracer. Likewise, 24-hr imaging has been suggested for visualization of inflammation in the thoracic cavity. Blood pooling in the chambers of the heart and lung uptake will have diminished by 24 hr. Osteomyelitis in the extremities may be demonstrated as early as 2 hr postinjection of ^{99m}Tc-leukocytes.

TUMOR IMAGING

OncoScint® CR/OV

OncoScint® CR/OV (Cytogen Corp., Princeton, NJ) (satumomab pendetide) is a monoclonal antibody to the tumor antigen TAG-72 that is associated with ovarian and colorectal cancer. After the antibody has been tagged with ^{111}In and injected into the patient, it binds to the tumor antigen at the site of the cancer. OncoScint® CR/OV is not used to diagnose ovarian or colorectal cancer, but rather to determine the location and extent of extrahepatic metastatic disease in patients with known disease.

OncoScint® is provided in kit form for labeling with 5–6 mCi (185–222 MBq) ^{111}In-chloride. Indium-111-chloride is first mixed with a buffering solution. The buffered ^{111}In is then added to the antibody. The mixture is incubated for 30 min. Since the antibody is a protein that can form particles, the preparation is filtered before intravenous administration to the patient.

No patient preparation is required prior to tracer administration. The tracer is infused slowly over a 5-min period. Adverse reactions are rare (occurring in less than 4% of patients), with the most frequent symptoms being fever, chills, hypotension, hypertension, itching, rash and sweating. Since monoclonal antibodies are produced from mouse spleen cells, the patient's immune system may identify the monoclonal antibody as a foreign protein. The patient's immune system then begins to produce antibodies against the monoclonal antibody. This response is called HAMA, human anti-murine (mouse) antibody. A HAMA response increases the possibility of an allergic response to a second administration of monoclonal antibody and decreases the likelihood of a second successful imaging procedure. For this reason, patients receiving a second administration of OncoScint® must be tested for this antibody before tracer administration.

Imaging may be performed as early as 2 days or as late as 5 days following tracer administration. Prior to imaging, a bowel preparation is recommended to remove tracer in the gastrointestinal tract that may obscure tumor uptake. Immediately before imaging, the patient should empty the urinary bladder and/or colostomy bag, as necessary. To aid the physician in interpretation, the technologist should note any recent surgical incisions or colostomy sites. Anterior and posterior planar images are obtained over the chest, abdomen and pelvis. SPECT images may be performed as indicated by information noted on the planar views.

Normal biodistribution of OncoScint® includes tracer uptake in the liver (greatest uptake), bone, blood pool in the heart (earlier images), colon, male genitalia, gluteal folds and the great vessels.

OctreoScan®

OctreoScan® (Mallinckrodt, St. Louis, MO) (^{111}In-pentetreotide) is a form of octreotide. Octreotide is an analog of the hormone somatostatin. OctreoScan® binds to somatostatin receptors on the surface of cells, concentrating in tumors with a high density of receptor sites. It is a peptide, which is the portion of an amino acid molecule that naturally binds to receptors on the cell surface.

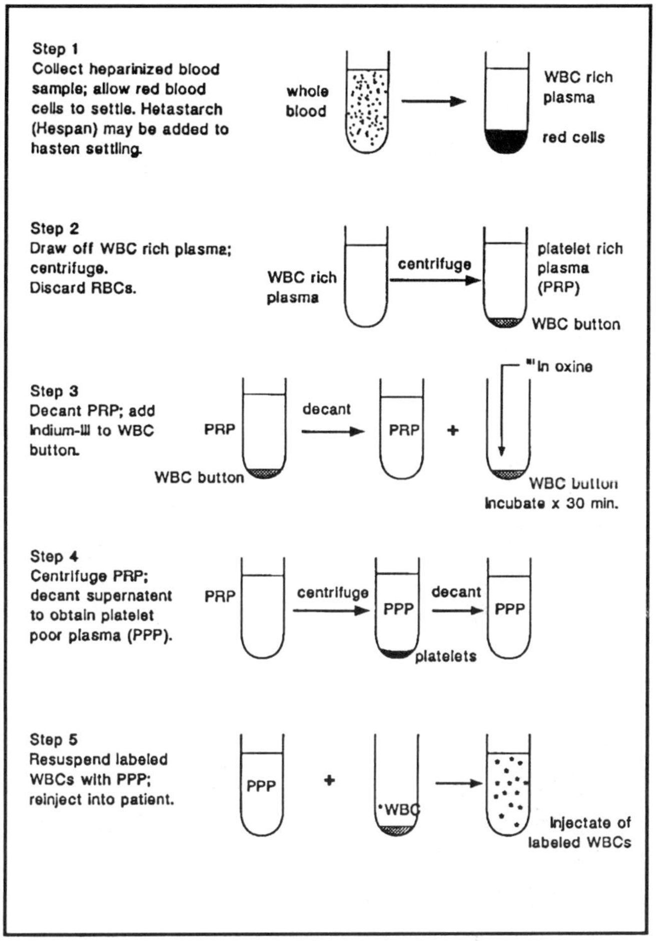

Figure 14.2 Leukocyte labeling technique.

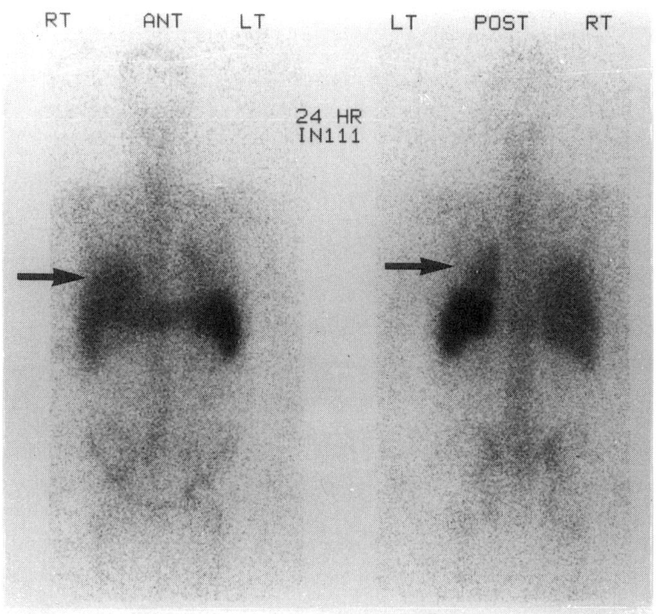

Figure 14.3 Infection in lower lobes of both lungs is visualized on ^{111}In-leukocyte images. Courtesy of Baptist Memorial Hospital East, Memphis, TN.

Somatostatin is a hormone concentrated in the hypothalamus, cerebral cortex, brain stem, gastrointestinal tract and pancreas. Its functions include neurotransmission and inhibition of the release of growth hormone, insulin, glucagon, gastrin and hormone production by certain types of tumors. Receptor sites for somatostatin are located in the anterior pituitary gland, pancreatic islet cells, lymphocytes and certain types of tumors (brain, breast, lung, lymphoma).

OctreoScan® is approved for localizing primary and metastatic tumors originating from neuroendocrine cells, cells that contain somatostatin receptor sites. This includes many types of tumors such as pituitary and endocrine tumors, paraganglioma, medullary thyroid carcinoma, carcinoids and small-cell lung cancer.

OctreoScan® is provided in kit form for labeling with 3.3 mCi (122 MBq) ^{111}In-chloride. Indium-111-chloride is mixed with the pentetreotide and incubated for 30 min at or below 77°F (25°C).

It is recommended that a mild laxative be given to the patient 24 hr before tracer administration and continue for 48 hr to remove any radioactivity in the gastrointestinal tract. The patient should void immediately before imaging because the tracer is eliminated from the body primarily through the genitourinary system. Imaging can begin 24–48 hr after tracer administration. Since the purpose of the procedure is to visualize the unknown primary site of the cancer or to demonstrate the extent of the disease, anterior and posterior whole-body imaging should be performed. Normal distribution of OctreoScan® includes tracer uptake in the pituitary and thyroid glands, liver, spleen and bladder and bowel (routes of tracer excretion).

Fewer than 1% of the patients in clinical trials with this agent have experienced any adverse effects; these effects were transient and mild because OctreoScan® is a peptide, not an antibody, and no HAMA effect occurs.

REFERENCES

1. Alazraki NP. Gallium-67 imaging in infection. In: Early PJ, Sodee DB. *Principles and practice of nuclear medicine,* 2nd ed. St. Louis: Mosby Year-Book; 1995:702–713.
2. Baker WJ, Datz FL. Preparation and clinical utility of ^{111}In-labeled leukocytes. *J Nucl Med Technol* 1984;12:131–136.
3. Ceretec® (technetium-99m exametazime injection). Package insert. Arlington Heights, IL: Amersham Healthcare; April 1995.
4. Kao CH, Wang YL, Wang SJ. Elution analysis and normal biodistribution of technetium-99m-HMPAO-labeled white blood cells. *J Nucl Med Technol* 1992;20:224–227.
5. Kipper MS, Williams RJ. Indium-111-white blood cell imaging. *Clin Nucl Med* 1983;8:449–455.
6. Krenning EP, Kwekkeboom DJ, Oei Y, et al. Octreotide agent shows peptide imaging potential. *Diagnostic Imaging* 1993;88–91.
7. OctreoScan® (kit for the preparation of indium-111-pentetreotide). Package insert. St. Louis, MO: Mallinckrodt Medical, Inc.; August 1994.
8. OncoScint® CR/OV (kit for the preparation of indium-111 satumomab pendetide). Package insert. Princeton, NJ: Cytogen Corp.; 1993.
9. Preston DF. Inflammatory process and tumor imaging. In: Bernier DR, Christian PE, Langan JK, eds. *Nuclear medicine technology and techniques,* 3rd ed. St. Louis: Mosby Year-Book; 1994:402–417.
10. Preston DF. Indium-111 label in inflammation and neoplasm imaging. In: Early PJ, Sodee DB. *Principles and practice of nuclear medicine,* 2nd ed. St. Louis: Mosby Year-Book; 1995:714–724.
11. Serafini AN. From monoclonal antibodies to peptides and molecular recognition units: an overview. *J Nucl Med* 1993;34(suppl):533–536.
12. Steffel FG, Rao SA. Rapid and simple methods for labeling white blood cells and platelets with indium-111-oxine. *J Nucl Med Technol* 1987;15:61–65.
13. Trembath L, Collier BD, Schulte WJ. A practical approach to monoclonal antibody imaging. *J Nucl Med Technol* 1993;21:171–176.
14. Wahl RL. Radiolabeled monoclonal antibodies. In: Early PJ, Sodee DB. *Principles and practice of nuclear medicine,* 2nd ed. St. Louis: Mosby Year-Book; 1995:678–701.

15 In Vivo Nonimaging Techniques

Helen H. Drew

Many nuclear medicine procedures are performed in which the patient receives radioactive material but is not imaged. Instead, the amount of radioactivity concentrated in a particular organ is quantified using an external counting device, usually an uptake probe. Alternatively, a blood or urine sample is collected from the patient and counted in a scintillation well counter. Diagnostic procedures such as these are referred to as in vivo nonimaging techniques.

HEMATOLOGIC STUDIES

Circulating blood is a complex mixture made up of the plasma compartment and the cellular compartment. Plasma is a watery fluid containing various ions and inorganic and organic molecules such as sodium (Na^+), potassium (K^+), chloride ion (Cl^-), magnesium (Mg^{++}), bicarbonate (HCO_3^-), calcium (Ca^{++}) and sugar. Plasma proteins, such as albumin, immunoglobulins, transport proteins, lipoproteins and clotting proteins, make up the solid portion and exert an osmotic force, which decreases the amount of fluid lost through the capillary pores.

When blood is collected with an anticoagulant (a substance that prevents normal clotting), the whole blood separates into plasma and the cellular components. If the blood is collected without an anticoagulant, the clot formed contains most of the cells and the coagulation proteins, leaving behind a straw-colored fluid called serum.

Red blood cells or erythrocytes make up the largest volume of the cellular compartment, about 5×10^6 per mm^3 of blood. Red cells are biconcave disks and measure 6 to 8 microns in diameter. The primary function of the red cell is to transport oxygen to the body's tissues and carry carbon dioxide, the byproduct of metabolism, back to the lungs for elimination from the body.

Red cells are produced from a bone marrow stem cell, which is initially a pro-erythroblast with the ability to synthesize hemoglobin. The cell matures into a normoblast and after extruding its nucleus becomes a reticulocyte. At this stage, the reticulocyte enters the peripheral circulation. The level of tissue oxygenation regulates red cell production. Tissue hypoxia stimulates erythropoietin production from the kidneys, which in turn stimulates bone marrow red cell production. Therefore, obese patients or those with cardiac failure or severe lung disease, which cause tissue hypoxia, exhibit increased red cell production. Red blood cells have a normal life span of 120 days; old red cells are destroyed primarily by the spleen.

Included in the cellular compartment, but not easily measured, are leukocytes and platelets. Leukocytes constitute a major defense system within our bodies and can be divided into granulocytes, lymphocytes and monocytes. These cells are present in a volume of 5×10^3 per mm^3 blood. The primary function of platelets is blood coagulation and clot retraction. Platelets also participate in hemostasis and in maintaining integrity of blood vessel walls by aggregating and sealing wall defects. Platelets are present in a volume of 3.5×10^5 per mm^3 blood. Each of these cell types, red blood cells, leukocytes and platelets, have different pathways within the open circulatory system.

A common method used to determine whether a patient has a normal number of red cells is to perform a hematocrit. This is done by placing a well mixed sample of anticoagulated blood into a capillary tube and centrifuging the tube for an appropriate period of time and g force. By definition, a hematocrit is the volume of packed red cells expressed as a percentage of the total volume (Fig. 15-1). When hematocrits are performed on normal blood, red cells make up the majority of the volume of packed cells. The grayish layer just above the packed red cells is made up of white cells; just above that layer is a cream-colored minute layer representing platelets. Readings of venous hematocrits, performed on individuals with normal blood, show red cell volumes of 35%–48%.

A simple hematocrit reading can sometimes yield misleading results when estimating red cell volume or plasma volume. If the patient is dehydrated and has a decreased plasma volume, the hematocrit will be falsely elevated. If the patient has an increased plasma volume, the hematocrit will be falsely low. Direct measurement of red cell volume and plasma volume is the only method to determine these values.

Total Blood Volume Determination

Determining total red cell volume (TRCV) and total plasma volume (TPV) through use of radiolabeled blood components is an accepted and widely practiced method performed by the nuclear medicine laboratory. Estimations of total blood volume (TBV) are clinically useful in the diagnosis and management of polycythemia or when changes in the venous hematocrit fail to reflect accurately changes in TRCV or TPV. When the venous hematocrit is increased, TRCV measurements distinguish absolute increases in red cell volume from decreases in plasma volume. In cases of gross splenomegaly, red cells pool in the spleen and increases in the plasma volume may give misleading venous hematocrit readings.

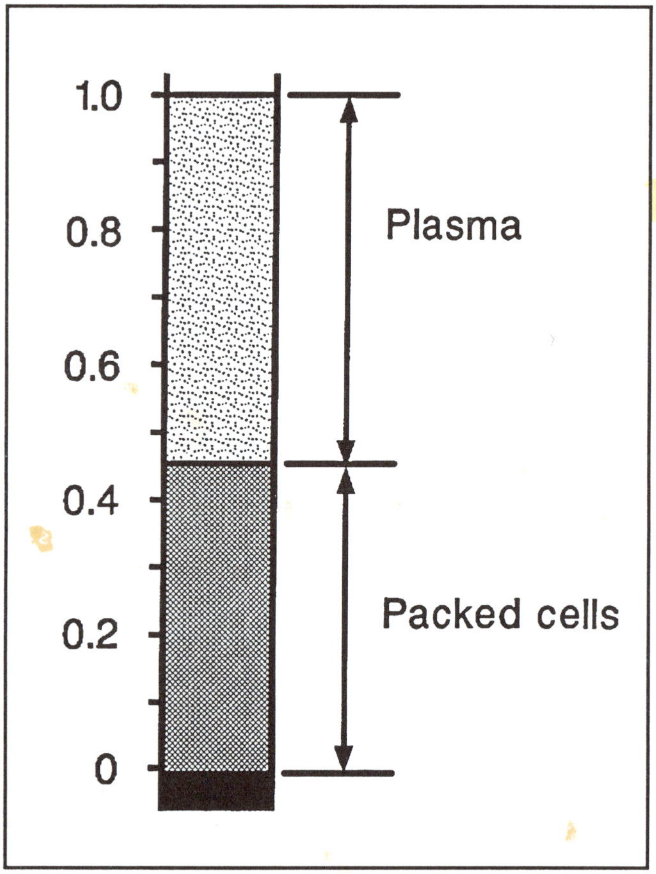

Figure 15.1 Hematocrit determination.

TBV measurements are calculated using the isotope dilution principle equation.

$$V = \frac{Q}{C},$$

where, V equals volume, Q equals dose administered in counts per minute and C equals concentration of dose after dilution in counts per minute. The larger the volume into which the label is mixed, the lower the counts in the sample withdrawn and, conversely, the smaller the volume, the higher the counts in the sample. The isotope dilution principle is only true when working with a closed system, where no radiopharmaceutical is allowed to leak out of the system being measured. Also, the volume of the unknown must not change significantly during the measurement. In most cases, red cell volume measurements are performed in a closed system using radiolabeled red blood cells.

Plasma Volume Determination

Plasma volume measurements are performed using radiolabeled albumin. Albumin does not remain within the intravascular space but diffuses rapidly into the extravascular compartments. Since this vascular space is now an open system, use of the closed system isotope dilution principle for calculations would cause errors in the plasma volume result. If the injected radiopharmaceutical leaves the open system at a slower rate than the uniform mixing rate within that system and samples are taken only after mixing has been completed, the volume can be obtained by an extrapolation procedure.

Plasma Volume Technique

Materials. The patient is administered ^{125}I-human serum albumin, 10 μCi (370 kBq), contained in 1.5 ml. Not more than 2% of the radioactivity can be in the free form. The free form is removed from the intravascular space more rapidly than the labeled albumin, which causes overestimation of the plasma volume. Technetium-99m-human serum albumin can also be used but labeling efficiency at time of injection must be performed and must be at least 98% bound. All equipment for collecting blood samples and injecting the radiopharmaceutical must be prepared in advance. This equipment includes gloves, 23-gauge needles, syringes and labeled heparinized blood collection tubes.

Patient Preparation. The patient should be at rest and supine for at least 15 to 20 min prior to starting the study. Plasma volume decreases when a person is standing because venous pressure increases in the legs and water moves from the intravascular to the extracellular nonvascular space.

Tracer Administration/Sample Collection. Prior to tracer administration, collect a background heparinized blood sample. Inject the radiolabeled albumin intravascularly, taking care to avoid infiltration of the dose. The exact volume injected must be known for the calculations; therefore, weighing the syringe on an analytical balance before and after injection is recommended. The difference between the preinjection and postinjection syringe weights is equivalent to the volume injected. Record the exact time of injection. Do not rinse the syringe with blood. Three 10-ml heparinized blood samples are collected at exactly 10, 20 and 30 min postinjection from a venous site different from the injection site.

Sample Handling. Centrifuge the samples and pipette 1-ml aliquots of plasma into labeled counting tubes. Prepare a standard by diluting a duplicate dose (10 μCi ^{125}I-human serum albumin in 1.5 ml) into a 500-ml volumetric flask. Again, the exact volume must be known, so the syringe should be weighed. Do not rinse the standard syringe in the water. Bring the volume in the flask up to the line using distilled water. Mix well by inverting and shaking the flask. Pipette duplicate 1-ml aliquots of the standard into labeled counting tubes.

Counting. Adjust the pulse-height analyzer of the scintillation spectrometer to count ^{125}I. Count each 1-ml sample for a time period that is long enough to assure a counting error of no greater than 1%. After counting, adjust all samples to net counts per minute by subtracting patient background from the patient samples and room background from the standard samples.

Calculations. The net counts per minute of each postinjection sample is plotted against time on semi-logarithmic graph paper. The best straight line is drawn through these points (Fig. 15-2). The zero-time activity is estimated by extrapolation; this value is used to calculate the total plasma volume (TPV) using the equation:

$$TPV = \frac{\text{volume injected} \times \text{net standard activity}}{\text{net patient activity at time zero}},$$

where TPV = total plasma volume.

Sources of Error. If the radiopharmaceutical is infiltrated, an erroneously high result will be obtained. If the patient contains a radiotracer from a previous diagnostic test and the count rate of the postinjection samples is not corrected for this contamination, an erroneously low result will be obtained. Inaccurate measurement of the injected volume and the standard volume can cause errors in the results.

Red Cell Volume Determination

Radiolabeling of red blood cells for red cell volume measurement is referred to as random labeling. The radionuclide labels erythrocytes circulating in the peripheral blood. This process labels all cells in the sample, from the youngest to the oldest erythrocytes or erythrocytes of random age.

The most commonly used radionuclides for random red cell labeling are [^{99m}Tc]pertechnetate and [^{51}Cr]sodium chromate. Due to the high elution rate of [^{99m}Tc]pertechnetate from the labeled red cells, this tracer is not recommended for red cell volume determinations.

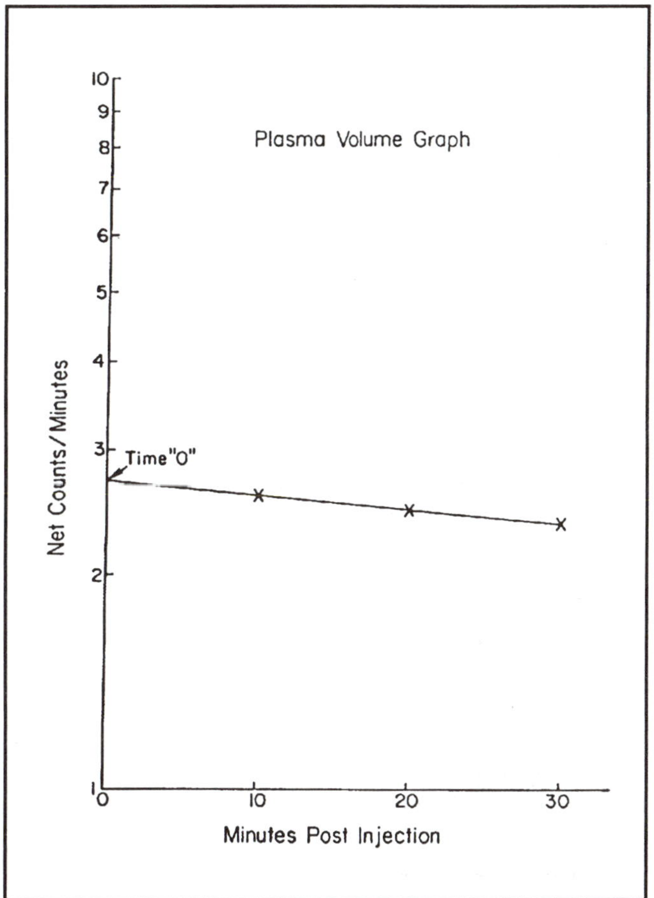

Figure 15.2 Extrapolation graph used to determine zero-time activity to calculate plasma volume.

Ascorbic Acid Method for Labeling Red Cells

Ten milliliters of whole venous blood is collected from the patient into a 20-ml syringe containing 2 ml of the anticoagulant acid-citrate-dextrose (ACD) solution. Heparin and ethylenediaminetetraacetic acid (EDTA) are unsatisfactory anticoagulants for use in this labeling procedure. After inverting to mix, transfer blood into a sterile vial. Add 30 μCi (1.11 MBq) ^{51}Cr to the vial. Gently mix and incubate for 30 min at room temperature. During this time, 80%–95% of the chromate ion is transported across the red cell membrane and binds to the beta chain of the hemoglobulin molecule. The hexavalent chromate ion is reduced to a trivalent chromic ion. Fifty milligrams of ascorbic acid are then added to reduce the free chromate to chromic ion. This prevents extracellular chromate from labeling circulating red cells following reinjection of the labeled red cell mixture. The reinjection mixture will contain both red cell-bound and free ^{51}Cr.

Wash Method for Labeling Red Cells

Ten milliliters of whole venous blood are collected from the patient into a 20-ml syringe containing 2 ml ACD anticoagulant. After mixing, transfer blood into a sterile vial. Centrifuge this mixture at 1000 to 1500 g for 5 to 10 min. Remove and discard the supernatant plasma, taking care not to remove any red cells. Add 30 μCi (1.11 MBq) ^{51}Cr to the packed red cells and mix gently. Allow this mixture to stand for 30 min at room temperature. Wash the labeled red cells in 4 to 5 ml isotonic saline, then centrifuge at 1,000 g for 5 to 10 min. Remove the supernatant saline, resuspend the labeled red cells in saline and recentrifuge. After the last centrifugation, resuspend the red cells in saline to the original volume. This method removes all of the free chromate ion so that the reinjection mixture contains only red cell-bound ^{51}Cr.

Red Cell Volume Technique

Materials. Use red cells labeled with 10–20 μCi (370–740 kBq) [^{51}Cr]sodium chromate. The exact volume must be known. Therefore, the syringe should be weighed on an analytical balance before and after injection. Equipment for collecting blood samples and injecting the radiopharmaceutical must be prepared in advance: this includes gloves, 20-gauge needles and heparinized blood collection tubes.

Patient Preparation. Patient should be at rest and supine for 15–20 min prior to the start of the study. A patient background sample must be collected.

Tracer Administration/Sample Collection. Inject intravenously 5 ml ^{51}Cr-labeled red cells, taking care not to infiltrate any of the dose. Record the exact time of injection. Do not rinse the dose syringe with the patient's blood. After waiting a sufficient length of time (usually 10–20 min) to ensure complete mixing of the labeled red cells within the circulation, withdraw 10 ml blood into a heparinized tube from a vein other than the one used for tracer injection. In seriously ill patients, a delay of up to 30 min for complete mixing may be necessary. For this reason, it is recommended that the postinjection sample be drawn at 30 min.

In certain disease states, such as severe polycythemia and splenomegaly, complete mixing of the labeled red cells may be greatly delayed. In such instances, serial postinjection samples at 30, 60 and 90 min should be collected.

Sample Handling. Perform a microhematocrit determination on the stock-labeled red cell mixture and on each postinjection blood sample.

Prepare a standard from the stock-labeled red cells by diluting 2 ml of the labeled cells into a 100-ml volumetric flask. Again, the exact volume must be known. Therefore, the syringe should be weighed pre- and postdilution on an analytical balance. Do not rinse the standard syringe into the water. Bring the volume in the flask up to the line using distilled water. Mix well by inverting and shaking. Pipette duplicate 1-ml aliquots of the standard into counting tubes labeled "standard whole blood." Pipette 1 ml whole blood from each postinjection sample into a counting tube labeled "sample whole blood."

If the ascorbic acid labeling method was used, centrifuge the remaining stock-labeled red cell mixture and each postinjection sample at 1500 g for 10 min. Pipette 1 ml plasma supernatant from each sample into labeled counting tubes. The standard counting tube should be labeled "standard plasma" and the sample counting tubes should be labeled "sample plasma."

Counting. Set the scintillation spectrometer to count ^{51}Cr. Count each 1-ml sample for sufficient time to ensure no more than a 1% counting error. Adjust all samples to net counts per minute by subtracting the patient background from the patient samples and room background from the standard samples.

Calculations. If the ascorbic acid labeling method was used, the following equation is used for the calculations:

$$\text{TRCV} = \frac{\begin{array}{c}\text{volume}\\\text{injected}\end{array}\left(\begin{array}{c}\text{net standard}\\\text{counts}\end{array} \times \begin{array}{c}\text{dilution}\\\text{factor}\end{array}\right)}{\text{net whole blood sample counts}} \times \text{decimal hematocrit},$$

where TRCV = total red cell volume. TRCV is calculated separately from each postinjection blood sample.

If the wash labeling method was used, the equation in Figure 15-3 is used for the calculations. Again, TRCV is calculated separately for each postinjection blood sample.

Sources of Error. Infiltration of the labeled red cells will cause erroneously high results. Likewise, damaged erythrocytes or excessive binding of the ^{51}Cr by leukocytes or platelets will yield spuriously high values. Falsely low results are caused by a failure to obtain a preinjection blood sample in a patient who has previously received radioactive tracers. All blood samples must be mixed well prior to hematocrit determinations and pipetting of samples. Chromium-51 should not be added to the ACD solution before the patient's blood is added to the vial. Dextrose contained in the ACD solution acts as a reducing agent and inhibits red cell labeling.

Normal Ranges. The interpretation of a red cell volume and plasma volume determination depends upon a comparison between the measured volumes and normal values. The most common method is to estimate the TRCV and TPV in terms of body weight (ml/kg). The normal values published by the International Panel on Standardization in Hematology are shown in Table 15-1.

Since fat is almost avascular, blood volume is closely related to lean tissue mass and not weight. Therefore, even in healthy normal individuals, there is considerable variation in blood volume among persons with identical height and weight. In patients with diseases such as cachexia, heart or renal failure with edema, ascites or obesity, an even greater variation in lean tissue mass must be taken into consideration.

Blood volume varies with body size, body type, sex, disease state, basal metabolic rate, nutritional state and amount of physical work because all of these factors affect the lean body mass. Also, blood volume varies with the season, arterial oxygen content and changes in body position.

In normal persons within the "ideal" weight range, lean body mass makes up a constant fraction of total body weight. In these individuals, blood volume correlates well with weight. When fat is excessive (obesity) or deficient (emaciation, cachexia), corrections must be made to obtain an adjusted ideal weight. Since fat has a vascularity of approximately 20%, adjustments can be calculated to permit a comparison of an individual's blood volume with normal values (Table 15-2).

From a precise measurement of red cell or plasma volume and the venous hematocrit, the volume of the other compartments and therefore total blood volume, can be calculated in normal individuals. Normally, there is a fixed relationship between the whole-body hematocrit and venous hematocrit, with a ratio of 0.89 to 0.92. The whole-body hematocrit is usually lower than the venous hematocrit due to variations in blood vessel size throughout the body.

Most patients referred to nuclear medicine for red cell and plasma volume measurements are ill and the predicted normal relationship between whole-body and venous hematocrits will most likely not be present. In patients with splenomegaly, the ratio of whole-body hematocrit to venous hematocrit may be unpredictably increased to greater than 1.0. In patients with polycythemia, plasma volume abnormalities as well as red cell volume abnormalities may be present. Therefore, in clinical situations, total blood volume can only be reliably measured by performing simultaneous independent measurements of red cell volume and plasma volume.

$$\text{TRCV} = \frac{\text{volume injected}\left[\left(\text{net whole blood counts} \times \text{dilution factor}\right) - \left(\text{net plasma standard counts} \times \text{standard plasmacrit}\right)\right]}{\text{net whole blood sample counts} - \left(\text{net plasma sample counts} \times \text{sample plasmacrit}\right)} \times \text{Decimal hematocrit}$$

Plasmacrit = 1 - decimal hematocrit

Figure 15.3 Total red cell volume calculation (wash labeling method).

Red Cell Survival

The red cell survival study determines the mean survival time of ^{51}Cr-labeled autologous red cells in patients with hemolytic anemia.

Materials. Chromium-51 is labeled to red blood cells with the ascorbic acid labeling technique. Chromium activity is adjusted to 1.5 μCi (55.5 kBq) per kg body weight, with a minimum activity of 50 μCi (1.85 MBq). Equipment for collecting blood samples and injecting the radiopharmaceutical must be prepared in advance and includes gloves, 20-gauge needles, syringes and labeled heparinized blood collection tubes.

Tracer Administration/Sample Collection. After labeling, the red cells are injected, and the first blood sample is obtained 24 hr later. This time period permits removal of cells that were damaged during the labeling procedure from the circulation, as well as clearance from the blood of any injected plasma activity. Heparinized blood samples are obtained from the patient, every other day, for the next 3 wk.

Sample Handling. On the day of collection, 5 ml well-mixed whole blood is pipetted into a labeled counting tube. A pinch of saponin powder is added to the tube and mixed to lyse the red cells. These samples are then stored at 4°C until the last day of the study. Hematocrit determinations also are made on each sample on the day of collection.

Table 15.1
Normal Blood Volume Values (ml/kg)

	Men	Women
Total blood volume	55–80	50–75
Total red cell volume*†	22–35	20–30
Total plasma volume	30–45	30–45

*95% confidence limits.
†Valid only at sea level.

Sample Counting. On the last day of the study, all samples are counted on a scintillation spectrometer with settings of 280 to 360 keV for ^{51}Cr. Samples are counted long enough to give a counting error of 1% or less.

Calculations. To calculate the mean half-time of disappearance of the labeled red cells, the net counts per minute of each sample is plotted on semilogarithmic paper as a function of time (Fig. 15-4). The best straight line is drawn through all the points. The half-time is obtained by extrapolating the line to time zero, which is the y intercept. Divide the y intercept value by 2. At this value on the y-axis, draw a straight line parallel to the x-axis until it intersects the best straight line drawn through the data points. Drop a perpendicular line to the x-axis. This value is the mean survival time of the labeled red blood cells.

Table 15.2
Adjustments for Fat Tissue

Ideal Weights

Male: 5-ft tall = 110 lb + 6 lb for every inch over 5 ft

Female: 5-ft tall = 100 lb + 5 lb for every inch over 5 ft

Calculated Weight*

Example: 6-ft man weighing 275 lb

Ideal weight calculations:

5 ft = 110 lb + 6 lb × 12 inches = 182 lb

Difference between ideal and actual weight

275 lb − 182 lb = 93 lb overweight

Twenty percent vascularity of amount overweight:

93 lb × 0.2 = 18.6 lb

Calculated Weight =

Ideal weight + 20% of amount overweight:

182 lb + 18.6 lb = 200.6 lb

*Includes 20% vascularity of fat.

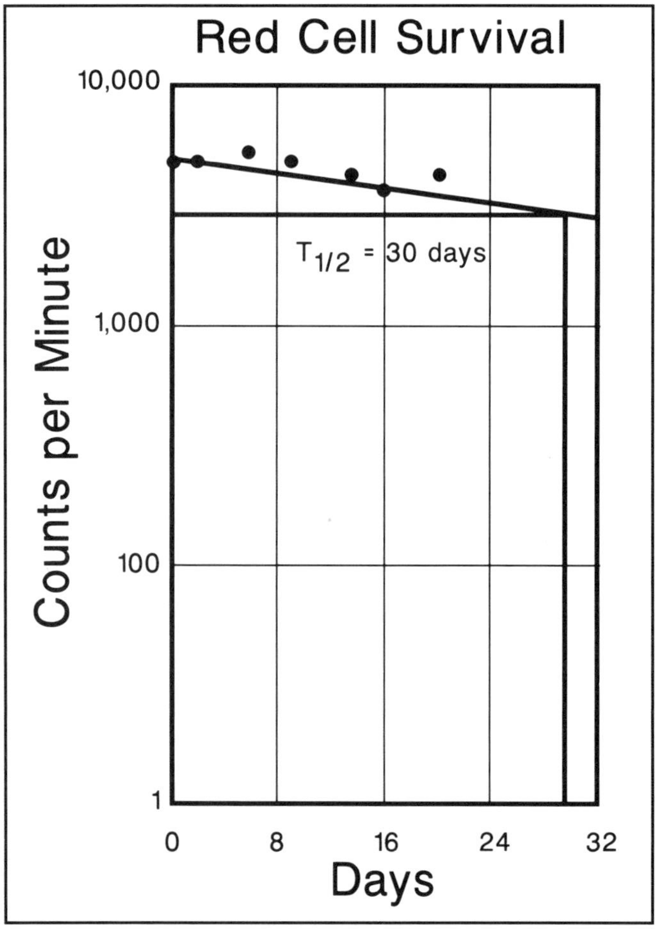

Figure 15.4 Red cell survival graph shows normal half-time of 30 days. Reprinted with permission from: McIntyre PA. Radioactive tracers in hematologic disease: I. *Hosp Pract* 1972;7:107.

Sources of Error. Determining the mean red cell life span is useful only in a patient who is in steady state with regard to the rate of production and destruction of red cells. Performing a hematocrit on each sample during the study provides an assessment of this steady-state condition. Chromium-51-red cell survival time will falsely appear to be shorter if the patient loses blood during the study. If the patient receives blood transfusions during the study, the mean survival time will appear shortened.

Normal Values. The mean half-time of normal ^{51}Cr-labeled red cells is from 25 to 35 days. As normal red cells age, they are removed from the circulation at a rate of 1% per day. Therefore, the true mean survival time of a normal random red cell population is 50 to 60 days. If this normal 1% per day removal is coupled with the 1% per day elution of the ^{51}Cr from the red cells, the combined mean half-time is 25 to 35 days. Tables are available for correction of this elution, but they are derived from studies in normal individuals. The elution rate is known to vary in disease states. Therefore, the use of these tables is questionable.

Splenic Sequestration

This test determines if the spleen is the site of red cell destruction in a patient who has evidence of increased red cell destruction. A splenic sequestration study is routinely performed in conjunction with a red cell survival study.

Materials. Use ^{51}Cr-red cells, 1.5 μCi (55.5 kBq) per kg body weight. A scintillation probe equipped with a flat-field collimator is used as the counting device.

Patient Preparation. Counting begins 24 hr after injection of the ^{51}Cr-labeled red cells. The patient is placed on the examining table, in the positions described below, and the skin is marked with indelible ink. Transparent tape is placed over each anatomical location and the patient is instructed not to remove or wash off the marks. Counting continues every other day for 3 wk.

Counting. The following anatomical locations are marked for counting:

- Precordium: With the patient in the supine position, the detector is centered over the left, third intercostal space at the sternal border.
- Liver: With the patient in the supine position, the detector is placed over the ninth and tenth ribs on the right midclavicular line.
- Spleen: With the patient in the prone position, the detector is placed two-thirds of the distance from the spinal process to the lateral edge of the body, at the level of the ninth and tenth ribs.

The same counting geometry must be present each time the patient is counted. Sufficient counts should be collected to give a counting error of 5% or less.

Calculations. Results are expressed as the ratio of the net organ counts per minute to the net precordium counts per minute for each day. These ratios are then plotted on linear graph paper as a function of time (Fig. 15-5).

Sources of Error. Inconsistent counting geometry from day to day will cause spurious results. Blood loss or transfusion during the counting interval also will affect results adversely.

Normal Values. The normal spleen-to-precordium ratio is between 0.5 and 1.0 and the normal liver to precordium ratio is 0.5. An initial spleen-to-precordium ratio greater than 2.0 indicates an increased splenic blood pool. A progressive, gradual increase over the course of the study indicates active splenic sequestration of the labeled red cells.

VITAMIN B_{12} ABSORPTION: (SCHILLING TEST)

The consequences of untreated vitamin B_{12} deficiency are extremely serious and include certain hematological abnormalities such as anemia, neurological defects and, if the condition is untreated, death. In the early stages, the symptoms of the deficiency are vague and insidious.

The most common causes of vitamin B_{12} deficiency are summarized in Table 15-3. Most cases of vitamin B_{12} deficiency are due to some disorder causing malabsorption. A deficiency in intrinsic factor, a protein secreted by the parietal cells of the stomach, is the most common cause of malabsorption.

Table 15-4 summarizes factors necessary for absorption of dietary vitamin B_{12} in humans. The absorption of this vitamin through the terminal ileum depends on the stomach's secretion of intrinsic factor, which exists as a dimer and binds two molecules of vitamin B_{12}. The intrinsic factor itself does not get absorbed at the sites in the terminal ileum but is required in an active transport mechanism. Ionic calcium and a pH of ileal contents greater than 6 are also required. Once absorption takes place, a normal transport protein, transcobalamin II, must be present in the blood to convey the B_{12} to areas of the body for utilization or storage.

Vitamin B_{12} Absorption Test: Stage I

Materials. The procedure requires 0.5–0.6 μCi (18.5–22.2 kBq) ^{57}Co-labeled vitamin B_{12}. It is important that this oral dose be in the range of 0.25–2.0 μg of vitamin B_{12}, the amount that might be present in a typical meal. Quantities above this level may be absorbed by a mechanism not dependent on the presence of intrinsic factor. Labeled urine containers large enough to hold a 24-hr sample are also needed.

Patient Preparation. The patient should have nothing to eat after midnight, the night before the test and should remain fasting for 2 hr following the oral dose of ^{57}Co-labeled vitamin B_{12}. The patient should not receive enemas or laxatives or be scheduled for a barium enema or intravenous pyelogram for the duration of the study. Due to the effects of hepatobiliary recirculation, treatment doses of vitamin B_{12} should be discontinued 2 to 3 days prior to starting the Schilling test.

Dose Administration/Sample Collection. The ^{57}Co vitamin B_{12} capsule is administered orally with water. Two hours later, 1 mg of stable cyanocobalamin (vitamin B_{12}) is given intramuscularly. Nonradioactive vitamin B_{12}, sometimes referred to as the "flushing dose," causes temporary saturation of the normal binding sites in the plasma and results in renal excretion of a portion of the absorbed tracer dose. Excretion of radioactive vitamin B_{12} is maximal between 8 and 12 hr after administration of the flushing dose. Two 24-hr urine collections are obtained, one for each 24-hr period. The patient should be instructed to collect all urine during this period.

Sample Handling. After mixing each 24-hr collection well, the total volume and specific gravity of each sample is measured. Two 5-ml aliquots are pipetted from each 24-hr urine collection into labeled counting tubes. A standard is prepared from the reference standard solution supplied with the capsules.

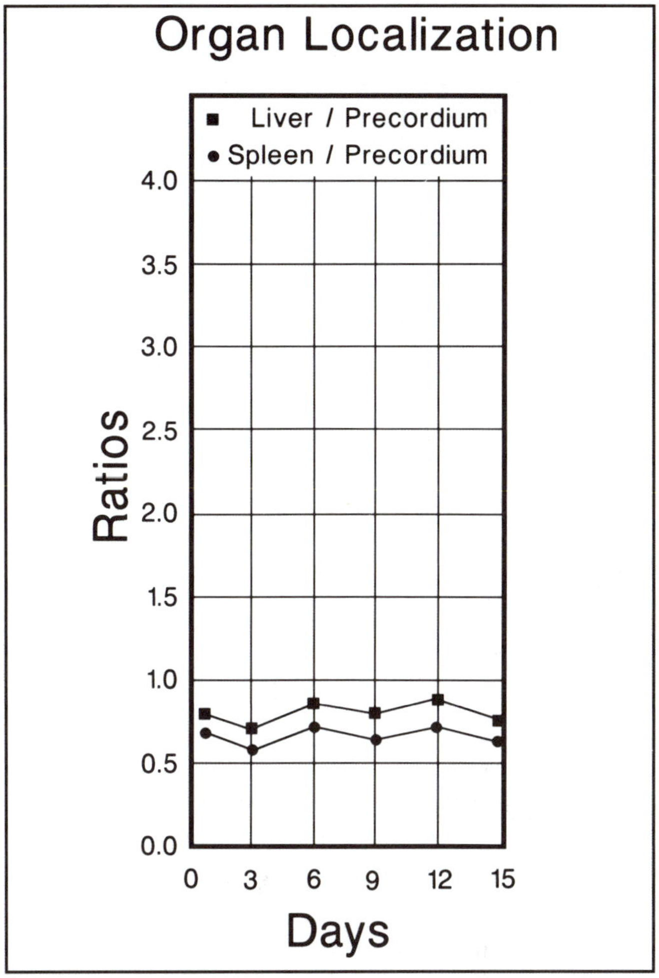

Figure 15.5 Organ localization of ^{51}Cr-red blood cells. Graph depicts normal liver-to-precordium and spleen-to-precordium ratios, which are about 1 : 1 or less. Reprinted with permission from: McIntyre PA. Radioactive tracers in hematologic disease: I. *Hosp Pract* 1972;7:107.

Sample Counting. All samples are counted with a scintillation spectrometer set to count ^{57}Co. Each sample is counted for a sufficient time to ensure no more than a 1% counting error. All sample counts are adjusted to net counts per minute by subtracting the room background radiation.

Calculations. The percentage of the administered dose excreted is calculated for each 24-hr urine sample using the following equation:

$$\% \text{ excreted} = \frac{\text{net cpm urine sample}}{\text{net cpm standard}} \times \frac{\text{urine sample/sample volume}}{\text{standard dilution factor}}.$$

Normal Values. Percent ^{57}Co excreted: Day 1: $\geq 9\%$; Day 2: $\leq 1\%$.

Sources of Error. The major problem encountered with this test is its dependence on complete 24-hr urine collections.

Table 15.3
Causes of Vitamin B_{12} Deficiency

I. Inadequate intake
II. Malabsorption
  A. 2° gastric abnormalities
    1. Absence of intrinsic factor
      a. Congenital
      b. Addisonian pernicious anemia
      c. Total gastrectomy
      d. Subtotal gastrectomy
    2. Excessive excretion of hydrochloric acid: Zollinger-Ellison syndrome
  B. 2° intestinal malabsorption
    1. Destruction, removal, or functional incompetence of ileal mucosal absorptive sites
    2. Competition with host for available dietary vitamin B_{12}
      a. *Diphylibothrium latum* (fish tapeworm)
      b. Small-bowel lesions associated with bacterial stagnation (jejunal diverticula, strictures, blind loops, etc.)
    3. Pancreatic insufficiency
    4. Drug therapy*
      a. Paraaminosalicylic acid (PAS)
      b. Neomycin
      c. Colchicine
      d. Calcium-chelating agents
  C. Genetic abnormality in transport protein transcobalamin II

*Although any of these agents may produce abnormalities in vitamin B_{12} absorption, only patients on long-term PAS therapy have been reported to develop clinical evidence of vitamin B_{12} deficiency.

Reprinted with permission from: McIntyre PA. Use of radioisotope techniques in the clinical evaluation of patients with megaloblastic anemia. *Semin Nucl Med* 1975;5:81.

The loss of just one urine collection may cause falsely low results. The test depends on normal urinary function. In patients with abnormal urinary retention, such as benign prostatic hypertrophy, the amount excreted in the first 24 hr will be reduced. Significant amounts of radioactivity will continue to be excreted for the next 24–48 hr, so that the total excretion will eventually be within normal limits. For this reason, it is recommended that two separate 24-hr urine specimens be collected following the "flushing" injection of cyanocobalamin.

Table 15.4
Parameters Involved in Absorption of Dietary Vitamin B_{12} in Humans

1. Available for human nutrition only in animal food sources.
2. Binding of vitamin B_{12} by intrinsic factor produced by gastric mucosa.
3. Normal ileal mucosal absorptive sites in the presence of ionic Ca^{++} and pH of ileal contents > 6.0.
4. Normal "transport" protein (transcobalamin II) to convey vitamin B_{12} from ileal absorptive sites to areas of active utilization and storage.

*Same parameters apply to absorption of tracer amounts of radioactive vitamin B_{12} used in absorption studies.

Reprinted with permission from McIntyre PA. Use of radioisotope techniques in the clinical evaluation of patients with megaloblastic anemia. *Semin Nucl Med* 1975;5:81.

Excretion of other previously administered radionuclides can cause erroneously high results.

Vitamin B_{12} Absorption Test: Stage II

If the absorption of ^{57}Co vitamin B_{12} is low when compared to normal individuals, then a second absorption test is performed by giving hog intrinsic factor along with the oral dose of labeled vitamin B_{12}. This test determines if the cause of the malabsorption is due to an absence of intrinsic factor.

Materials. In addition to the materials described in Stage I, a 10-mg dose of intrinsic factor is needed; it is usually provided with the commercially available Schilling test kit.

Patient Preparation. See Stage I.

Dose Administration. The ^{57}Co-labeled vitamin B_{12} and intrinsic factor are administered orally with water simultaneously. The remainder of the test is the same as described for Stage I.

Normal Values. Percent ^{57}Co excreted: Day 1: $\geq$9%; Day 2: $\leq$1%.

Sources of Error. When the radioactive vitamin B_{12} and the intrinsic factor are given in separate capsules, there may be incomplete binding of the two in the stomach, which gives a false-negative Stage II Schilling test. It is recommended that prior to administration, the radioactive vitamin B_{12} and intrinsic factor be mixed together in water.

If hog intrinsic factor is used, a negative result does not completely rule out intrinsic factor-dependent malabsorption, since some patients who have been previously exposed to hog intrinsic factor (present in many multivitamin preparations) may have antibodies against it.

Vitamin B_{12} deficiency can produce small bowel megaloblastosis with atrophy, which may cause ileal malabsorption. If a Stage II study is performed before vitamin B_{12} therapy is started, and the ileum is allowed to heal, a false-negative result will be obtained.

Vitamin B_{12} Absorption: Stage III

Having determined that the Stage II Schilling test is truly abnormal, other causes of malabsorption must be investigated. If bacterial overgrowth is suspected, treatment with a broad spectrum antibiotic followed by a repeat Stage I Schilling test is performed. If pancreatic insufficiency is suspected, a repeat Stage I Schilling test can be performed after the administration of pancreatic extract.

Dual-Isotope Method for Measuring Vitamin B_{12} Absorption

The conventional Schilling test of vitamin B_{12} absorption just described is done in two stages, requiring at least 1 wk for a final result if Stage I is abnormal. A modified Schilling test is available in which vitamin B_{12}, labeled with two different isotopes of cobalt, is administered. One form, ^{57}Co-labeled vitamin B_{12}, is already bound to intrinsic factor by prior incubation with normal human gastric juice, and the other contains nonprotein-bound ^{58}Co-labeled vitamin B_{12}.

The two capsules are ingested orally, followed by the injection of nonradioactive vitamin B_{12} and two 24-hr urine collections. Differential isotope counting is then performed to determine the percent administered dose of each isotope that has been excreted in the urine. A patient with normal vitamin B_{12} absorption will excrete the same amount of both isotopes, while a patient lacking intrinsic factor will excrete greater quantities of the intrinsic factor-bound ^{57}Co-labeled vitamin B_{12}. In patients with bacterial overgrowth or small bowel lesions resulting in vitamin B_{12} malabsorption, both isotopes will be excreted in abnormally low quantities.

The dual-isotope Schilling test has several advantages over the conventional method. The practical advantage of taking only 2 days, instead of 1 wk, to obtain results leads to earlier diagnosis and treatment and saves money. The use of ^{57}Co bound to human gastric juice eliminates the use of hog intrinsic factor preparations, against which some patients may have developed antibodies. Also, while an incomplete urine collection is undesirable, some information can often be salvaged from the ^{57}Co : ^{58}Co ratio.

Although the same patient conditions are present in this method, small bowel changes caused by vitamin B_{12} deficiency are not considered in the comparison of the absorption of "free" and "bound" vitamin B_{12}. The absorption of the ^{57}Co-labeled vitamin B_{12} bound to gastric juice will be falsely low, along with a low ^{58}Co-labeled vitamin B_{12} absorption. This will lead to a false-negative result.

THYROID UPTAKE

One of the earliest clinical nuclear medicine procedures was the measurement of radioiodine uptake by the thyroid gland. Thyroid uptake measures the amount of radioactive iodide taken up and retained within the thyroid gland. Different aspects of thyroid iodine metabolism are reflected in the uptake value, depending upon how long after tracer administration the uptake is measured. Under normal conditions, thyroid uptake at 2–6 hr following tracer administration reflects iodide trapping and organification within the gland. Uptake values at 24–48 hr are affected by the rate at which iodine is lost from the gland.

Radioiodine uptakes are useful in patients with hyperthyroidism in whom ^{131}I therapy is indicated and in patients with organification defects, which are seen in instances of congenital organification defect and certain types of thyroiditis.

Materials. The radiopharmaceutical used is an ^{123}I capsule, 100 μCi (3.7 MBq). A thyroid uptake probe with a 2-inch diameter sodium iodide crystal and a cylindrical straight-bore collimator, connected to a pulse-height analyzer and scaler is used.

Patient Preparation. The patient should be questioned about prior thyroid history, medications and recent radiographic procedures. The patient should be instructed not to eat after midnight on the night before the test and to remain fasting for 2 hr following capsule administration.

Dose Administration. The capsule is administered orally with a small amount of water.

Standard Counting. If the dose capsule is to be used as the standard, the ^{123}I capsule is placed in a neck phantom and counted. The thyroid probe is positioned perpendicular to the capsule, at a distance of 10–20 cm from the face of the collimator to the capsule. The exact distance will need to be determined in each laboratory. The capsule is counted for 1 min using ^{123}I energy settings. Each time an uptake measurement is performed on a patient, a correction factor must be applied to correct for physical decay.

Some laboratories use a duplicate capsule as a standard. After being placed in a neck phantom, this standard capsule is counted with a thyroid probe each time an uptake measurement is performed on the patient. The phantom is positioned at the previously calibrated distance from the face of the collimator.

Patient Background Counting. Nonthyroid background measurements are collected over the thigh for 1 min on ^{123}I energy settings. It is important to exclude bladder activity. Therefore, the probe is positioned vertically over one leg, at a distance slightly above the patient's knee.

Some laboratories estimate nonthyroid background by placing a lead thyroid shield over the patient's neck to cover the thyroid. The probe is then placed in the uptake position and counts are collected for 1 min with ^{123}I energy settings.

Thyroid Gland Counting. The patient is positioned supine with the neck hyperextended. The probe is positioned above the neck with the center line of the probe between the thyroid cartilage and the suprasternal notch at the calibrated distance between the face of the collimator and the surface of the neck. Counts are collected for 1 min using ^{123}I energy settings.

Calculations. Thyroid uptake is calculated using the following equation:

$$\%\text{ uptake} = \frac{N - T}{(S \times D_f) - B} \times 100,$$

where N = patient neck counts per minute, T = patient background counts per minute, S = standard counts per minute, D_f = decay factor (to account for elapsed time from initial standard count to time uptake measurement is performed) and B = room background counts per minute.

Sources of Error. Medications containing iodine and radiographic procedures using iodinated contrast media will expand the patient's iodide pool, resulting in a low radioiodine uptake. Thyroid medications containing T_4 and antithyroid drugs will suppress the thyroid uptake. Table 15-5 gives a partial list of factors influencing radioiodine uptake.

The presence of food in the patient's stomach may impede gastric emptying and intestinal absorption of iodide, causing a falsely low uptake value.

Since ^{123}I has a low energy photon of 159 keV, correction for attenuation by soft-tissue absorption should be considered. Patients with extremely large goiters or heavy necks may attenuate the photons, due to variable thyroid depths, thereby causing erroneous results.

Table 15.5
Factors Influencing Thyroidal Iodine Uptake

Increased uptake	Decreased uptake
Iodine deficiency	Suppression by exogenous thyroid hormone
Pregnancy (normal)	Renal failure or severe congestive heart failure
Lithium	Excess iodine (including radiographic contrast agents and iodine-containing drugs)
Rebound following suppression with thyroid hormone	Other drugs including thionamides and glucocorticoids
Rebound following cessation of antithyroid drugs	

Reprinted with permission from Drew HH, LaFrance ND, Chen J. Thyroid imaging studies. *J Nucl Med Technol* 1987;15:83.

Each time an uptake measurement is performed, the patient's prior positioning must be reproduced to ensure constant geometry. Standardized distances between the detector and the patient's neck or the neck phantom should be maintained.

To account for residual activity, patients who have received previous radioactive tracers must have a count taken over their thyroid gland to correct for this activity before the iodine capsule is administered. Failure to perform a residual count will result in a falsely increased thyroid uptake value.

Normal Values. Normal values should be established by each department for its geographical area. In Baltimore, Maryland, for example, the following normal values have been established: 2-hr uptake equals 5%–12%, 6-hr uptake equals 8%–25% and 24-hr uptake equals 12%–35%.

REFERENCES

1. Wright RR, T'no M, Pollycove M. Blood volume. *Semin Nucl Med* 1975;5:63–77.
2. Langan JK, McIntyre P. The hematopoietic system. In: Bernier DR, Langan JK, Wells LD, eds. *Nuclear medicine technology and techniques*, 1st ed. St. Louis: CV Mosby; 1989:403–414.
3. International Committee for Standardization in Hematology (ICSH) Standard techniques for the measurement of red cell and plasma volume. *Br J Haematol* 1973;17:71–73.
4. Huff RL, Feller DD. Relation of circulating red cell volume to body density and obesity. *J Clin Invest* 1956;35:1–4.
5. Fudenberg H, Baldini M, Mahoney JP, Dameshek W. The body hematocrit/venous hematocrit ratio and the "splenic reservoir." *Blood* 1961;17:71–73.
6. International Committee for Standardization in Hematology (ICSH). Recommended methods for radioisotope red cell survival studies. *Br J Haematol* 1971;21:241–250.
7. McIntyre P. Radioactive tracers in hematologic disease: I. *Hosp Pract* 1972;7:94–108.
8. McIntyre P. Use of radioisotope techniques in the clinical evaluation of patients with megaloblastic anemia. *Semin Nucl Med* 1975;5:79–94.
9. International Committee for Standardization in Hematology. Recommended methods for the measurement of vitamin B_{12} absorption. *J Nucl Med* 1981;22:1091–1093.
10. McDonald JW, Barr RM, Barton WB. Spurious Schilling test results obtained with intrinsic factor enclosed in capsules. *Ann Intern Med* 1975;83:827–829.
11. Haurani FI, Sherwood N, Goldstein F. Intestinal malabsorption of vitamin B_{12} in pernicious anemia. *Metabolism* 1964;13:1342–1348.
12. Drew HH, LaFrance ND, Chen JJ. Thyroid imaging studies. *J Nucl Med Technol* 1987;15:79–87.
13. Martin PM, Rollo FD. Estimation of thyroid depth and correction of I-123 uptake measurements. *J Nucl Med* 1977;18:919–924.

16 Radionuclide Therapy

Ann M. Steves

The most commonly used radionuclides for therapy are ^{131}I, ^{32}P and ^{89}Sr (Table 16-1). The technologist's primary involvement in radionuclide therapy is to ensure that radiation safety practices are implemented. This chapter will address those practices.

RADIOIODINE THERAPY FOR THYROID CARCINOMA

Patients receiving more than 30 mCi (1.11 GBq) ^{131}I must be hospitalized. In the case of thyroid carcinoma treatment, doses range from 50–150 mCi (1.85–5.55 GBq). Before radioiodine administration, the patient, nursing staff and the isolation room must be prepared to minimize radioactive contamination and unnecessary radiation exposure.

Patient Preparation

Patient cooperation is essential, so the time taken to explain what the patient can expect is well spent. The patient should be informed that any necessary nursing care will be provided, but that nursing personnel will minimize the amount of time spent in contact with the patient. Rules about the amount of time visitors may remain in the patient's room and the distance that must be maintained between them and the patient should be thoroughly explained. Children and pregnant women should not be allowed to visit patients.

Some patients may have difficulty being confined to a small area. They should be encouraged to bring materials to provide some diversion during their confinement. However, patients should also be informed that these materials may become contaminated so that it may be necessary to hold them for decay in storage following the patient's discharge. Access to a television and telephone can lessen the feelings of isolation patients may experience. It is also important to stress that the patient must remain in the isolation room until it has been determined that the emitted radiation levels are within acceptable limits. The technologist should be wary of predicting when the patient will be released from isolation.

Large amounts of the radioiodine will be excreted in the urine. Human excreta may be disposed of through the sewer system. The patient should be instructed to flush the toilet three or four times after each use to remove and dilute the radioactivity.

The patient should fast before the radioiodine is administered to enhance its absorption from the stomach. The technologist should ascertain that the patient has no difficulty swallowing by asking the patient to drink a small amount of water.

Preparation of the Isolation Room

Sources of contamination include airborne ^{131}I and radioactivity in the patient's urine, perspiration and saliva. To facilitate decontamination of the treatment room, floors, countertops and other porous surfaces should be covered with plastic backed absorbent paper. Plastic covers should be placed over chairs. The use of a plastic mattress cover is recommended. Plastic wrap can be used to cover knobs, handles, telephone receiver and the toilet. Most of the radioactive contamination will be present on the bathroom fixtures and floor, so these should receive special attention.

The patient's linen should be kept in a container in the isolation room and monitored for contamination before it is sent to the hospital laundry. Likewise, the patient's disposable eating utensils and uneaten food should be collected for monitoring before disposal.

After administration of the radioiodine, the isolation room should be posted with a "Caution: Radioactive Material" sign. When the patient is discharged, the isolation room should be decontaminated and monitored before housekeeping personnel prepare the room for another patient.

Instructions to Hospital Personnel

All nursing personnel should be issued film badges and instructed on how to wear them. No pregnant personnel should be assigned to care for the therapy patient. Safe exposure times for other assigned personnel should be determined and posted in the patient's chart or on the patient's door. Personnel should be instructed to wear shoe covers and gloves when entering the isolation room.

The names and telephone numbers of the nuclear medicine physician and the radiation safety officer should be included with detailed instructions placed in the front of the patient's chart. Hospital personnel should be encouraged to call on these individuals should any question or unusual circumstance arise.

Patient Monitoring

The patient is monitored with a portable ionization chamber to determine safe exposure times for personnel, exposure to nearby patients and when the patient can be released from isolation.

According to NRC regulations, the radiation exposure of visitors and nursing personnel (nonoccupational individuals) must be limited to 2 mrem in any one hour. If the measured dose rate exceeds 2 mrem/hr, the length of time that visitors or nursing personnel can remain in the room must be calculated.

Table 16.1
Radioactive Therapeutic Agents

Agent	Principal use
Sodium iodide ^{131}I solution/capsules	Hyperthyroidism Thyroid carcinoma
Sodium phosphate ^{32}P solution	Polycythemia vera Certain leukemias Skeletal metastases
Chromic phosphate ^{32}P suspension	Peritoneal and pleural effusions
[^{89}Sr] strontium chloride	Skeletal metastases

For example, if the survey meter measurement at the bedside is 15 mrem/hr, how long can a visitor or nurse remain at the point where the reading was made? Since 2 mrem in any one hour is the exposure limit for nonoccupational individuals:

$$\frac{15 \text{ mrem}}{60 \text{ min}} = \frac{2 \text{ mrem}}{x}$$

$$x = \frac{2 \text{ mrem } (60 \text{ min})}{15 \text{ mrem}}$$

$$x = 8 \text{ min.}$$

The radiation dose rate will decrease with increasing distance. Therefore, the farther visitors stand from the bedside, the longer they will be able to remain in the room.

To ensure that patients in adjacent rooms do not receive more than 2 mrem in an hour, measurements should be made to ascertain that exposure limits for nearby patients are not exceeded. This requires that a therapy patient be placed in a private room.

To determine when a patient can be released from isolation, daily radiation measurements are compared to the initial measurement recorded immediately after the patient receives the radioiodine. The dose rate at the time of administration is measured at a distance of at least 3 m. Subsequent measurements are made at the same distance. The dose rate measurements are related to the number of millicuries retained in the patient.

$$\frac{\text{initial dose rate}}{\text{mCi administered}} = \frac{\text{subsequent dose rate}}{\text{mCi retained}}.$$

For example, a patient receives 100 mCi (3.7 GBq) of ^{131}I. Immediately following the administration, the dose rate at 3 m measures 150 mrem/hr. Twenty-four hr later, the dose rate at 3 m measures 50 mrem/hr. How many millicuries remain in the patient?

$$\frac{150 \text{ mrem/hr}}{100 \text{ mCi}} = \frac{50 \text{ mrem/hr}}{x \text{ mCi}}$$

$$x = \frac{100 \text{ mCi } (50 \text{ mrem/hr})}{150 \text{ mrem/hr}}$$

$$x = 33.3 \text{ mCi } (1.23 \text{ GBq})$$

Therefore, the patient must remain in isolation.

Discharge Instructions

Therapy patients continue to excrete radioiodine into their saliva, urine and perspiration for about 1 wk following discharge from the isolation room. NRC regulations require that patients be instructed in techniques that will minimize the radiation dose to family members or other individuals with whom therapy patients may come in contact. The most likely routes of radioiodine transfer should be reviewed with the patient, along with the following guidelines.

1. Intimate personal contact should be avoided. The patient should not share a bed with anyone. Close contact with children, such as holding or kissing, should be avoided.
2. The patient should use a separate bathroom, if one is available, from other household members. The toilet should be flushed twice after each use.
3. The patient should not share eating utensils, cups, glasses or towels.
4. The patient should wash hands thoroughly after using the bathroom.

RADIOIODINE THERAPY FOR HYPERTHYROIDISM

Since amounts of ^{131}I administered to treat hyperthyroidism are less than 30 mCi (1110 MBq), patients being treated for this condition typically are not hospitalized. The patient is prepared in a manner comparable to what has previously been described, with the exception of the need for isolation. Similar instructions designed to minimize radiation exposure to other household members should be given as well.

PHOSPHORUS-32 THERAPY

Phosphorus-32 is a pure beta emitter. Beta particles are effectively shielded by the glass vial or plastic syringe containing the radionuclide. Once the radionuclide has been introduced into the patient, there is no external radiation hazard. Therefore, ^{32}P therapy does not require that the patient be placed in isolation.

Sodium Phosphate ^{32}P

Sodium phosphate ^{32}P is a clear, colorless solution intended for intravenous administration. Doses range from 1 to 20 mCi (37–740 MBq), depending on the pathology being treated. Sodium phosphate ^{32}P is used for the treatment of polycythemia vera and the control of bone pain resulting from metastatic disease in the skeleton. Technical considerations similar to those for ^{89}Sr therapy should be adhered to during sodium phosphate ^{32}P therapy. These considerations are discussed in the section on ^{89}Sr therapy.

Chromic Phosphate ^{32}P

Chromic phosphate ^{32}P suspension is a blue-green colloidal solution intended for intracavitary use only. If this agent is mistakenly administered intravenously, the colloidal particles will be taken up by the Kupffer cells of the liver, thereby causing severe localized radiation damage. Doses range from 6 to 20 mCi (222–740 MBq).

Colloidal ^{32}P is introduced into the peritoneal or pleural cavities. Once administered, the agent remains in the cavity into which it was introduced. However, drainage from the instillation site or dressings covering the site should be considered radiation hazards and handled appropriately. Likewise, materials used during the instillation (gloves, needles, tubing) should be disposed of as radioactive material.

STRONTIUM-89 THERAPY

Strontium-89-chloride is administered to treat bone pain caused by metastatic bone disease. The goal of this type of therapy is to relieve pain and restore the patient's ability to resume the activities of daily living.

Strontium-89 is an analog of calcium that is rapidly cleared from the blood and localizes in the bone. Greater uptake of the tracer occurs in sites of osteogenesis, which means that areas of bony metastases will concentrate ^{89}Sr to a greater extent than areas of normal bone. It also remains in the metastatic sites longer than in normal bone (about 50 days compared to 14 days).

Strontium-89-chloride is administered intravenously. The recommended unit dose is 4 mCi (148 MBq) or 40–60 μCi/kg (1.5–2.2 MBq/kg) based on the patient's body weight. Depending on the patient's response to therapy, ^{89}Sr may be administered at 3-mo intervals. The nuclear medicine technologist's responsibilities occur primarily at the time of radiopharmaceutical administration.

The technologist should be aware of several technical considerations. Strontium-89 is a beta emitter with a 50-day half-life. Appropriate shielding material, plastic rather than lead, should be used to avoid the production of brems-strahlung radiation. Infiltration of ^{89}Sr during intravenous administration could lead to localized irradiation of soft tissue at the injection site. (Recall that beta particles have short ranges in tissue.) Therefore, it may be prudent to establish an intravenous line and confirm its patency prior to introducing the tracer through it. Approximately two-thirds of the administered dose is excreted in the urine and the remainder in the feces. Urinary excretion is greatest in the first two days following administration. Incontinent patients should be catheterized to minimize contamination of bed linens, clothing and other areas of the environment.

Accurate assay of ^{89}Sr before its administration is complicated by the fact that it is a pure beta-emitter. The NRC requires that radiopharmaceutical doses be assayed prior to administration to the patient. It is not, however, possible to directly assay a beta-emitter in a dose calibrator. Therefore, the NRC does not require that patient doses containing pure beta-emitters be measured before administration if the doses are supplied as unit doses from a manufacturer or licensed radiopharmacy. If, however, the beta-emitting radiopharmaceuticals are not received in unit dose form, the licensee must assay them directly, using special instrumentation capable of the assay or assay them indirectly, using a combination of measurements and calculations, with available instrumentation. The reader is referred to the references at the end of this chapter addressing the method by which beta-emitters may be assayed.

REFERENCES

1. Bender JM, Dworkin HJ. Iodine-131 as an oncology agent. *J Nucl Med Technol* 1993;21:14–150.
2. Clarke MT, Galie E. Radionuclide therapy of osseous metastatic disease. *J Nucl Med Technol* 1993;21:3–6.
3. Dickinson CZ, Hendrix NS. Strontium-89 therapy in painful bony metastases. *J Nucl Med Technol* 1993;21:133–137.
4. Early PJ, Sodee DB. *Principles and practice of nuclear medicine*, 2nd ed. St. Louis: Mosby Year-Book; 1995:331–333, 752–756.
5. Herold TJ, Gross GP, Hung JC. A technique for measurement of strontium-89 in a dose calibrator. *J Nucl Med Technol* 1995;23:26–28.
6. Instrumentation meets NRC beta-emitter assay requirements. *Radiology & Imaging Letter* 1995;15:84.
7. *Issues associated with use of strontium-89 and other beta-emitting radiopharmaceuticals.* IN 94-70. Nuclear Regulatory Commission, September 29, 1994.
8. LaRoque L. Whole-body ^{131}I metastatic survey as an aide in determining functional thyroid metastases. *J Nucl Med Technol* 1979;7:36–39.
9. Miller KL, Bott SM, Velkley DE, Cunningham DE. Review of contamination and exposure hazards associated with therapeutic uses of radioiodine. *J Nucl Med Technol* 1979;7:163–166.
10. Porter WC, Eck L. A technique for measurement of strontium-89 in a dose calibrator [Letter]. *J Nucl Med Technol* 1995;23:217–218.
11. *Precautions in the management of patients who have received therapeutic amounts of radionuclides, NCRP Report No. 37.* Washington, DC: National Council on Radiation Protection and Measurements; October 1970.
12. Steves AM. Radiation protection in nuclear medicine. In: Dowd SB. *Practical radiation protection and applied radiobiology.* Philadelphia: WB Saunders; 1994:217–221.

Appendix A

Solutions to Exercises

Chapter 1

1.

$$\frac{I_1}{I_2} = \frac{(d_2)^2}{(d_1)^2}$$

$$\frac{6 \text{ mR/hr}}{I_2} = \frac{(1.5 \text{ m})^2}{(4.5 \text{ m})^2}$$

$$I_2 = \frac{(6 \text{ mR/hr})(4.5 \text{ m})^2}{(1.5 \text{ m})^2}$$

$$I_2 = \frac{(6 \text{ mR/hr})(20.25 \text{ m}^2)}{2.25 \text{ m}^2}$$

$$I_2 = 54 \text{ mR/hr}$$

2.

$$\frac{I_1}{I_2} = \frac{(d_2)^2}{(d_1)^2}$$

$$\frac{2.6 \text{ mR/hr}}{1.3 \text{ mR/hr}} = \frac{(d_2)^2}{(0.4 \text{ m})^2}$$

$$(d_2)^2 = \frac{(2.6 \text{ mR/hr})(0.4 \text{ m})^2}{1.3 \text{ mR/hr}}$$

$$(d_2)^2 = 0.32 \text{ m}^2$$

$$d_2 = \sqrt{0.32 \text{ m}^2} = 0.57 \text{ m}$$

3.

$$\frac{I_1}{I_2} = \frac{(d_2)^2}{(d_1)^2}$$

$$\frac{175 \text{ mR/hr}}{I_2} = \frac{(12 \text{ in.})^2}{(0.5 \text{ in.})^2}$$

$$I_2 = \frac{(175 \text{ mR/hr})(0.5 \text{ in.})^2}{(12 \text{ in.})^2}$$

$$I_2 = 0.30 \text{ mR/hr}$$

Example 3 illustrates the power of distance as a quick and inexpensive way to reduce radiation exposure.

4.

$$\frac{I_1}{I_2} = \frac{(d_2)^2}{(d_1)^2}$$

$$\frac{96 \text{ mR/hr}}{2 \text{ mR/hr}} = \frac{(d_2)^2}{(1 \text{ m})^2}$$

$$(d_2)^2 = \frac{(96 \text{ mR/hr})(1 \text{ m})^2}{2 \text{ mR/hr}}$$

$$d_2 = \sqrt{48 \text{ m}^2} = 6.9 \text{ m}$$

5.

$$\frac{I_1}{I_2} = \frac{(d_2)^2}{(d_1)^2}$$

If the initial exposure rate is reduced by 75%, the second exposure rate is 25% of the original. Therefore, $I_2 = 0.25(200 \text{ mR/hr})$. Thus,

$$\frac{200 \text{ mR/hr}}{0.25\,(200 \text{ mR/hr})} = \frac{(d_2)^2}{(3 \text{ m})^2}$$

$$(d_2)^2 = \frac{(200 \text{ mR/hr})(9 \text{ m}^2)}{50 \text{ mR/hr}}$$

$$(d_2)^2 = 36 \text{ m}^2$$

$$d_2 = \sqrt{36 \text{ m}^2} = 6 \text{ m}$$

6. a. 1 HVL = 2.6 mm
2 HVL = 2.6 mm × 2 = 5.2 mm.

Since each HVL absorbs 50% of the photons and transmits the remaining 50%, 2 HVLs transmit 25% of the original photons.

6. b.

# HVL	Exposure rate (mR/hr)	Lead thickness (mm)
0	30	0
1	15	2.6
2	7.5	5.2
3	3.75	7.8
4	1.87	10.4

Therefore, 10.4 mm of lead are needed to reduce the exposure rate to not more than 2 mR/hr.

7. a.

# HVL	Exposure rate (mR/hr)	Lead thickness (cm)
0	40	0
1	20	1.25
2	10	2.5
3	5	3.75

7. b.

# HVL	Lead thickness (cm)	% Photons transmitted
0	0	100
1	1.25	50
2	2.50	25
3	3.75	12.5

If 12.5% of the original photons were transmitted, then 87.5% was absorbed.

Chapter 3

1.

$$\text{Concentration} = \frac{\text{activity}}{\text{unit volume}}$$

$$C = \frac{378 \text{ mCi}}{20 \text{ ml}} = 18.9 \text{ mCi/ml}$$

2.

$$\frac{10.6\ \mu\text{Ci}\ ^{99}\text{Mo}}{598 \text{ mCi}\ ^{99m}\text{Tc}} = 0.018\ \mu\text{Ci}\ ^{99}\text{Mo/mCi}\ ^{99m}\text{Tc}$$

3. Decay correct the initial ^{99}Mo and ^{99m}Tc measurements for 10 hr (0600 to 1600 = 10 hr) using the appropriate decay factors.

^{99}Mo: $6.1\ \mu\text{Ci} \times 0.9 = 5.49\ \mu\text{Ci}$

^{99m}Tc: $279 \text{ mCi} \times 0.316 = 88.2 \text{ mCi}$

At 1600, the ^{99}Mo concentration is:

$$\frac{5.49\ \mu\text{Ci}\ ^{99}\text{Mo}}{88.2 \text{ mCi}\ ^{99m}\text{Tc}} = 0.062\ \mu\text{Ci}\ ^{99}\text{Mo/mCi}\ ^{99m}\text{Tc}.$$

This eluate may be used in patients at 1600 because the ^{99}Mo concentration is below the limit set by the NRC.

4. Based on the maximum reconstituting volume (5 ml), 4.6 GBq can be prepared.

$$925 \text{ MBq/ml} = 5 \text{ ml} = 4625 \text{ MBq}$$

$$4625 \text{ MBq} \times \frac{\text{GBq}}{1000 \text{ MBq}} = 4.6 \text{ GBq}$$

This amount does not exceed the maximum activity that can be prepared from one kit or the maximum reconstituting volume.

5. The maximum activity that can be prepared with this kit is equal to:

$$\frac{\text{maximum}}{\text{reconstituting volume}} \times\ ^{99m}\text{Tc concentration}$$

$$\text{maximum activity} = 3 \text{ ml} \times 38.5 \text{ mCi/ml} = 115.5 \text{ mCi}$$

$$\text{Concentration} = \frac{\text{total activity}}{\text{total volume}}$$

$$C = \frac{\text{maximum activity prepared}}{\text{Tc volume + kit reagents}}$$

$$C = \frac{115.5 \text{ mCi}}{3 \text{ ml} + (3 \text{ ml} + 2 \text{ ml} + 2 \text{ ml})} \approx 11.6 \text{ mCi/ml}$$

6. At 0900, there are 300,000 particles/ml and 3 mCi/ml. After 6 hr (1 $T_{1/2}$), there are 300,000 particles/ml and 1.5 mCi/ml. Therefore, 2 ml of the preparation must be administered to obtain 3 mCi.

$$2 \text{ ml} \times 300{,}000 \text{ particles/ml} = 600{,}000 \text{ particles administered}$$

7. Based on the *Rf* values, the counts on the top half of the chromatography strip are free pertechnetate ($^{99m}TcO_4^-$) in the preparation; the counts on the lower half are the radiopharmaceutical ^{99m}Tc-pentetate (DTPA).

$$\%\text{ radiochemical purity} = \frac{\text{counts on bottom half of strip}}{\text{counts on bottom and top halves of strip}} \times 100$$

$$\%\text{ radiochemical purity} = \frac{27{,}695 \text{ cpm}}{27{,}695 \text{ cpm} + 1563 \text{ cpm}} \times 100 = 94.7\%.$$

8. The free pertechnetate impurity is calculated from solvent 1, where it is separated from the other two components in the preparation. The HR-^{99m}Tc impurity is calculated from solvent 2.

$$\%\text{ Free } ^{99m}\text{TcO}_4^- = \frac{1550 \text{ cpm}}{1550 \text{ cpm} + 26{,}750 \text{ cpm}} \times 100 \approx 5.5\%$$

$$\%\text{HR-}^{99m}\text{Tc} = \frac{850 \text{ cpm}}{40{,}139 \text{ cpm} + 850 \text{ cpm}} \times 100 \approx 2.1\%$$

$$\%\text{ Tagging efficiency} = 100\% - (5.5\% + 2.1\%) \approx 92.4\%.$$

9. The initial concentration must be decay-corrected for July 15 (72 hr). From a decay factor table for ^{111}In, the decay factor for 72 hr (3 days) is 0.480:

$$74 \text{ MBq/ml} \times 0.480 \approx 35.5 \text{ MBq/ml}$$

$$\text{Volume} = \frac{29.6 \text{ MBq}}{35.5 \text{ MBq/ml}} = 0.83 \text{ ml}$$

10. The elapsed time between calibration and dose administration is 70 hr (1400, September 7 to 1200, September 10). Using the decay factor for 70 hr, the concentration on September 7 is:

$$C_0 = \frac{3.0 \text{ mCi/ml}}{0.517} = 5.8 \text{ mCi/ml}.$$

In this instance, the concentration is divided by the decay factor because the assay date is later than the time of use.

The volume to be administered is:

$$V = \frac{1.0 \text{ mCi}}{5.8 \text{ mCi/ml}} = 0.17 \text{ ml}.$$

Appendix B

Federal Regulations

Department of Transportation (DOT), Title 49, Code of Federal Regulations

TOPIC	DOT REGULATION
Packaging radioactive materials	§170–178. For shipping purposes, radioactive material is defined as any material spontaneously emitting ionizing radiation with specific gravity greater than 0.002 μCi/g uniformly distributed. (Therefore, the return of radioactive materials and/or their residues to a radiopharmacy or manufacturer are subject to DOT regulations.) Packaging procedure: 1. Survey package and verify absence of surface contamination with a wipe test. 2. Attach appropriate category of "RADIOACTIVE" label and indicate Transport Index. 3. Prepare shipping papers.

Nuclear Regulatory Commission (NRC), Title 10, Code of Federal Regulations (1/1/95)

TOPIC	NRC REGULATION
Packaging radioactive materials	§71. DOT regulations must be adhered to whenever radioactive materials are shipped, whether or not such shipments are interstate.
Area posting	§20.1003/20.1902. Radiation areas should be posted appropriately. **1. GRAVE DANGER: VERY HIGH RADIATION AREA** An area in which an individual could receive an absolute radiation dose in excess of 500 rads (5 grays) in 1 hr. **2. CAUTION: HIGH RADIATION AREA** An area in which radiation levels could result in an individual receiving a dose equivalent exceeding 0.1 rem (1 mSv) in an hr. **3. CAUTION: RADIATION AREA** An area in which radiation levels could result in an individual receiving a dose equivalent exceeding 0.005 rem (0.05 mSv) in an hour. **4. CAUTION: RADIOACTIVE MATERIAL** Post in areas where radioactive materials are used or stored in amounts exceeding 10 times the quantity of material specified in NRC Appendix C (see Table 1-4, p. 4).
Radiation safety and protection records	§20.2103/20.2108. Length of time records must be kept. Personnel radiation exposure and bioassay records: indefinitely; room and package surveys: 3 yr, others indefinitely; waste disposal (release into sanitary sewer, incineration, transfer for burial): indefinitely. §35.33. Misadministration records to include names of those involved (prescribing physician, allied health personnel, patient, referring physician), patient's social security or ID number, brief description of event, effect on patient and any actions taken to prevent recurrence: 5 yr.

TOPIC	NRC REGULATION
	§35.53. Measurement of patient dose records to include radiopharmaceutical name, lot number, expiration date, radionuclide, patient's name, patient ID number, prescribed dosage, activity of dose at time of administration or notation that total administered activity was less than 30 μCi (1.1 MBq), date and time of measurement, initials of record maker: 3 yr.
	§35.70. Records of surveys for contamination and radiation exposure rate to include date of survey, plan of area surveyed, trigger level established for each area, detected dose rates at several points in area or removable contamination, instrument used for survey, initials of record maker: 3 yr.
	§35.92. Records of disposal by decay-in-storage to include date of disposal, date material placed in storage, radionuclides disposed, survey instrument used, background dose rate, dose rate measured at surface of waste containers, name of individual performing disposal: 3 yr.
	§35.315. Surveys following therapeutic dose administration to include time and date of survey, plan of area or list of points surveyed, measured dose rates expressed in mrem/hr, instrument used to make survey, initials of surveyor: 3 yr.
Patient monitoring	§35.75. Following radioiodine therapy, patients may be released from isolation if the activity in the patient is less than 30 mCi or the measured dose rate is less than 5 mrem/hr at 1 m.
Occupational dose limits	§20.1201. See Table 1-3, p. 3.
Syringe shields	§35.60. Use of syringe shields is required during radiopharmaceutical kit preparation and administration (except when contraindicated for the patient).
Vial shields	§35.61. Radiopharmaceutical vials must be shielded.
Notification regarding excessive radiation exposure	For staff technologists, the appropriate reporting authority is the chief technologist or radiation safety officer. These individuals are responsible for implementing the regulations. Regulations concerning the type of incident that needs to be reported, the information that should be included in the report and the reporting mechanism (telephone or written report) are found in 10CFR, 20.2203. [Examinees are not responsible for these regulations.]
Radiopharmaceutical misadministration	§35.2/35.33. [For staff technologists, the appropriate reporting authority is the chief technologist or nuclear medicine physician.] A reportable misadministration is defined as the administration of: 1. More than 30 μCi [^{125}I] or [^{131}I]sodium iodide involving the wrong patient or the wrong radiopharmaceutical, or when the administered dosage differs from the

TOPIC	NRC REGULATION
	prescribed by more than 20% of the prescribed and the difference between administered and prescribed dosages exceeds 30 μCi. 2. Any other therapeutic radiopharmaceutical involving the wrong patient, wrong radiopharmaceutical, or wrong route of administration, or when the administered dosage differs from the prescribed by more than 20% of the prescribed. 3. A diagnostic radiopharmaceutical involving the wrong patient, wrong radiopharmaceutical, wrong route of administration, or when the administered dosage differs from the prescribed dosage, *and* the dose to the patient exceeds 5 rem effective dose equivalent or 50 rem dose equivalent to any individual organ. These misadministrations must be reported to the NRC by telephone no later than the next day after their discovery and in writing within 15 days of discovery.
Radiopharmaceuticals that pose special hazards	§35.205. Aerosols/gases must be administered in a room that directly vents to the atmosphere *or* that provides for collection of aerosol/gas in a shielded container *and* that has negative pressure compared to surrounding areas.
Radiation safety instructions to patient, family and hospital staff	§35.310. Personnel dealing with therapy patients must receive radiation safety instruction concerning: visitor and patient control, waste management, contamination control, notification of radiation safety officer in case of emergency. §35.315. Therapy patients must be given radiation safety guidance and advised how to implement the ALARA principle before their release from isolation.
Wipe tests and area radiation surveys	§20.1302. Permissible levels of radiation in unrestricted areas: if an individual is continuously present, the dose may not exceed 0.002 rem (0.02 mSv) in an hour or 0.05 rem (0.5 mSv) in a year. §35.70. Surveys are required daily in areas where radiopharmaceuticals are administered or prepared *and* weekly in areas where stored. Wipe tests must be performed weekly in the same areas. §35.315. Materials removed from a therapy patient's room must be monitored and handled as radioactive waste if contaminated. Survey therapy patient's room following discharge. Decontaminate until removable contamination < 200 dpm/100 cm^2.
Receipt of radioactive materials	§20.1906. Wipe tests must be performed on the external surfaces of packages. External monitoring for radiation levels is required only for packages containing quantities of radioactive material greater than or equal to Type A quantities. [This exempts

TOPIC	NRC REGULATION
	essentially all packages received in a nuclear medicine department.]
	Monitor any package for radioactive contamination and radiation levels if there is evidence of leakage or damage to the package.
Generator eluate quality control	§35.204. A licensee may not administer to humans a radiopharmaceutical containing more than 0.15 μCi ^{99}Mo per mCi ^{99m}Tc.
	Each elution must be assayed for ^{99}Mo.
	Records of ^{99}Mo assays must be maintained for 3 yr.
Verification of activity administered to patients	§35.50. Patient doses must be measured with a dose calibrator prior to administration.
Radiopharmaceutical preparation and administration records	§35.204. Concentration records for ^{99}Mo must include for each elution the measured activity of ^{99m}Tc expressed in mCi, measured activity of ^{99}Mo expressed in μCi, the ratio of the measures expressed as μCi ^{99}Mo/mCi ^{99m}Tc, time and date of measurement and the initials of individual making measurement.
Disposal of radioactive material	§20.1904. Deface or remove radioactive label from containers that no longer contain radioactive materials.
	§20.2001. Dispose of licensed material by transfer to an authorized recipient, by decay in storage, by release in effluents (certain wastes and limits apply).
	§20.2003. Patient excreta may be discarded into sanitary sewer (no limits).
	§20.2004. Disposal by incineration by NRC special approval only.
Storage area for decay of radioactivity	§35.92. Physical half-life must be less than 65 days: hold for decay a minimum of 10 half-lives; monitor before disposal to determine waste has reached background levels; deface labels; separate generator column from shielding to monitor.
Instrumentation quality control records	§35.50. Dose calibration quality control records to be retained for 3 yr unless directed otherwise and to include: 1. Constancy checks: model and serial number of instrument, radionuclide used as test source, date of test, activity measured, initials of individual performing test. 2. Accuracy checks: model and serial number of instrument, model and serial number of each source used, radionuclide and its activity, date of test, results of test, identity of individual performing test. 3. Activity linearity check: model and serial number of dose calibrator, calculated activities, measured activities, date of test, identity of individual performing test.

TOPIC	NRC REGULATION
	4. Geometry dependence check: model and serial number of dose calibrator, configuration of source measured, activity measured for each volume measured, date of test, identity of individual performing test. This record must be maintained for the life of the instrument.
	§35.51. Survey meter calibration records to be retained for 3 yr and to include description of calibration procedure, date of calibration, description of source used and certified exposure rates from source, rates indicated by the instrument being calibrated, correction factors, signature of individual performing calibration.
Dose calibrator linearity	§35.50. Linearity check required upon installation, quarterly, and following repair. Test over a range of activities from the highest dosage that will be administered to 30 μCi. Correct readings if error is greater than 10%.
Dose calibrator accuracy	§35.50. Accuracy check required upon installation, annually, and following repair. Assay at least two different sources, one of which has a principal photon energy between 100 and 500 keV. Repair or replace if error is greater than 10%.
Dose calibrator constancy	§35.50. Constancy check required daily and following repair on frequently used settings. Repair or replace if error greater than 10%.
Reference check source test on survey meters	§35.51. Calibrate survey instruments annually and following repair. Check source daily to ensure proper operation. No records required.

United States Pharmacopoeia XXII, 1995

Topic	Standard
Generator eluate quality	No more than 0.15 μCi ^{99}Mo per mCi ^{99m}Tc. No more than 10 μg Al^{+3}/ml of eluate.
MAA particle size	At least 95% of particles in preparation must have diameter between 10 and 90 microns; none may be greater than 150 microns.

Preparing and Taking a Certification Examination

Preparation

The first step in preparing for a certification exam is to review the task analysis, which is a list of all tasks that individuals in the field should be able to perform. Questions on these tasks will be included on the exam. Candidates should compare their knowledge to those tasks on the list. For instance, nuclear medicine technologists who work in departments that use commercial radiopharmacies to supply radiopharmaceuticals may not feel confident about the tasks concerning radiopharmacy practice. These technologists should devote time to reviewing the radiopharmacy practice topics.

Equally important is to note what topics are emphasized. For example, the Nuclear Medicine Technology Certification Board (NMTCB) exam is divided into two content areas: the critical domain (CD) and the associated domain (AD). Tasks that are judged to be important, performed frequently or with the greatest medical consequences are included in the CD. Questions on each of these tasks are included on every NMTCB exam. Although AD tasks are important to entry-level practice, knowledge of them is only randomly sampled on any given test. Questions concerning AD tasks appear on every exam, but there will not be a question on every AD task on every exam.

The NMTCB exam is based on entry-level, job-related skills: this type of exam is sometimes referred to as competency-based testing. This means that the exam material is directly applicable to everyday clinical practice. Therefore, recall of knowledge is not tested, but the application of that knowledge to nuclear medicine technology practice is. For instance, examinees are not questioned about collimator characteristics, but they may be asked to choose which collimator in a given group will best perform a particular imaging procedure.

Since the NMTCB exam is given nationally, knowledge of federal regulations (NRC, DOT and FDA) only is tested and only FDA-approved radiopharmaceuticals and diagnostic procedures are included. Likewise, great effort has been made to ensure that geographical differences in nuclear medicine technology practice are not evident in the test questions. Certain topics, such as radiation biology and medical internal radiation dosimetry, may not be included on the exam although they are taught in nuclear medicine technology programs.

In summary, the individual is the best judge of her or his weakness. Reviewing the task analysis familiarizes the candidate with the content of the exam and permits the candidate to prepare more effectively.

Lastly, during publication of this text, the NMTCB was considering changing the testing format: from a traditional "paper and pencil" to the more advanced testing tool of Computer Adaptive Testing (CAT). If the NMTCB does change the testing tool, the steps described below may need to be revised in accordance with the CAT.

Test-taking Techniques

The following tips are designed to help you with the mechanics of taking a multiple choice examination. They will help you avoid making mistakes (that can cost you points), even when you know the correct answer.

1. Begin the test at question number one and work in order through the entire exam. Starting in the middle of the exam or at the end and working backward are not good ideas. Should you begin marking the answer sheet in the wrong space, all subsequent answers will be placed in the wrong space.
2. Answer all questions in order; do not skip a question, planning to come back to it later. If you are unsure of an answer, circle the question number in the test booklet, not on the answer sheet and come back to the question later, if there is time. This technique will help ensure that you do not waste time pondering certain items and no blank spaces will be left on the answer sheet.
3. If there is no penalty for guessing, it is to your advantage to provide an answer for every item on the exam. There is, however, a technique to making an educated guess. First, eliminate any choices that are obviously incorrect. Then, review the remaining choices to see if any contain clues that might indicate the correct answer or that rule out other choices as incorrect. If the question deals with a topic that you are totally unfamiliar with, an "educated guess" may be impossible. In that instance, choose any answer. If there are five possible answers, you have a 20% chance of guessing the correct one. If you leave the question unanswered, your chances are zero.
4. Certain types of responses are often the correct answer: all of above; none of the above; or the longest of the five choices.
5. Incorrect answers offered for calculations are often chosen to mimic frequently made mistakes. Be certain that you have done the complete calculation and are not choosing an intermediate answer.
6. Be careful of negative answers (those containing the words *not* or *except*). Read carefully.

Appendix D

Sample Certification Examination Questions

The following 46 certification examination questions have been graciously supplied by the NMTCB. These questions are representative of those that appear on current NMTCB exams. Each question is referenced to the appropriate task from the NMTCB Task Analysis. The task analysis is a list of 93 tasks that individuals who have recently entered NMT practice should be able to perform; it is divided into four categories: Radiation Safety, Instrumentation, Clinical Procedures, Radiopharmacy.

Sample questions for all tasks included in the NMTCB Task Analysis could not be included here. However, a complete list of all tasks included in the task analysis is available from the NMTCB, 2970 Clairmont Road, Suite 610, Atlanta, GA 30329, (404)315-1739. Although the sample items are grouped by category here, on the examination, questions from the four groups are randomly arranged.

Answers to the questions appear on page 131.

Group I: Radiation Safety

Task: *Post appropriate signs in designated areas to comply with NRC regulations.*

1. According to the NRC, an unrestricted area is one in which a person would receive a radiation dose of less than:

a. 2 mrem/hr.
b. 5 mrem/hr.
c. 10 mrem/hr.
d. 20 mrem/hr.
e. 50 mrem/hr.

Task: *Take appropriate measures to reduce radiation exposure when necessary.*

2. A patient hospitalized in a private room receives 200 mCi of Na^{131}Iodide. A monitor shows that the patient in the adjacent room is receiving a radiation exposure of 3 mR/hr. To comply with the ALARA philosophy, the technologist should:

a. contact the referring physician.
b. send home the patient receiving therapy.
c. continually monitor the adjacent room.
d. contact the NRC for guidance.
e. move the adjacent patient's bed to the opposite side of the room.

Task: *Notify the appropriate authority of misadministration, when applicable.*

3. Due to the manufacturer's mislabeling, a patient received 1 mCi [^{99m}Tc]pertechnetate intravenously instead of the prescribed 10 mCi. The resulting image is technically satisfactory. According to the NRC regulations, which of the following statements is TRUE?

a. This is a reportable misadministration because the administered activity differs by 50% from the prescribed activity.
b. This is a nonreportable misadministration because the patient received a smaller activity than prescribed.
c. This is a nonreportable misadministration because the image is technically satisfactory.
d. This is a nonreportable misadministration because the manufacturer mislabled the patient dose.
e. This is a nonreportable misadministration because the dose to the patient or to an individual organ does not exceed the limits stated in the regulations.

Task: *Perform wipe tests and area radiation surveys following a standardized schedule and format.*

4. Which of the following instruments is most appropriate for monitoring a ^{99m}Tc spill of 50 μCi?

a. film badge
b. thin-end window Geiger counter
c. a cutie pie ionization chamber
d. direct-reading dosimeter
e. liquid scintillation counter with a millipore filter

Task: *Appropriately dispose of radioactive material.*

5. What must be done before vials previously containing radioactive material can be discarded?

a. The radioactive label must be removed or defaced.
b. Appropriate disposal seals must be affixed to the vials.
c. The vials must be shipped to an appropriate disposal site.
d. The liquid contents of each vial must be removed.
e. Wipe tests must be performed to ensure that the vials are not contaminated.

Task: *Use proper procedures for managing a radioactive spill.*

6. The first action of a technologist who accidentally spills a radioactive solution should be to:

a. leave the area quickly because the substance may be toxic.
b. disregard the spill and let housekeeping take care of it.
c. notify the supervisor and all coworkers.
d. prevent the spread of the spill by covering it with absorbent materials.
e. notify the radiation safety officer and let the officer take care of it.

Group II: Instrumentation

Task: *Calibrate a scintillation spectrometer.*

7. Electrical power to a scintillation counter is suddenly interrupted. When power is restored 1 hr later, the radionu-

clide standards are measured immediately and found to be outside of the acceptable range. The next step should be to:

a. correct for the decay of the standards.
b. arrange for the counter to be repaired.
c. measure a radionuclide standard of another energy.
d. repeat the measurement of the radionuclide standards after 30–60 min.
e. record the discrepancy in the quality control log and continue the daily routine.

Task: *Obtain background counts on a scintillation spectrometer.*

8. A thyroid uptake probe used to measure the background count in the room should be:

a. aimed at the floor.
b. pointed at the ceiling.
c. covered with a lead apron.
d. positioned so that it is not aimed at a window.
e. positioned as it would be for a patient neck count.

Task: *Adjust the pulse-height analyzer (PHA) on the scintillation spectrometer or camera for the appropriate photopeak.*

9. A comparison of image A to image B (Fig. D-1), which was obtained on the same instrument, reveals that the quality of image B most likely is degraded due to:

a. incorrect photopeaking.
b. an incorrect intensity setting.
c. contact with a phototube.
d. a faulty image recording device.
e. a malfunctioning photomultiplier tube.

Task: *Perform field uniformity check on the scintillation camera on a routine basis.*

10. The flood correction image used in emission computed tomography requires a minimum of how many counts?

a. 500,000
b. 1 million
c. 2 million
d. 5 million
e. 30 million

Task: *Perform spatial resolution check on the scintillation camera on a routine basis.*

11. Clinical images obtained from a scintillation camera have recently deteriorated in quality, but routine flood and bar phantom images appear unchanged. Which of the following statements best explains this discrepancy?

a. The liquid in the flood field was inadequately mixed.
b. The narrowest bar spacing in the phantom was too wide to detect changes.
c. The correction circuitry of the camera was in the "on" position.
d. The flood image was obtained for 10 million rather than 50 million counts.
e. The flood image was collected with the camera pointing up.

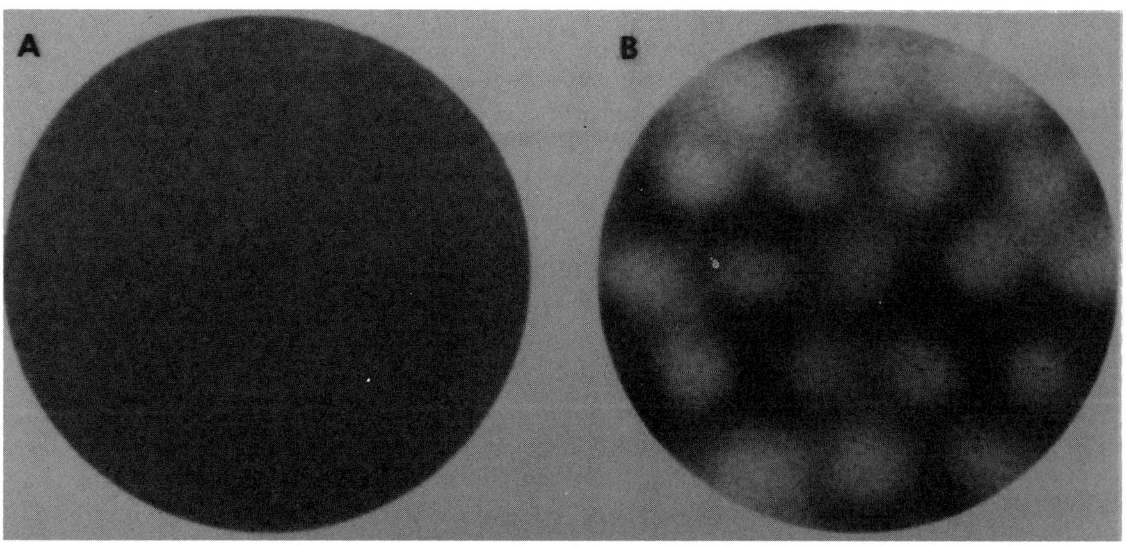

Figure D.1

Task: *Assess performance of image recording equipment.*
12. A series of ^{99m}Tc flood images are acquired for a constant number of counts on a properly functioning multiformatter. Which of the following image characteristics will NOT remain constant?

a. size
b. time
c. shape
d. density
e. uniformity

Task: *Perform reference check on survey meters.*
13. Periodic check source tests on survey instruments are performed to determine:

a. consistency of response.
b. energy resolution.
c. dead time.
d. spatial resolution.
e. decay factors.

Task: *Test accuracy of dose calibrator for commonly used radionuclides.*
14. The most important reason for using ^{57}Co as a reference standard to check the accuracy of a dose calibrator is that:

a. its photon energy is close to the photon energy of ^{99m}Tc.
b. its half-life is close to the half-life of ^{99m}Tc.
c. it has the same decay mode as ^{99m}Tc.
d. it has no beta emissions.
e. it is readily available.

Task: *Check for constancy of dose calibrator using a long-lived radionuclide standard.*
15. The constancy of a dose calibrator is best monitored by measuring:

a. ^{57}Co and ^{137}Cs standards at installation.
b. ^{57}Co and ^{137}Cs standards daily.
c. ^{99m}Tc and ^{201}Tl standards daily.
d. ^{125}I and ^{137}Cs standards weekly.
e. ^{131}I and ^{111}In standards weekly.

Task: *Perform basic computer operations.*
16. Which of the following would NOT allow the technologist to form a region of interest of irregular shape and size?

a. mouse
b. light pen
c. joy stick
d. track ball
e. cursor lines

Group III: Clinical Procedures

Task: *Schedule patient studies, ensuring appropriate sequence for multiple procedures and interact with hospital staff regarding special orders.*
17. Immediate postexercise ^{201}Tl images reveal normal myocardial uptake and markedly increased uptake in the nearby gastrointestinal organs. Which of the following is the most likely cause of these findings?

a. The patient had a recent myocardial infarct.
b. The radiopharmaceutical was infiltrated.
c. The patient was injected in the upright position.
d. The patient was not in a fasting state.
e. This is the normal distribution of ^{201}Tl.

Task: *Receive patient and provide proper nursing care during nuclear medicine procedure.*
18. When imaging a patient who has a urine drainage bag, the technologist should:

a. place the bag on the floor.
b. hang the bag at the level of the bladder.
c. hang the bag above the level of the bladder.
d. hang the bag below the level of the bladder.
e. clamp the catheter tubing.

Task: *Recognize emergency conditions and determine patient's vital signs when necessary.*
19. A patient who slumps over in the chair during an injection most likely has experienced:

a. shock.
b. syncope.
c. anaphylaxis.
d. paresthesia.
e. a seizure.

Task: *Administer cardiopulmonary resuscitation and first aid when necessary.*
20. During two-person cardiopulmonary resuscitation, the technologist providing breaths is not able to feel the patient's carotid pulse. This is most likely because the:

a. sternum is being compressed 4 cm.
b. patient is on a hard, flat surface.
c. ventilations are inadequate.
d. compressions are inadequate.
e. airway is obstructed.

Task: *Administer cardiopulmonary resuscitation and first aid when necessary.*
21. What should a technologist do when a patient suddenly has a seizure?

a. Restrain the patient so that he will not injure himself.
b. Force a padded tongue blade between the patient's teeth to protect his tongue.
c. Take the patient's vital signs, including pulse rate, blood pressure and temperature.
d. Administer oxygen to ease the patient's labored breathing.
e. Protect the patient from injury without restraint or other interference.

Task: *Receive patient and verify patient identification and written orders for study.*
22. When an imaging procedure is requested, the best source of verifying the order is to check:

a. the daily log book.
b. the physician's written order.
c. the consultation request.
d. with the patient.
e. with the nursing staff.

Task: *Check procedural contraindications for study and obtain pertinent patient history.*
23. A computed tomography scan using iodinated contrast media is performed on a patient. What effect would this study have on a [^{123}I]sodium iodide thyroid uptake study and image obtained 3 days later?

a. increase the radiopharmaceutical uptake
b. decrease the imaging time
c. decrease the radiopharmaceutical uptake
d. decrease the background counts
e. no effect

Task: *Prepare patient for procedure as required. Note: This applies to preparations that occur in the nuclear medicine department and are normally performed by the technologist.*
24. The best reason for checking a patient's clothing before performing imaging is to:

a. make the study more sensitive.
b. detect objects that may attenuate radiation.
c. prevent buttons and zippers from being caught in the equipment.
d. make certain the patient is comfortable during the examination.
e. make certain the detector head is in close contact with the patient.

Task: *Administer the appropriate radiopharmaceutical by the proper route.*
25. Before performing an indirect cystogram, the technologist should:

a. inject ^{99m}Tc-DMSA intravenously.
b. inject ^{99m}Tc-DTPA intravenously.
c. inject ^{111}In-DTPA intrathecally.
d. administer ^{99m}Tc-sulfur colloid orally.
e. infuse $^{99m}TcO_4$ in saline solution directly into the bladder.

Task: *Wait appropriate length of time after administration of the radiopharmaceutical to begin imaging.*
26. Following the administration of ^{99m}Tc-sulfur colloid, imaging is begun immediately. What is the most likely cause of the cardiac blood-pool activity on the first image?

a. poor radiopharmaceutical preparation
b. hepatocellular dysfunction
c. insufficient delay after injection
d. congestive heart failure
e. recent myocardial infarction

Task: *Place the patient in correct position using supportive materials and immobilizers, at appropriate distance from the detector, for obtaining each view.*
27. A physician's order for a patient to undergo bone imaging indicates a need to rule out a stress fracture in the left metatarsal region. To demonstrate the pathology, the technologist should obtain which of the following views of the feet?

a. anterior
b. posterior
c. lateral
d. medial
e. plantar

Task: *Indicate appropriate anatomical landmarks for each view of a procedure.*
28. What labels are appropriate for these 24-hr ^{67}Ga images?

	Image A	Image B
a.	RT ANT LT	LT POST RT
b.	LT ANT RT	RT POST LT
c.	LT POST RT	LT ANT RT
d.	RT POST LT	RT ANT LT
e.	LT ANT RT	LT POST RT

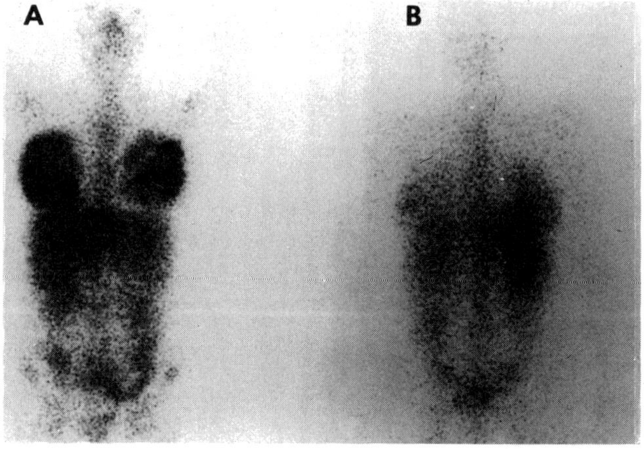

Figure D.2

Task: *Analyze image appearance or computer information for normal structure and artifacts, making adjustments, if necessary, and assuring correct information is supplied.*

29. The largest area of increased radiopharmaceutical uptake in the bone images most likely demonstrates:

a. osteomyelitis.
b. defects in the collimator surface.
c. attenuation artifacts.
d. avascular necrosis of the humeral head.
e. extravasation of the radiopharmaceutical.

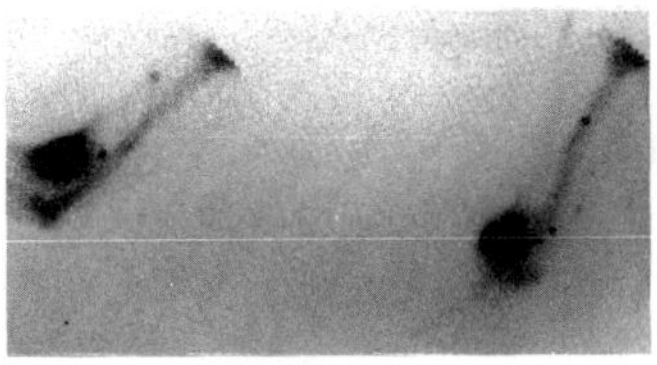

Figure D.3

Task: *Perform any special views as required.*

30. When hepatobiliary imaging is performed, which of the following views should be obtained to distinguish gallbladder activity from bowel and kidney activity?

a. posterior
b. left lateral
c. right lateral
d. left posterior oblique
e. right posterior oblique

Task: *Record information relative to any special circumstances affecting the procedure as needed.*

31. The anterior bone images of a patient's chest reveal abnormalities. These abnormalities are most likely associated with:

a. a breast prosthesis.
b. arthritis.
c. recent fever.
d. recent trauma to the area.
e. the possibility of contamination.

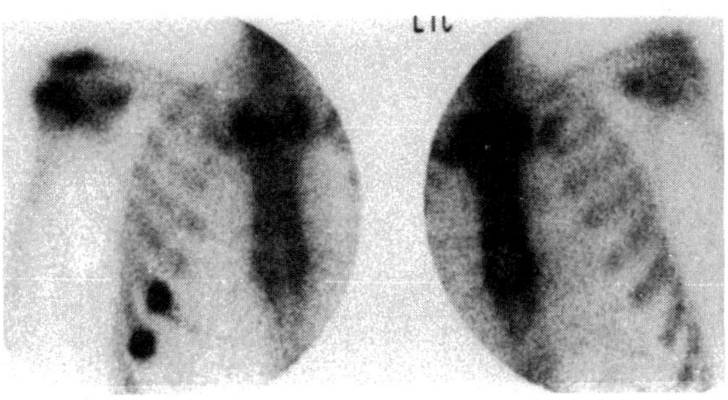

Figure D.4

Task: *Prepare a standard dilution.*

32. A standard is prepared by diluting 1 ml of activity to a volume of 10 ml. A 100-μl aliquot of this preparation is diluted to a volume of 4 ml for counting. What is the final dilution?

a. 1:10
b. 1:40
c. 1:100
d. 1:400
e. 1:4000

Task: *Store and maintain adequate supplies including kits to assure timely completion of patient studies.*

33. If a technologist has the following materials available to tag white blood cells, what is the last day that the procedure can be performed?

Reagent	Expiration date
^{111}In-oxine	February 15
Heparin	January 26
Normal saline	August 1

a. January 26
b. January 31
c. February 15
d. July 31
e. August 1

Task: *Choose correct detector-patient distance for external counting and count for a statistically significant number of counts.*

34. When a thyroid uptake is performed, a standard is measured in a phantom to:

a. equalize the scattered radiation among patients.
b. standardize the spectrum of ^{123}I.
c. equalize tissue absorption among patients.
d. simulate the counting geometry of the thyroid.
e. determine the background.

Task: *Choose correct detector-patient distance for external counting and count for a statistically significant number of counts.*

35. Why are probe positions marked with indelible ink over the patient's heart, liver and spleen when a red cell sequestration study is to be performed?

a. to assure patient comfort
b. to accurately count the standard
c. to reproduce probe geometry
d. to increase the count rate
e. to reproduce the count rate

Task: *Choose correct detector-patient distance for external counting and count for a statistically significant number of counts.*

36. A thyroid uptake was performed with an uptake probe 4 hr after administration of the radiopharmaceutical . The technologist obtained two successive counts of the patient's neck, 56,000 cpm and 24,000 cpm, respectively. What is the most likely cause for the discrepancy in the count rates?

a. detector-to-patient distance
b. collimator selection
c. iodine turnover
d. radiopharmaceutical decay
e. septal wall penetration

Task: *Review nonimaging procedures for possible technical errors that may alter results.*

37. Inadvertently damaged red cells are injected when a red cell mass determination is being performed. This can result in:

a. serious danger to the patient.
b. no effect on the red cell mass.
c. underestimation of the plasma volume.
d. underestimation of whole-body hematocrit.

Group IV: Radiopharmacy

Task: *Assemble and elute a radionuclide generator using aseptic technique.*

38. After eluting a new ^{99}Mo/^{99m}Tc generator, the technologist finds no activity in the elution vial. The technologist should:

a. attempt elution using a second vial.
b. change the outlet line of the generator.
c. return the generator to the manufacturer.
d. empty the saline reservoir of the generator.
e. try to elute the generator with a syringe and needle.

Task: *Check the generator eluate for radionuclide and chemical contamination.*

39. A technologist using indicator paper impregnated with aluminum ion reagent observes no color change after spotting the paper with ^{99m}Tc eluate. This result indicates:

a. the lack of excess aluminum ions.
b. the presence of ^{99}Mo breakthrough.
c. that the eluate should not be used in the preparation of kits containing stannous ions.
d. there is alumina breakthrough that exceeds limits set by the NRC.
e. that the solution of known Al^{+3} concentration used for comparison purposes contains insufficient aluminum ions.

Task: *Determine the total volume and radioactivity to be added to a radiopharmaceutical kit within activity limits.*

40. A radiopharmaceutical kit is prepared at 1100 with 3 ml pertechnetate from generator eluate that is calibrated for 600 mCi in 10 ml at 0600. How much activity, in mCi, will the kit contain? (5-hr decay factor is 0.561.)

a. 72
b. 90
c. 96
d. 101
e. 113

Task: *Calculate the concentration of radioactivity of a compound and label vial as to date, time of preparation, lot number, concentration and volume.*

41. On April 4, a radiopharmaceutical is received and calibrated at 150 μCi/ml. What is the concentration, in μCi/ml, on April 20? ($T_{1/2}$ = 8 days.)

a. 18.3
b. 37.5
c. 75.0
d. 112.5
e. 300.0

Task: *Check all radiopharmaceutical preparations for proper pH, color, clarity and particle size, as appropriate.*

42. During routine lung imaging with ^{99m}Tc-macroaggregated album (MAA), liver accumulation is observed. Which of the following quality control parameters would best explain this finding?

a. radiochromatography
b. color of the solution
c. pH of the ^{99m}Tc eluate
d. particle size in the solution
e. breakthrough of ^{99}Mo in the eluate

Task: *Determine the radiochemical purity of radiopharmaceutical preparations by chromatography.*

43. A preparation of ^{99m}Tc-Sn DTPA contains 5% free pertechnetate with 10% ^{99m}Tc bound to stannous oxide. The radiochemical purity of the ^{99m}Tc-Sn DTPA would be:

a. 95%
b. 85%
c. 70%
d. 60%
e. 50%

Task: *Verify label on radiopharmaceutical vial, including concentration, specific activity, total activity, lot number, assay time and date.*

44. The label on a radiopharmaceutical states that the total activity is 25 mCi on December 1 at noon. The dose cali-

brator reading of this shipment is 12.3 mCi on December 1 at noon. Because the label information is not confirmed, the technologist should first:

a. notify the radiation safety officer.
b. use the radiopharmaceutical as if it contained 25 mCi.
c. use the radiopharmaceutical as if it contained 12.3 mCi.
d. return the shipment to the radiopharmaceutical supplier.
e. perform quality assurance on the dose calibrator.

Task: *Determine the volume or number of capsules of the radiopharmaceutical required for diagnostic and therapeutic procedures.*

45. A radiopharmaceutical calibrated for 0900 on November 2 contains 5 mCi in 1 ml. A patient weighing 43 kg is to receive 30 μCi/kg of activity at 0900 on November 5. What is the correct total activity and volume to be administered to this patient? (1-day decay factor is 0.783.)

a. 6.3 mCi in 2.60 ml
b. 2.8 mCi in 0.85 ml
c. 2.8 mCi in 1.20 ml
d. 1.3 mCi in 0.26 ml
e. 1.3 mCi in 0.54 ml

Task: *Verify that radionuclide impurity limits are not exceeded in the dispensed preparation.*

46. The ^{124}I contaminant in an ^{123}I-labeled radiopharmaceutical used for imaging does NOT affect the:

a. shelf life of the drug.
b. choice of gamma camera collimator.
c. percentage of drug uptake by the target organ.
d. absorbed radiation dose to the patient.
e. radiation levels at the surface of the shipping container.

Table D-1
Answers to Sample Test Questions

Answers	Answers
1. a	24. b
2. e	25. b
3. e	26. c
4. b	27. e
5. a	28. a
6. d	29. e
7. d	30. c
8. e	31. d
9. a	32. d
10. e	33. a
11. b	34. d
12. b	35. c
13. a	36. a
14. a	37. e
15. b	38. a
16. e	39. a
17. d	40. d
18. d	41. b
19. b	42. d
20. d	43. b
21. e	44. e
22. b	45. e
23. c	46. c

Appendix E

Table of Chi Square

Degrees of freedom* (n − 1)	0.99	0.95	0.90	0.50	0.10	0.05	0.01
	There is a probability of … that the calculated value of chi-square will be equal to or greater than						
2	0.020	0.103	0.211	1.386	4.605	5.991	9.210
3	0.115	0.352	0.584	2.366	6.251	7.815	11.345
4	0.297	0.711	1.064	3.357	7.779	9.488	13.277
5	0.554	1.145	1.610	4.351	9.236	11.070	15.086
6	0.872	1.635	2.204	5.348	10.645	12.592	16.812
7	1.239	2.167	2.833	6.346	12.017	14.067	18.475
8	1.646	2.733	3.490	7.344	13.362	15.507	20.090
9	2.088	3.325	4.168	8.343	14.684	16.919	21.666
10	2.558	3.940	4.865	9.342	15.987	18.307	23.209
11	3.053	4.575	5.578	10.341	17.275	19.675	24.725
12	2.571	5.226	6.304	11.340	18.549	21.026	26.217
13	4.107	5.892	7.042	12.340	19.812	22.362	27.688
14	4.660	6.571	7.790	13.339	21.064	23.685	29.141
15	5.229	7.261	8.547	14.339	22.307	24.996	30.578
16	5.812	7.962	9.312	15.338	23.542	26.296	32.000
17	6.408	8.672	10.085	16.338	24.769	27.587	33.409
18	7.015	9.390	10.865	17.338	25.989	28.869	34.805
19	7.633	10.117	11.651	18.338	27.204	30.144	36.191
20	8.260	10.851	12.443	19.337	28.412	31.410	37.566
21	8.897	11.591	13.240	20.337	29.615	32.671	38.932
22	9.542	12.338	14.041	21.337	30.813	33.924	40.289
23	10.196	13.091	14.848	22.337	32.007	35.172	41.638
24	10.856	13.848	15.659	23.337	33.196	36.415	42.980
25	11.534	14.611	16.473	24.337	34.382	37.382	44.314
26	12.198	15.379	17.292	25.336	35.563	38.885	45.642
27	12.879	16.151	18.114	26.336	36.741	40.113	46.963
28	13.565	16.928	18.939	27.336	37.916	41.337	48.278
29	14.256	17.708	19.768	28.336	39.087	42.557	49.588

*The number of degrees of freedom is usually one less than the number of observations n.

Reprinted with permission from: Early PJ, Sodee DB. *Principles and practice of nuclear medicine.* St. Louis: CV Mosby Co., 1985:348.

Appendix F

Système International (SI) Unit Conversions

Quantity	CGS units	SI (MKS) units	Equivalents
Length	centimeter (cm)	meter (m)	1 cm = 0.01 m
Mass	gram (g)	kilogram (kg)	1 g = 0.001 kg
Time	second (s)	second (s)	1 s = 1 s
Energy	erg	Joule (J)	1 erg = 10^{-7} J
Radioactivity	Curie (Ci)	Becquerel (Bq)	1 Ci = 3.7×10^{10} Bq
Radiation absorbed dose	rad	Gray (Gy)	1 rad = 0.01 Gy
Exposure	Roentgen (R)	Coulomb/kilogram (C/kg)	1 R = 2.58×10^{-4} C/kg
Dose equivalent	rem	Sievert (Sv)	1 rem = 0.01 Sv

Common Prefixes Used in SI

Prefix	Symbol	Numerical equivalent
giga	G	10^9 = 1,000,000,000
mega	M	10^6 = 1,000,000
kilo	k	10^3 = 1,000
deci	d	10^{-1} = 0.1
centi	c	10^{-2} = 0.01
milli	m	10^{-3} = 0.001
micro	μ	10^{-6} = 0.000001
nano	n	10^{-9} = 0.000000001
pico	p	10^{-12} = 0.000000000001

To convert CGS units to SI units, multiply the CGS value by the SI equivalent.

Example: Convert 20 mCi → MBq

$$1{,}000 \text{ mCi} = 1 \text{ Ci}$$

$$20 \text{ mCi} = 0.02 \text{ Ci}$$

$$0.02 \text{ Ci } (3.7 \times 10^{10} \text{ Bq/Ci}) = 0.074 \times 10^{10} \text{ Bq}$$

$$(0.074 \times 10^{10} \text{ Bq}) \left(\frac{10^{-6}\text{MBq}}{\text{Bq}}\right) = 0.074\ 3\ 10^{4}\text{MBq}$$

$$= 740 \text{ MBq}$$

To convert SI units to CGS units, divide the SI value by the CGS equivalent.

Example: Convert 100 Gy → rad

$$\frac{100 \text{ Gy}}{0.01 \text{ Gy/rad}} = 10{,}000 \text{ r}$$

CGS = centimeter-gram-second; MKS = meter-kilogram-second.

Index